RESEARCH IN
NURSING, MIDWIFERY
& ALLIED HEALTH

EVIDENCE FOR BEST PRACTICE

7E

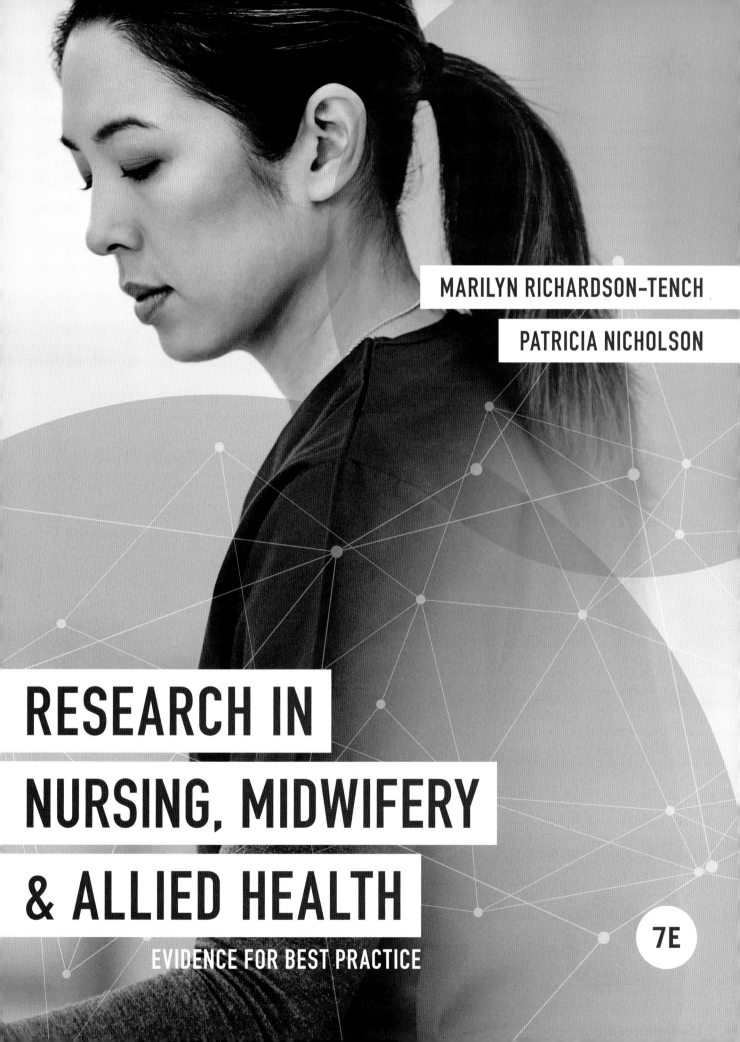

MARILYN RICHARDSON-TENCH

PATRICIA NICHOLSON

RESEARCH IN NURSING, MIDWIFERY & ALLIED HEALTH

EVIDENCE FOR BEST PRACTICE

7E

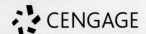

Research in Nursing, Midwifery & Allied Health
7th Edition
Marilyn Richardson-Tench
Patricia Nicholson

Portfolio lead: Fiona Hammond
Product manager: Michelle Aarons
Developmental editor: Talia Lewis/Christin Quirk/James Cole
Project editor: Alex Chambers
Cover designer: Nikita Bansal
Text designer: Jenki (Jennai Lee Fai)
Editor: Leanne Peters
Permissions/Photo researcher: Liz McShane
Indexer: Nikki Davis
Proofreader: Carolyn Leslie
Cover: Getty Images/The Good Brigade
Typeset by KnowledgeWorks Global Ltd.

Any URLs contained in this publication were checked for currency during the production process. Note, however, that the publisher cannot vouch for the ongoing currency of URLs.

6th edition published 2018

© 2022 Cengage Learning Australia Pty Limited

For product information and technology assistance,
in Australia call **1300 790 853**;
in New Zealand call **0800 449 725**

For permission to use material from this text or product, please email **aust.permissions@cengage.com**

National Library of Australia Cataloguing-in-Publication Data
ISBN: 9780170452007
A catalogue record for this book is available from the National Library of Australia.

Cengage Learning Australia
Level 7, 80 Dorcas Street
South Melbourne, Victoria Australia 3205

Cengage Learning New Zealand
Unit 4B Rosedale Office Park
331 Rosedale Road, Albany, North Shore 0632, NZ

For learning solutions, visit **cengage.com.au**

Printed in China by 1010 Printing International Limited.
1 2 3 4 5 6 7 26 25 24 23 22

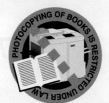

BRIEF CONTENTS

CONTENTS

Chapter 7:   Qualitative research methodologies   166

Chapter 8:   Collection, management and analysis of qualitative data   198

Chapter 9:   Mixed methods   224

Chapter 13: Evidence-based practice   341

PREFACE

When the first edition of this book was published in 1998, for the first time students were able to access a research text written by Australian nurse-researchers. The success of the first edition reflected the warm reception of the Australian nursing context and content. The second edition was published in 2002. Beverley Taylor and Kathryn Roberts continued the use of Australian nursing research examples, with equal space devoted to quantitative and qualitative research approaches.

The third edition was published in 2006 and welcomed as a co-author Stephen Kermode, who was invited to undertake the rewriting of Kathryn's chapters. Kathryn retired in 2004 but her name remained on this book in honour of her initial role as first author on two editions and the fact that some of her reworked content appeared in the third edition. The title of the third edition was changed to be more inclusive of other health professionals and in view of the international readership of the book. The content reflected a multidisciplinary approach to health research, with research examples from nursing and other professional healthcare groups.

The fourth edition was published in 2011 and welcomed Marilyn Richardson-Tench, who was invited to undertake the rewriting of the book. All the above authors' names remained on the book in recognition of their roles in previous editions. The fourth edition was a significant rewrite in response to reviewers and consumers, with the content focused on nursing and the provision of updated information suitable for undergraduate, honours and postgraduate students. A new chapter on mixed methods was contributed by Malcolm Elliot, who also revised the chapter on literature reviews.

The fifth edition was published in 2014 and included the provision of additional case studies covering practical paramedic and midwifery applications of research, as well as clinical and research nursing environments. There was also a special focus on the use of evidence-based practice and ethics. Additionally, the text was made student-friendly with the inclusion of diagrams that were more helpful.

The sixth edition welcomed Patricia Nicholson as co-editor/author and underwent an extensive revision in response to comments by reviewers. Evidence-based practice was highlighted by the inclusion of research that has impacted on clinical practice or has implications for evidence-based practice. Case studies were updated to include allied health professional examples. The edition was also revised to include chapter body features signposting important facets that are relevant to research and evidence-based practice.

New to this edition

This new edition has undergone further change in response to reviewer feedback. The previous edition's new features have been retained with the addition of visual cues to highlight key information in the chapter and assist students in using the textbook more efficiently. Case studies have been revised, as have the review questions, to illustrate the many contexts of research in healthcare and provide students with a sense of where research can be applied in their clinical practice. The research framework diagram, which can be found at the beginning of each chapter, has been reimagined to illustrate the multiple stages in the process of conducting a research project: think and plan, discover, research methodologies, gather and analyse, write and publish, and share/impact. The redesign prompted a reorder of the chapters to match the stages of conducting a research project.

We hope that the seventh edition will be informative and engaging for all nursing, midwifery and allied health students.

Marilyn Richardson-Tench and Patricia Nicholson

Guide to the text

As you read this text you will find a number of features in every chapter to enhance your study of nursing research and help you understand how the theory is applied in the real world.

CHAPTER OPENING FEATURES

CHAPTER

1 RESEARCH IN NURSING AND HEALTH

Chapter learning objectives

The material presented in this chapter will assist you to:
1 differentiate between conducting research, the critical appraisal of research and the clinical use of research in practice
2 appreciate the value of collaborative research within the multidisciplinary health team
3 understand why research in nursing is important
4 describe the research paradigms
5 distinguish between quantitative and qualitative research processes
6 describe the relationship between research, practice and theory
7 explain the use of a theoretical–conceptual framework in a research project.

Identify the key concepts that the chapter will cover with the **Learning Objectives** at the start of each chapter.

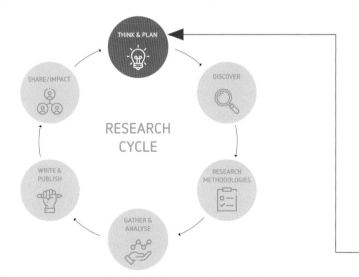

Research cycle

This book introduces research and encompasses all areas of the research cycle as shown in the above diagram. The process of research is cyclical, commencing with thinking and planning about a research topic and concluding with sharing the results of the research. The primary focus of this chapter is to provide an introduction to research and relates to thinking and planning.

1

The chapter-opening **Research Framework Diagram** illustrates the multiple stages in the process of conducting a research project: think and plan, discover, research methodologies, gather and analyse, write and publish, and share/impact. The highlighted stage identifies **the stage of the process** explored in the chapter.

FEATURES WITHIN CHAPTERS

EVIDENCE FOR BEST PRACTICE

CLINICAL USE OF RESEARCH

Research undertaken by Durkin and colleagues (2020) explored the effect of a mass media campaign on the participation rates in home bowel screening. A significant increase in completed home faecal occult blood tests during the campaign was discovered, although results did not differ significantly by age, sex or socioeconomic status when compared to the control group. Findings were consequential for planning future public health campaigns.

A five-year study by Marriott and colleagues (2020) investigated the experiences of Aboriginal women giving birth and receiving maternity care on Country versus in the suburban setting. Recommendations from the study provided guidance on midwifery practice and education in meeting Aboriginal women's expectations.

A randomised control trial was undertaken in a group of nursing homes to ascertain which intervention was the most effective in managing urinary incontinence in elderly female residents. Findings were significant for improving the quality of care for this population (Hödl et al., 2019).

A study in Finland sought to identify acute care nurses's views on practicing in environmentally responsible ways. Using a Delphi study, results focused on using materials efficiently (such as minimising waste and using sustainable products) and actively reducing energy consumption.

Evidence-based practice boxes highlight the importance of applying research to clinical practice and assists you to identify where and how you can use research to guide your own clinical decision making.

Evidence-based practice (EBP) margin icons indicate where clinical decision making has been guided by evidence.

EBP

ACTIVITY

Access the following articles and identify the different search strategies that have been used to support the literature review. Discuss these findings with your colleagues.

- Reardon, M., Abrahams, R., Thyer, L., & Simpson, P. (2020). Prevalence of burnout in paramedics: A systematic review of prevalence studies. *Emergency Medicine Australasia*, *32*(2), 182–9. https://doi.org/10.1111/1742-6723.13478
- Coleman, R., Hartz, D., & Dahlen, H. (2020). The experiences of Aboriginal and Torres Strait Islander Bachelor of Midwifery students: An integrative literature review. *Women and Birth*. https://doi.org/10.1016/j.wombi.2020.02.008
- Thornton, R., Nicholson, P., & Harms, L. (2019). Scoping review of memory making in bereavement care for parents after the death of a newborn. *Journal of Obstetric, Gynecologic and Neonatal Nursing*, *48*(3), 351–60. https://doi.org/10.1016/j.jogn.2019.02.001

Engage actively and personally with the material by completing the practical activities in the **Activity boxes**. These help you to assess your own knowledge, beliefs, traits and attitudes.

FOR EXAMPLE

WAS THE DATA COLLECTED IN A WAY THAT ADDRESSED THE RESEARCH ISSUE?

Data were collected using extended digitally-recorded semi-structured interviews. Parents were offered a choice of in-person, telephone or Skype interviews ... In keeping with the tenets of grounded theory, an initial interview guide was developed with several broad, open-ended questions. ... The interview guide was updated after each interview, enabling exploration of emergent categories and subcategories ... Sampling continued until no new categories or subcategories were emerging from subsequent interviews, and until the categories and subcategories were well developed in terms of their properties and dimensions, adding to the theoretical rigour of the emerging grounded theory.

Source: Thornton, R., Nicholson P., & Harms, L. (2020). Creating evidence: Findings from a grounded theory of memory-making in neonatal bereavement care in Australia. *Journal of Pediatric Nursing*, *53*, 29–35.

For example boxes showcase examples of real research writing to help you understand research theory in practice.

FEATURES WITHIN CHAPTERS

TIP The following are 10 simple rules for writing a literature review (Golash-Boza, 2015; Pautasso, 2013).
1 Define the research topic and the audience.
2 Search the literature using a structured process.
3 Make notes about emerging themes while reading the articles.
4 Select the type of literature review required.
5 Keep the review focused.
6 Be critical and consistent.
7 Develop a logical structure.

Tip boxes in each chapter give you helpful hints for successful research.

Defining epistemology and ontology

In understanding how knowledge is generated, two words are unavoidable: **epistemology** and **ontology**.

Epistemology is the study of knowledge and how it is judged to be 'true'; however, truth is, and has always been, an uncertain concept in philosophy. Over time, the search for what counts as truth has accounted for the various interpretations of new knowledge. It has always been important to argue the veracity of ideas before claiming their validity in counting towards the development of new or amended knowledge (Coleman, 2019).

Ontology is the study of existence itself (Monsen et al., 2018); that is, how things can or do exist. Various authors have given their versions of the meaning of life and their views have been thoroughly debated. The philosopher Martin Heidegger, for example, believed that there is no discernible difference between ontology and epistemology; he believed in the philosophy of existence. For Heidegger, knowing is extrapolated from interpretation and understanding. In other words, he argued that we construct our reality, and therefore

Important **Key terms** are marked in bold when they are used in the text for the first time. A full list of key terms is also available in the glossary, which can be found at the back of the book.

Ethics margin icons highlight important coverage of ethics in research.

Ethics

END-OF-CHAPTER FEATURES

At the end of each chapter you will find several tools to help you to review, practise and extend your knowledge of the key learning objectives.

SUMMARY

This chapter discussed the critical appraisal of research and outlined how to critique both quantitative and qualitative research articles.

1 Provide a rationale for undertaking a critique of research evidence	• Undertaking a critique of research evidence:
	  – promotes learning and develops critical thinking skills as a requirement of an assignment
	  – enables students to discriminate what should be included in a literature review
	  – determines the suitability of the evidence for a literature review in a research proposal or article

2 Explain how critically appraising the literature examines the value, trustworthiness and relevance of research evidence	• To judge the trustworthiness, value and relevance in a particular context • To make an informed decision about the value of the research to clinical practice
3 Analyse and evaluate the quality of research articles using critical appraisal criteria	• Standard critical appraisal tools and checklists include those designed by the Critical Appraisal Skills Programme (CASP, 2018), CONSORT (2017) and Joanna Briggs (n.d.) • When critiquing a research article the following questions need to be answered: – What is the clinical question that needs to be answered?

Review your understanding of the key chapter topics with the **Summary**.

END-OF-CHAPTER FEATURES

REVIEW QUESTIONS

1 Explain the three foundational factors when appraising a research article.
2 Explain the process of critiquing a research article.
3 Explain why it is important for clinicians to be able to critically review research articles.
4 Identify the differences when critiquing quantitative and qualitative research articles.
5 Describe the process for critiquing the ethical components of a research article.

Test your knowledge and consolidate your learning through the **review questions** and **challenging review questions**.

CHALLENGING REVIEW QUESTIONS

1 You have been asked to review the literature and make recommendations about evidence-based practice in relation to sustainability and recycling in the healthcare setting. Explain how you will approach reporting on the current evidence and recommendations for clinical practice.
2 Explain how critiquing research articles is linked to evidence-based practice.
3 Explain how engagement in research activities can be promoted in clinical settings.

CASE STUDY 1

Analyse in-depth **Case studies** that present issues in context, encouraging you to integrate and apply the concepts discussed in the chapter to the workplace. These case studies cover **nursing**, **midwifery**, **paramedicine** and **other allied health professions**, giving you the full scope of how research can be applied to all areas of practice.

Prisha is an undergraduate nursing student beginning third year. Prisha is considering her options for a graduate position after she completes her course. As a student nurse, Prisha is aware that stress and burnout are important considerations for hospital nurses and would like to ensure she is fully prepared.

Prisha has found a research paper that she found to be interesting, one published by Kim (2019) that employed a descriptive cross-sectional design when examining emotional labour strategies, stress from emotional labour and burnout in nurses.

Kim, J-S. (2019). Emotional labor strategies, stress, and burnout among hospital nurses: A path analysis. *Journal of Nursing Scholarship, 52*(1), 105–12. https://doi:10.1111/jnu.12532

1 Why is it important to critically appraise the research evidence Prisha is about to read?
2 How do the concepts of validity, reliability and applicability relate to the critical appraisal of the research evidence Prisha is reviewing in relation to her future?
3 There are a variety of tools available to critically appraise research evidence. Can you help Prisha by suggesting an appropriate tool she could use to critically appraise the Kim (2019) research article?

FURTHER READING

Extend your understanding through the suggested **Further reading** relevant to each chapter.

Cooper, H. (2009). *Research Synthesis and Meta-Analysis: A Step-by-Step Approach* (4th edn). London: SAGE.
Crombie, I. (2008). *The Pocket Guide to Critical Appraisal* (2nd edn). Oxford, UK: Wiley.
Day, R., & Gastel, B. (2006). *How to Write and Publish a Scientific Paper* (6th edn). Westport, CT: Greenwood Press.
Fineout-Overholt, E., Melnyk, B. M., Stillwell, S., & Williamson, K. (2010). Evidence-based practice, step by step: Critical appraisal of the evidence part III. *American Journal of Nursing, 110*(11), 43–51. https://doi.org/10.1097/01.NAJ.0000390523.99066.b5
Greenhalgh, T. (2014). *How to Read a Paper. The Basics of Evidence-Based Medicine* (5th edn). Oxford, UK: Wiley.
Livingstone, W., van de Mortel, T., & Taylor, B. (2011). A path of perpetual resilience: Exploring the experience of a diabetes-related amputation through grounded theory. *Contemporary Nurse, 39*(1): 20.
Malloch, K., & Porter-O'Grady, T. (2010). *Introduction to Evidence-Based Practice in Nursing and Health Care.* Sudbury, MA: Jones and Bartlett.
Pain, E. (2016). How to review a paper. https://www.sciencemag.org/careers/2016/09/how-review-paper
Polgar, S., & Thomas, S. A. (2013). *Introduction to Research in the Health Sciences.* Edinburgh: Churchill Livingstone.
Ridley, D. (2012). *The Literature Review. A Step-by-Step Guide for Students* (2nd edn). Los Angeles, CA: SAGE.
Polit, D., & Beck, C. (2006). *Essentials of Nursing Research: Methods, Appraisal and Utilization* (6th edn). Philadelphia, PA: Lippincott.

Guide to the online resources

FOR THE INSTRUCTOR

Cengage is pleased to provide you with a selection of resources
that will help you to prepare your lectures and assessments,
when you choose this textbook for your course.
Log in or request an account to access instructor resources at
au.cengage.com/instructor/account for Australia or
nz.cengage.com/instructor/account for New Zealand.

INSTRUCTOR'S MANUAL

The **Instructor's manual** includes:

- A chapter overview
- Key topics
- Learning objectives
- Connecting key concepts to student experience activities

- Adjunct teaching tips and warm up activities
- Answers to the chapter activities, case studies, review questions and search me! activities

WORD-BASED TEST BANK

This bank of questions has been developed in conjunction with the text for creating quizzes, tests and exams for your students. Deliver these though your LMS and in your classroom.

POWERPOINT™ PRESENTATIONS

Use the chapter-by-chapter PowerPoint slides to enhance your lecture presentations and handouts by reinforcing the key principles of your subject.

ARTWORK FROM THE TEXT

Add the digital files of graphs, tables, pictures and flow charts into your course management system, use them in student handouts, or copy them into your lecture presentations.

SELECTED SOLUTIONS

Solutions to the Review questions from the end of the book.

CASE STUDY ARCHIVE

Additional case studies for students to analyse issues in context, encouraging them to integrate the concepts discussed in the chapter and apply them to the workplace.

ABOUT THE AUTHORS

Main authors

Marilyn Richardson-Tench (PhD) is a casual academic at James Cook University, Queensland, Australia. She is a Fellow of the Australian College of Perioperative Nurses (ACORN). She is an experienced researcher and has presented her research at national and international conferences. Dr Richardson-Tench was the inaugural International Research Visiting Fellow at the University of Glamorgan, Wales, to develop collaborative research on the use of simulation in undergraduate education and perioperative/day surgery practice development. Her current research projects cover areas such as day surgery, nursing ethics and perioperative care of the elderly. Dr Richardson-Tench is also a member of the editorial team and a reviewer for a number of national and international nursing journals.

Patricia Nicholson (PhD) is an Associate Professor and Higher Degree by Research Director at the School of Nursing and Midwifery, Deakin University, Burwood, Australia. She is a Senior Fellow at the University of Melbourne (Nursing), Honorary Research Fellow (Nursing) at Peter MacCallum Cancer Centre and Fellow of the Australian College of Perioperative Nurses (ACORN). She is an experienced academic and researcher and has presented her research both nationally and internationally. Her current research includes higher education, nursing competencies, pressure injuries in surgical patients and medication compliance and postoperative complications. Associate Professor Patricia Nicholson is an ACORN Faculty Member and Standards Lead Reviewer and member of the ACORN journal subcommittee and journal reviewer.

Contributors

This seventh edition has been enhanced by excellent new case studies.
- For the paramedic case studies, featured in Chapters 1, 4, 5, 6 and 11, Cengage would like to thank **Helen Webb**, Associate Professor in Paramedicine at Australian Catholic University, Ballarat campus.
- For the midwifery case studies, featured in Chapters 3, 7, 8, 9 and 10, Cengage would like to thank **Kristen Graham**, lecturer and coordinator (midwifery programs) at Flinders University, Adelaide.
- For the new and updated nursing case studies featured in Chapters 4, 7, 12 and 13, Cengage would like to thank **Sam Edwards**, lecturer in nursing at the University of the Sunshine Coast.
- For the new and updated nursing case studies featured in Chapters 3, 8, 10, 12 and 13, Cengage would like to thank **Sandra Leathwick**, lecturer and coordinator (clinical nursing) at the Australian Catholic University.

ACKNOWLEDGEMENTS

The authors and Cengage would like to thank the following reviewers for their incisive and helpful feedback:

- Sandra Leathwick – Australian Catholic University (Brisbane)
- Melissa Carey – University of Southern Queensland
- Annabel Matheson – Charles Sturt University
- Jacqueline Randle – Australian Catholic University
- Sam Edwards – University of the Sunshine Coast
- Emily Tomlinson – Deakin University
- Natasha Morris – The University of Melbourne
- Nicholas Ralph – University of Southern Queensland
- Fiona Dillon – Flinders University
- Helena Anolak – Flinders University
  The authors would also like to thank the following people.
- Marilyn Richardson-Tench: to my husband Edward and my son Matthew for their support and belief in me, and most of all, their love. And to all the nurses and professional health carers everywhere who have undertaken research for the purpose of advancing the knowledge base of their discipline.
- Patricia Nicholson: to my husband Grenville, and children Jessica and Matthew, for teaching me to persevere and providing me with the courage to strive for excellence in my career. To the nurses who attended my research lectures, and to the students I had the privilege of supervising while undertaking a research degree, they have inspired me with their commitment to providing quality care for their patients that is evidence-based.

RESEARCH IN NURSING AND HEALTH

Chapter learning objectives

The material presented in this chapter will assist you to:

1 differentiate between conducting research, the critical appraisal of research and the clinical use of research in practice
2 appreciate the value of collaborative research within the multidisciplinary health team
3 understand why research in nursing is important
4 describe the research paradigms
5 distinguish between quantitative and qualitative research processes
6 describe the relationship between research, practice and theory
7 explain the use of a theoretical – conceptual framework in a research project.

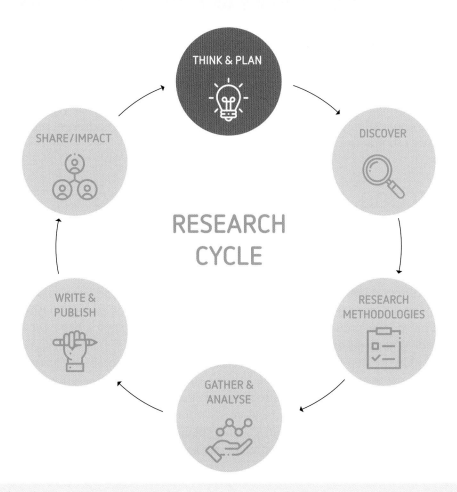

Research cycle

This book introduces research and encompasses all areas of the research cycle as shown in the above diagram. The process of research is cyclical, commencing with thinking and planning about a research topic and concluding with sharing the results of the research. The primary focus of this chapter is to provide an introduction to research and relates to thinking and planning.

Introduction

Health research includes any study addressing the understanding of human health, health behaviours or health services (Sand et al., 2020). **Research** literally means 'looking carefully again'. In the simplest interpretation of the word, when researchers undertake projects, they are searching again for new or adapted knowledge to inform them about areas of interest so they can begin or add to a body of knowledge. Those who carry out nursing research are interested in developing the profession; what patients and clients feel and experience, advancing clinical practice, technological development, health promotion and the outcomes of nursing practice (Hopia & Heikkilä, 2020). Whether it be **quantitative research**, **qualitative research** or a combination of these two main approaches to inquiry, research is systematic in its approach to finding and adapting knowledge.

It is acknowledged that not all nurses want to contribute to the science of nursing by initiating and conducting research projects; however, all nurses need to be consumers of research (Nursing and Midwifery Board of Australia, 2016).

This chapter introduces fundamental ideas relating to research in nursing and health. The importance of collaborative, multidisciplinary research is emphasised, as is the nature of nursing and why research is integral to its practice. Research paradigms are identified as quantitative or qualitative, and both processes are described. Additionally, the three major categories of research used in this book – empirico-analytical, interpretive and critical – are introduced.

Research can be basic or applied. **Basic research** develops fundamental knowledge and tests **theory**; for example, studies of clients' health states, their ability to care for themselves, and their perceptions of phenomena pertaining to health and illness. **Applied research** concerns the application of knowledge to specific situations, and addresses problems such as the best way to practise healthcare.

Conducting, appraising and using research in practice

Conducting research

The purpose of conducting research is to generate new knowledge or to validate existing knowledge. The process begins with compelling questions about a particular phenomenon, such as: What do we know about the phenomenon? What evidence has been developed and reported? What gaps exist in the knowledge base?

A final important step in the research process is the publication of study results with a description of how they contribute to the body of knowledge. Examples of potential nursing research include: conducting a systematic review of studies on the impacts of interdisciplinary team training on patient outcomes, a randomised controlled trial exploring new technology in telehealth, or a qualitative study to investigate the lived experiences of patients from non-English speaking backgrounds in the Australian oncology system (Im et al., 2020).

Critical appraisal of research

Every nurse needs to be a consumer of research, and in order for research results to be implemented in practice, the practitioner must critically appraise research to broaden understanding, summarise knowledge for practice and provide a knowledge base for future studies. Critical appraisal allows the consumer of research to make an assessment of a study and determine its contribution to the discipline and to patient care (Gray, Grove & Sutherland, 2017). It is crucial to determine not only what was done and how, but also how well it was done. An easy method for conducting critical appraisal is to answer the following three key questions.

1   What were the results of the study? (What is the evidence?)
2   How valid are the results? (Can they be trusted?)
3   Will the results be helpful in caring for other patients? (Are they transferable?)
    Critical appraisal of research is covered in more detail in Chapter 4.

Clinical use of research

The clinical use of research is to apply the best evidence available to make patient care decisions; that is, **evidence-based practice (EBP)**. While most of the best evidence stems from research, EBP is about translating the evidence and applying it to clinical decision making, which includes clinical expertise as well as patient preferences and values. The use of EBP takes into consideration that sometimes the best evidence is that of opinion leaders and experts, even though no definitive knowledge from research results exists. EBP involves innovation in terms of finding and translating the best evidence into clinical practice; it is not about developing new knowledge or validating existing knowledge.

EBP

EVIDENCE FOR BEST PRACTICE

CLINICAL USE OF RESEARCH

Research undertaken by Durkin and colleagues (2020) explored the effect of a mass media campaign on the participation rates in home bowel screening. A significant increase in completed home faecal occult blood tests during the campaign was discovered, although results did not differ significantly by age, sex or socioeconomic status when compared to the control group. Findings were consequential for planning future public health campaigns.

A five-year study by Marriott and colleagues (2020) investigated the experiences of Aboriginal women giving birth and receiving maternity care on Country versus in the suburban setting. Recommendations from the study provided guidance on midwifery practice and education in meeting Aboriginal women's expectations.

A randomised control trial was undertaken in a group of nursing homes to ascertain which intervention was the most effective in managing urinary incontinence in elderly female residents. Findings were significant for improving the quality of care for this population (Hödl et al., 2019).

A study in Finland sought to identify acute care nurses's views on practicing in environmentally responsible ways. Using a Delphi study, results focused on using materials efficiently (such as minimising waste and using sustainable products) and actively reducing energy consumption. Participants shared that embracing environmentally friendly nursing required training, guidance and inducements, as well as multidisciplinary collaboration (Kallio et al., 2020).

Research was undertaken to investigate the psychosocial outcomes after bariatric surgery, from the perspective of the patient. Data from semistructured interviews highlighted that patients needed accessible and holistic long-term care; these findings will inform the design of patient-centred follow-up care (Coulman et al., 2020).

The origins of EBP, the definitions and criteria used in judging levels of evidence, and how to implement research are discussed in Chapter 13.

Research is linked with theory in a reciprocal relationship within the **theoretical framework** of a study. This chapter also describes the nature of theory and discusses the use of a **conceptual framework** in all stages of the research project.

Collaborative research

Nurses and other health professionals can participate in research in various ways.

- *Independent level:* a researcher can conduct the whole project alone, but to do so takes a considerable amount of training, preferably to doctoral level.
- *Interdependent level:* a researcher can participate in a research project in collaboration with other researchers. Interdependence implies that the researcher makes a contribution to the conceptualisation, implementation, evaluation and dissemination of the project.
- *Dependent level:* a researcher could be a data collector for another researcher's project but not make a significant contribution to the conceptual part of the project.

Nursing research provides many opportunities to collaborate with other researchers in a multidisciplinary team. Nurses are rapidly breaking down barriers to multidisciplinary research, creating new meanings and interpretations that can expose improved findings to establish optimum care and satisfactory patient outcomes (Adhikari et al., 2014). Nurses working in practice, administration and education have opportunities to collaborate with other researchers on research projects. They may work across various wards or units in the same healthcare facility or collaborate on a larger project that requires more research participants and the expertise of multiple researchers.

Healthcare requires the expertise of many workers qualified in different fields of practice, such as medical practitioners, nurses, midwives, paramedics, physiotherapists, pharmacists, speech therapists, nutritionists, occupational therapists and so on. The complexity of human problems when body dysfunction is present means that the overall needs of patients are often best met by multidisciplinary teams in hospitals and community organisations. Many research questions that can directly benefit patient care can be raised within such multidisciplinary teams.

Research collaboration is possible between researchers in nursing and researchers from other disciplines. It may take time, energy, opportunities and organisational skills before projects commence, but the rewards can be great for the respective disciplines and for those with whom the researchers collaborate (Roberts & Goodhand, 2018). Research collaboration between educational organisations, healthcare agencies and the community can also be used to achieve mutual outcomes and amalgamate theory and practice (Babl et al., 2020).

FOR EXAMPLE

COLLABORATIVE RESEARCH

Research collaboration has brought together diverse teams, such as nurses nationally and abroad, psychologists and the community.

- McCullough and colleagues (2020) worked with nurses who shared their knowledge and experience of working in very remote communities. Participants described healthcare access issues, such as a lack of resources, and needing to making compromises to provide healthcare when support is unavailable.

- Bampoh and colleagues (2020) led a team of international researchers, government officials and academics with the aim of improving the healthcare provided to refugees, using nurse-centred initiatives. Key findings from this public healthcare initiative were aimed at improving the nursing care of refugees through standardisation of clinical practices and enhancement of nurse leadership. Nurses themselves were also empowered through this study, as their role in caring for vulnerable and marginalised populations was given a spotlight.
- Ruiz (2020) examined an emergency department's attitudes towards an advanced nurse practitioner role. Findings indicated that the multidisciplinary team in the emergency department believed the role would improve patient care, waiting times and the quality of patient experience. Further, funding was identified as an issue, as was the availability for supervision by a senior doctor when required.
- Carter and colleagues (2020) carried out a feasibility study for a randomised controlled trial to assess the effectiveness of a peer support program for women with antenatal depression. Women assigned to the control group had routine midwifery and general practitioner care, and women in the intervention group had additional regular visits from a peer support worker. Data analysis showed that the peer support worker had a positive impact, reducing feelings of alienation, stigma and isolation, and improving feelings of confidence and self-esteem.

ACTIVITY

Think of three areas of healthcare that involve a multidisciplinary team and provide one research question for each area. Who could be involved in researching these questions?

Why research?

Practice and research in health professions

Occupations become professions by attaining the credentials of professionalism. Lifelong learning and inquiry is essential to professionalism, and practitioners are responsible for maintaining currency in practice and updating their knowledge (Dickerson & Graebe, 2020). Nurses identify themselves as professionals, having moved in their practice evolution from occupational to professional status.

Fundamental to the development of professional research is the tertiary education system, which promotes systematic inquiry and scholarship development. In Australia, academic nursing began in the 1950s and continues to this day. In the late 1980s, the move of basic nursing education into the tertiary education sector was an important influence on the development of Australian nursing research. Individuals in health professions, such as medicine, have been educated in the tertiary sector for much longer, which is reflected in the strong professional status of doctors as clinicians and the prioritisation of government support for biomedical research into health and illness.

Research as a means of generating knowledge

The basic reason for conducting research is to find new knowledge and adapt existing knowledge. The history of research is basically the history of ideas, or philosophy. From the time of Plato, Socrates and their contemporaries to the rebirth of knowledge in the Renaissance, humans have progressed through phases of observation and conjecture about people, their planet and the universe. Since the 17th century and the work of Descartes, the scientific model has been the established approach. However, there has been a reaction to that model as the benchmark of all research in the last century or so, with the generation of multiple qualitative research approaches.

The reason for raising these ideas about research as a means of generating knowledge is to have you consider the possibility that there may be many approaches to finding knowledge through research that have merit, and that one kind should not necessarily be seen as being superior to another (Rutberg & Bouikidis, 2018). The debate about the essence, role and relationships of nursing knowledge retains significance as it defines the professional status of the discipline, regulates intellectual and/or technical nursing activities and determines the degree of emphasis given to research, theory, practice development and teaching (Borbasi & Jackson, 2016).

Defining epistemology and ontology

In understanding how knowledge is generated, two words are unavoidable: **epistemology** and **ontology**.

Epistemology is the study of knowledge and how it is judged to be 'true'; however, truth is, and has always been, an uncertain concept in philosophy. Over time, the search for what counts as truth has accounted for the various interpretations of new knowledge. It has always been important to argue the veracity of ideas before claiming their validity in counting towards the development of new or amended knowledge (Coleman, 2019).

Ontology is the study of existence itself (Monsen et al., 2018); that is, how things can or do exist. Various authors have given their versions of the meaning of life and their views have been thoroughly debated. The philosopher Martin Heidegger, for example, believed that there is no discernible difference between ontology and epistemology; he believed in the philosophy of existence. For Heidegger, knowing is extrapolated from interpretation and understanding. In other words, he argued that we construct our reality, and therefore our comprehension, from our experience of being in the world; and we are the only beings to examine our human 'being' through enquiry about our daily lives (Takkal et al., 2018). While a diversion into ontological thought is not warranted now, it is a central focus of human thought and has relevance for nursing research.

Nurses and other healthcare workers need to ask questions about knowing and existing because the answers to such questions form the substance of their disciplines. Whenever researchers raise questions about what they know and how they know it is trustworthy knowledge, they are asking epistemological questions. Whenever researchers ask about the nature of the existence of something or someone, they are asking ontological questions, which is what makes these words relevant and integral to nursing and health research.

Overview of research paradigms

A **paradigm** is a broad view of, or perspective on, something; some may even say that it is a world view; that is, a comprehensive approach to a particular area of interest. The paradigm of a profession not only concerns the content of the professional knowledge but also the **processes** by which that knowledge is produced, and as a result is flexible in application. Carrying out research is not a value-free exercise. Research paradigms are the tools through which researchers ask 'why' questions. Different paradigms produce different questions, and focus on different parts of a research topic (Nairn, 2019).

FOR EXAMPLE

RESEARCH ON PARADIGMS

Brown and colleagues (2009) demonstrated a shift in paradigm surrounding the delivery of care for individuals with intellectual disabilities from a deficit-based approach to a support-based approach. These changes have a profound effect on the delivery of care to the individual client.

Lamont and Waring (2015) identified a paradigm shift in nursing research to study safety as a relational property which they argue would bring to the fore relationships of accountability. Further, these studies may highlight the interdependencies between different care providers, specifically in admissions and discharge.

Regan, Carol and Vorderer (2018) demonstrated a paradigm shift in the inpatient psychiatric care of children to that of child- and family-centred care. These changes have shown a decrease in some practices such as restraint and seclusion.

Various approaches to doing research can be classified paradigmatically. Researchers may, for example, speak of quantitative or qualitative research, or they may refer to certain paradigms across all the possible kinds of knowledge that can be generated through research.

A paradigmatic view provides overall, overarching categories in which certain kinds of research and ways of knowledge generation and verification can be placed.

A student who is new to research will find that there is a great deal of detail to be learned about the various research approaches. This can be very confusing for novice researchers who are trying to acquire an overview of the possibilities and problems confronting them. With this in mind, we have organised this book into distinct chapters that give information on quantitative and qualitative research. We have also maintained the concept of two forms of qualitative inquiry, to help sort out the differences between qualitative research methodologies. The three major categories of research we have used to structure this book generate and verify empirico-analytical (quantitative), interpretive (mostly qualitative) and critical (mostly qualitative) forms of knowledge.

Empirico-analytical (quantitative) research

All research needs a foundation for its inquiry. This foundation is provided by world views and scientific or **positivist** paradigms. The positivist paradigm provides an objective reality against which researchers can compare their claims and ascertain truth to find a relationship between certain variables. The positivist position is grounded in the theoretical belief that there is an objective reality that can be known to the researcher if he or she uses the correct **methods** and applies those methods in the correct manner (Coleman, 2019).

Empirico-analytical research employs the scientific method (and is sometimes referred to by this term) in observation and **analysis**. The scientific method is basically a set of rules for how to do research, which can be considered to be rigorous in the sense that it can be shown to test something over and over again and be consistently accurate (reliability). It also shows that it is testing what it actually intends to test (validity) rather than other things that are unnoticed (extraneous variables). To achieve this, the scientific method demands that research be as free as possible from the distorting influences of people, such as their ideas, intentions and emotions (**subjectivity**). In other words, research needs to show that due consideration has been given to achieving objectivity. This process is common to all disciplines that produce scientific knowledge, and has traditionally been regarded as the best way to build knowledge. The scientific method comprises induction (a theory-building approach) and deduction (a theory-testing approach).

Another requirement of the scientific method is that the only research questions that can be legitimately asked are ones that are structured in ways that can be observed and analysed (by empirico-analytical means), and can be measured by numbers, percentages and statistics (quantified). This is why research using the scientific method is also referred to as empirico-analytical and/or quantitative research.

Empirico-analytical and/or quantitative researchers want to reduce things of interest to their most focused and smallest parts (reductionism) in order to study them. They do this based on an underlying assumption that there are cause-and-effect links between certain objects and subjects (variables). It is assumed that these cause-and-effect relationships have a far greater chance of being discovered if the variables in a study are carefully controlled and manipulated. Researchers take a great deal of care to design their projects to ensure that they are observing and analysing the effects of what they intend to study so that they can demonstrate to the scientific community that the results are statistically significant. This means they try to confirm or dispute the degree of certainty they can place in cause-and-effect relationships through mathematical explanations.

Research (typically undertaken using quantitative and experimental methods) is evaluated using three criteria.

- *Validity*: the extent to which a measurement approach or procedure gives the correct answer (allowing the researcher to measure or evaluate an objective reality).
- *Reliability*: the extent to which a measurement approach or procedure gives the same answer whenever it is carried out.
- *Generalisability*: the extent to which the findings of a study can be applied externally or more broadly outside of the study **context**.

Health professions have been identified as sciences because they primarily use the empirical method for their research inquiry. Nurses, for example, adopted the empirical scientific method because they believed that it was the best way of developing nursing knowledge and of promoting the acceptance of nursing as a valid discipline. The classification of any health profession as a science allies it with empirical science, especially where decisions about research funding and research **ethics** are concerned.

The quantitative research process

The steps of the quantitative scientific research process are depicted in Figure 1.1. This process generally completes one phase entirely before going on to the next.

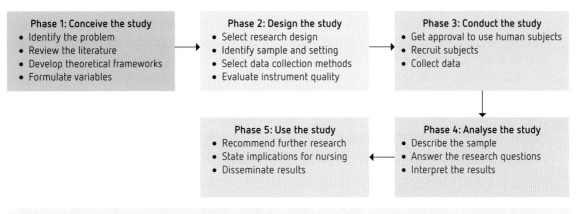

Phase 1: Conceive the study
- Identify the problem
- Review the literature
- Develop theoretical frameworks
- Formulate variables

Phase 2: Design the study
- Select research design
- Identify sample and setting
- Select data collection methods
- Evaluate instrument quality

Phase 3: Conduct the study
- Get approval to use human subjects
- Recruit subjects
- Collect data

Phase 5: Use the study
- Recommend further research
- State implications for nursing
- Disseminate results

Phase 4: Analyse the study
- Describe the sample
- Answer the research questions
- Interpret the results

▶ **Figure 1.1** The qualitative research process

Source: This figure was published in *Navigating the Maze of Nursing: Enhancing Nursing and Midwifery Practice* (4th edn), Sally Borbasi, & Debrah Jackson, p. 18, copyright Elsevier 2016.

The quantitative research process attempts to discover scientific knowledge through the **measurement** of elements, at four possible levels.

1 *Description*: elements of a phenomenon are counted.
2 *Correlation*: relationships of two or more elements are investigated.
3 *Explanation*: one element explains another.
4 *Prediction*: the activity of one element can be predicted from that of another.

The quantitative research process may involve an inductive process in which a lot of **data** are collected and described. If, for example, you wanted to find out the average occurrence of some characteristic of people, you could go out and measure a certain number of people and calculate the mean, but you would then have to test your findings to see if they hold up. You would do this by measuring a lot more people of varying kinds and seeing if most of the measurements fell near the average. Many quantitative designs involve testing relationships between phenomena, usually by proposing a hypothesis or statement about the relationship between the variables; then, data are gathered, findings analysed and conclusions drawn about the findings.

EVIDENCE FOR BEST PRACTICE

EBP

QUANTITATIVE RESEARCH

Mwakanyanga and Tarimo (2018) undertook a study to quantify the skill of intensive care nurses when providing suctioning to intubated patients. Using a questionnaire and observation, the researchers found that a significant number of participants did not perform the skill in line with current recommendations. This has implications for training and further research.

Qualitative research

Qualitative research involves questions that focus on human consciousness and subjectivity, and value humans and their experiences in the research process. It involves finding out about the changing (relative) nature of knowledge, which is seen to be special and centred on the people, place, time and conditions in which it finds itself (unique and context dependent). Qualitative research uses thinking that starts from the specific instance and moves to the general pattern of combined instances (inductive), so it grows from the ground up to make larger statements about the nature of what is being investigated.

Rather than starting with a statement (hypothesis), qualitative research begins a project with a statement of the area of interest.

FOR EXAMPLE

QUALITATIVE RESEARCH USING A THEORETICAL FRAMEWORK

Slemon and colleagues (2018) explored the experiences of nursing students in a mental health placement. Students shared that they witnessed nursing practices that were not congruent with their beliefs, such as purposefully avoiding patients, giving medication rather than counselling patients and not guiding the students themselves in this specialty area. Results were analysed through a theoretical power and resistance framework by Foucault. Nurses held power over clients, and the students were drawn into a complex situation where they met this power with resistance. By actively engaging in conversation or activities with clients, and seeking support from each other, they were able to navigate the challenges. The students also perceived themselves as being a disempowered group, but the clinical educator was fundamental in providing support via debrief and empowering students to resist some dominant practices in the unit.

The measures for ensuring validity in qualitative research involve asking participants to confirm that the interpretations represent faithfully and clearly what the experience was/is like for them. Reliability is often not an issue in qualitative research as it is based on the idea that knowledge is relative and is dependent on all the features of the people, place, time and other circumstances (context) of the setting. People are valued as sources of information and their expressions of their personal awareness (subjectivity) are valued as being integral to the meaning that comes out of the research. Rather than saying that something can be claimed to be statistically significant, qualitative research makes no claims to generate knowledge that can be confirmed as certain (absolute).

A distinction is made in this book between qualitative interpretive research and qualitative critical research. Interpretive research aims mainly to generate meaning. It tries to explain and describe in order to make sense of items of interest. Qualitative critical research overtly aims to bring about change to the status quo. By working collaboratively with participants as co-researchers to address research problems systematically, qualitative researchers try to find answers and use them to bring about change (see Chapter 8 for a more detailed discussion). The principal difference between interpretive and critical research is that interpretive forms are concerned mainly with creating meaning, while critical forms focus on causing sociopolitical change. Postmodern influences on research can be considered as extending combinations of qualitative interpretive and critical research, taking a highly eclectic view of knowledge generation and validation methods and processes.

The qualitative research process

There are similarities between the processes for quantitative and qualitative research. All projects need: a well-planned beginning; a careful middle section in which the data are collected, analysed and interpreted; and a thoroughly executed end stage in which the results are written up and disseminated. However, there are also differences between quantitative and qualitative research processes.

Qualitative research tends to define the word 'process' differently from the accepted dictionary usage, which is synonymous with a set of steps or methods. Qualitative research defines *process* as the 'how' of research, especially in relation to how the people in the research relate to one another.

There are features of research processes that identify qualitative research projects as being different from quantitative research projects. The differences lie in the use of language, the degree of involvement and collaboration of the research participants, and the ownership of the project, as can be seen in Figure 1.2.

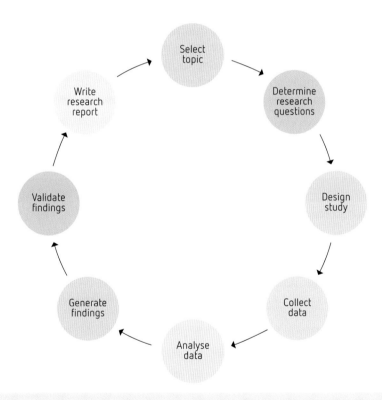

▶ **Figure 1.2** The qualitative research process

TIP

Quantitative researchers tend to refer to the people they have accessed in the research as 'subjects'. Qualitative researchers tend to refer to the people they have accessed in the research as 'participants'.

By objective means, subjects are exposed to carefully prepared methods and instruments in quantitative research such as surveys, questionnaires, clinical trials and so on. When doing qualitative research projects, researchers claim to work with participants by means that value the subjectivity of participants.

There are variations in the degree of participant involvement in qualitative research. Critical forms of qualitative research, for example, pay far more attention to ensuring a high degree of participant involvement and collaboration, evidenced by the tendency of many of the researchers who use critical methodologies to refer to participants as co-researchers. Critical researchers also try to minimise the effects of power differences between the researcher and the participants or co-researchers. Friendships that last throughout the life of the project and beyond sometimes develop between the people involved in the research.

In qualitative critical methodologies such as feminist and action research approaches, there is a tendency for participants or co-researchers to have an influential **voice** in the overall conduct of the project. The project may run according to the wishes and directions of the group, which may develop a strong sense of joint ownership of the project. This sense of ownership may be reflected in the acknowledgement in the **research report** of all the people involved in its direction. Ownership may also manifest in the publication of jointly authored journal articles and the presentation of jointly prepared papers at professional conferences.

Differences between quantitative and qualitative research

It is a major oversimplification to say that efforts to explain human knowledge and existence have gone into two main streams; that is, quantitative and qualitative inquiry. However, this claim will be asserted here to prevent the need for following each and every detail and detour in past and present philosophical debate. Table 1.1 will help you to consider some differences between quantitative and qualitative research.

The reason for caution in thinking of quantitative and qualitative research as being categorically different is that there may be some remnants of one in the other. Both approaches can use deductive and inductive thinking, and both require a scientific design in the sense that each must show it is systematic and rigorous. Caution is necessary in trying to set up both approaches as irreconcilable alternatives.

▶ Table 1.1   Differences between quantitative and qualitative research

Quantitative research	Qualitative research
Focuses on a small number of specific concepts and their relationship and differences	Attempts to understand the entirety or whole of some phenomenon within a prescribed context
Is set on a predefined theoretical foundation – 'educated guesses' made about the relationship between concepts and study outcomes	No preconceived theoretical boundaries or preconceived notions about study outcomes
The researcher controls and interprets data	Focuses on people's interpretations of events and circumstances rather than the researcher's
Tends to use larger samples	Uses smaller samples
Describes people in the study as subjects	Describes people in the study as participants, informants or sometimes co-researchers
Uses language in such a way that implies neutrality, such as writing in the third person	Can be written using the first person
Uses structured procedures and formal instruments to collect information	Collects information without formal structured instruments
Collects information under conditions of control and manipulation	Doesn't attempt to control the context of research, but attempts to capture it in its entirety
Emphasises objectivity in the collection and analysis of information Attempts to exclude all forms of subjective bias	Attempts to capitalise on the subjective as a means of understanding and interpreting human experiences Is comfortable with the notion of bias
Uses objective tools to collect data	The researcher is the instrument of data collection

Source: This table was published in *Navigating the Maze of Nursing: Enhancing Nursing and Midwifery Practice* (4th edn), Sally Borbasi, & Debrah Jackson, p. 18, copyright Elsevier 2016.

The following is a practice situation that may be analysed using both a quantitative and a qualitative approach.

FOR EXAMPLE

QUANTITATIVE AND QUALITATIVE QUESTIONS

A 65-year-old man with advanced chronic obstructive pulmonary disease has been frequently hospitalised in the last three months for shortness of breath. During his current admission, he reported that he has been anxious and is frightened of suffocating. Despite maximal therapy, the palliative care team suggests a trial of opioids.

- *Quantitative question:* What is the most effective pharmacological therapy to manage dyspnoea in this situation?
- *Qualitative question:* What is it like for families who provide home care for relatives who are suffering from dyspnoea?

In summary, the features of empirico-analytical or quantitative research are to attain **rigour** in the reliability and validity of projects by using observational and analytic means to control and manipulate variables, and to produce objective data that can be quantified to demonstrate the degree of statistical significance in cause-and-effect relationships. This sounds like a good idea, and it is for research in which the rules of the scientific method can be applied uniformly. Problems become apparent when researchers decide that they want to ask questions about human knowledge and existence that are outside the observe-and-analyse domain, and when they want to value people's intentions, ideas and emotions as part of the research process.

ACTIVITY

Write two research questions each for imaginary quantitative and qualitative projects and explain what the main intentions of both sets of questions are. Can any of these questions be approached by mixed methods? Why?

A shifting paradigm

Research in the quantitative paradigm has long attracted major funding because it often produces clear and concise findings that can be generalised. But mixed-methods research projects increasingly have been adopted to broaden the scope of findings using both quantitative (science-oriented) and qualitative (humanities-oriented) designs, underpinning the importance of human sciences in exploring the experiences of people.

Relationship between research, practice and theory

Research is linked with theory in a reciprocal relationship. Research findings are 'incorporated into theory by human scientists … to describe, explain, predict and prescribe important aspects of our lives' (Greenwood, 1996). Research can lead to the revision of existing practice theories by testing them using quantitative approaches. Conversely, research using qualitative methodologies, such as grounded theory, can lead to the development of useful theories for any health profession. Both approaches can lead to the development of knowledge in the discipline of nursing.

Research into the health status of the client and professional practice can lead to the development of useful theories for health and nursing.

Deriving theory from research data is an inductive approach. Many instances of data are collected and then a theory is proposed that fits the observations. This approach is associated with qualitative research designs, such as grounded theory and **phenomenology**.

Theory can stimulate research when a researcher has ideas that are based in a theory. These ideas about the potential outcomes of the study form its framework. The conceptual framework of a research study is like the skeleton of the body in that it gives structure. This structure helps to plan the work, to know how the parts fit together, to know where to add parts and to provide a place to attach the other parts. All parts of the research project are linked to the theory, thus forming a coherent whole. Using theory as a conceptual framework is a deductive approach that is associated primarily with quantitative research methodology.

Research can also answer questions about theory through theory testing. A researcher might, for example, decide to test one of the propositions of an existing theory against a new group of clients, or in a healthcare situation in which previous research on that proposition has not been carried out.

TIP

Theory testing is a deductive approach primarily associated with quantitative research design.

Using a theoretical – conceptual framework

A framework comprises the conceptual underpinnings of a study and is used in all stages of the research project. Polit and Beck (2017) suggest that in a study based on a theory, the framework is referred to as a theoretical framework, while in a study that has its roots in a specified conceptual model, such as a nursing model, the framework is often called the conceptual framework (Polit & Beck, 2017, p. 119).

The first step in using a conceptual or theoretical framework is to choose a theory or model that is suited to the research question. It is important to examine the relationship between the question asked and the conceptual or theoretical framework. The methodology of the study, including data analysis, should be congruent with the theory or model. You can use the theory or model as a guide to interpreting the findings and judging their significance. In writing up the report, you can use the model to provide a structure for organising the literature review, the presentation of the results and the discussion, which, if used appropriately, lead to an integration of the parts of the study. Chapter 8 provides more information on theoretical models.

TIP

The terms 'conceptual framework', 'conceptual model' and 'theoretical framework' are often used interchangeably.

FOR EXAMPLE

USE OF A THEORETICAL FRAMEWORK

Richardson-Tench (2008) used the theoretical framework of Foucauldian feminist poststructuralism in 'The scrub nurse: Basking in reflected glory'.

SUMMARY

This chapter established this research textbook's foundation by introducing some fundamental ideas relating to research in nursing.

1	Differentiate between conducting research, the critical appraisal of research and the clinical use of research in practice	• Critical appraisal skills are needed by all nurses in practice to determine the application of research findings to practice • Nurses need to implement the recommendations of clinical research to ensure their practice is evidence-based • Not all nurses need to conduct research
2	Appreciate the value of collaborative research within the multidisciplinary health team	• Nursing research provides many opportunities to collaborate with other researchers in a multidisciplinary team
3	Understand why research in nursing is important	• Research in nursing is important because it: – is essential to professionalism – generates new knowledge and adapts existing knowledge
4	Describe the research paradigms	• Various approaches to research can be classified paradigmatically, such as: – quantitative and qualitative – empirico-analytical (quantitative) – interpretive (mostly qualitative) – critical (mostly qualitative)
5	Distinguish between quantitative and qualitative research processes	• The quantitative research process attempts to find out scientific knowledge by the measurement of elements • The qualitative research process involves finding out about the changing (relative) nature of knowledge, which is seen to be special and centred in the people, place, time and conditions in which it finds itself (unique and context dependent)
6	Describe the relationship between research, practice and theory	• Research, practice and theory are linked in a relationship that connects knowledge generation and validation and applies them to solve practice problems and to create deeper insights into how people experience health disruptions and how health professionals can give them the best possible care
7	Explain the use of a theoretical–conceptual framework in a research project	• A theoretical–conceptual framework is used in all stages of the research project to give it structure

REVIEW QUESTIONS

1 Why is it essential for nurses to be active in research?
2 What research questions are best suited to a quantitative approach?
3 What research questions are best suited to a qualitative approach?
4 Identify some areas of research that could be undertaken collaboratively.

CHALLENGING REVIEW QUESTIONS

1 Discuss the varying research paradigms and identify where each may be used.
2 How do the qualitative, interpretive and critical approaches differ in their research intentions?
3 Discuss the use of a conceptual or theoretical framework in a qualitative study.

CASE STUDY 1

Katie, an experienced registered nurse with a master qualification, works in the dementia ward in a large aged-care facility. Katie has observed that some dementia patients have a positive response to music being played in the ward.

This observation led Katie to undertake a literature search for any current research that might help in the care of these residents. While she found research on the use of music as a treatment to improve cognitive function in people with dementia, there was a lack of standardised methods for music therapy interventions and the effect on quality of life was inconclusive. Katie has decided to undertake some research herself on music therapy interventions to see if these have any effect on the quality of life for residents with dementia.

Realising that her research will need to involve the expertise of the multidisciplinary team in her unit, Katie decided to formulate a research proposal to present to its members during an aged-care team meeting.

Can you help Katie to brainstorm ideas for the project? Respond to the following questions that Katie should consider before she begins to write the proposal.

1 What members of the multidisciplinary team could be involved in the research?
2 What clinical expertise can they offer?
3 What research paradigms are they likely to favour?
4 How can the research team ensure that its research provides the best evidence for practice?

CASE STUDY 2

Chloe is a paramedic at a busy metropolitan ambulance branch. She attended a motor vehicle collision and sustained a significant back and shoulder injury while assisting in the extrication of a 110-kilogram patient from the vehicle. Chloe has been on WorkCover for 18 months. Every aspect of her life has changed, and she is unlikely to be able to return to on-road paramedic work. She has had three surgical procedures, her rehabilitation is not progressing, she is in constant pain and she feels depressed. Chloe has found out that many of her colleagues, both male and female, have sustained similar workplace injuries. Chloe has enrolled in a research master's degree and wants to investigate workplace injury in paramedicine, as she has found published research in this area to be scant.

1 Which research paradigms could be used to study workplace injury in paramedicine?
2 Is there opportunity for collaborative research? Which other health disciplines could be involved in the study?
3 Develop one or more research questions for each research paradigm you identified for question one.

REFERENCES

Adhikari, R., Tocher, J., Smith, P., Corcoran, J., & Macarthur, J. (2014). A multi-disciplinary approach to medication safety and the implication for nursing education and practice. *Nurse Education Today, 34*(2), 185–90. https://doi.org/10.1016/j.nedt.2013.10.008

Babl, F. E., Dalziel, S. R., & Borland, M. L. (2020). Establishing a research network. *Journal of Paediatrics and Child Health, 56*(6), 857–63. https://doi.org/10.1111/jpc.14896

Bampoh, V., Thongkhamkitcharoen, M., Dicker, S., Dalal, W., Frerich, E., Mann, E., Porta, C., Siddons, N., Stauffer, W. M., & Hoffman, S.J. (2020). Nursing practice and global refugee migration: Initial impressions from an intergovernmental-academic partnership. *International Nursing Review, 67*(3), 334–40. https://doi.org/10.1111/inr.12588

Borbasi, S., & Jackson, D. (2016). *Navigating the Maze of Research. Enhancing Nursing and Midwifery Practice* (4th edn). Sydney: Elsevier.

Brown, H. K., Ouellette-Kuntz, H., Bielska, I., & Elliott, D. (2009). Choosing a measure of support need: Implications for research and policy. *Journal of Intellectual Disability Research, 53*(Part 11), 949–54.

Carter, R., Cust, F., & Boath, E. (2020). Effectiveness of a peer support intervention for antenatal depression: A feasibility study. *Journal of Reproductive and Infant Psychology, 38*(3), 259–70. https://doi.org/10.1080/02646838.2019.1668547

Coleman, P. (2019). An examination of positivist and critical realist philosophical approaches to nursing research. *International Journal of Caring Sciences, 12*(2), 1–7. http://search.proquest.com/docview/2303668683/

Coulman, K., MacKichan, F., Blazeby, J., Donovan, J., & Owen-Smith, A. (2020). Patients' experiences of life after bariatric surgery and follow-up care: A qualitative study. *BMJ Open, 10*(2), e035013. https://doi.org/10.1136/bmjopen-2019-035013

Dickerson, P., Graebe, J., & Shinners, J. (2020). Nursing continuing professional development – a paradigm shift. *The Journal of Continuing Education in Nursing, 51*(7), 297–9. https://doi.org/10.3928/00220124-20200611-02

Durkin, S., Broun, K., Guerin, N., Morley, B., & Wakefield, M. (2020). Impact of a mass media campaign on participation in the Australian bowel cancer screening program. *Journal of Medical Screening, 27*(1), 18–24. https://doi.org/10.1177/0969141319874372

Gray, J. R., Grove, S. K., & Sutherland, S. (2017). *Burns and Grove's The Practice of Nursing Research: Appraisal, Synthesis, and Generation of Evidence* (8th edn). St Louis, MO: Elsevier.

Greenwood, J. (1996). Nursing research and nursing theory. In J. Greenwood (ed.), *Nursing Theory in Australia: Development and Application* (pp. 20–37). Sydney: Harper Educational Australia.

Hödl, M., Halfens, R. J. G., & Lohrmann, C. (2019). Effectiveness of conservative urinary incontinence management among female nursing home residents – a cluster RCT. *Archives of Gerontology and Geriatrics*, 81, 245–51. https://doi.org/10.1016/j.archger.2019.01.003

Hopia, H., & Heikkilä, J. (2020). Nursing research priorities based on CINAHL database: A scoping review. *Nursing Open, 7*(2), 483–94. https://doi.org/10.1002/nop2.428

Im, E.-O., Sakashita, R., Lin, C.-C., Lee, T.-H., Tsai, H.-M., & Inouye, J. (2020). Current trends in nursing research across five locations: The United States, South Korea, Taiwan, Japan, and Hong Kong. *Journal of Nursing Scholarship: An Official Publication of Sigma Theta Tau International Honor Society of Nursing, 52*(6), 671–9. https://doi.org/10.1111/jnu.12592

Kallio, H., Pietilä, A.-M., & Kangasniemi, M. (2020). Environmental responsibility in nursing in hospitals: A modified Delphi study of nurses' views. *Journal of Clinical Nursing*. https://doi.org/10.1111/jocn.15429

Lamont, T., & Waring, J. (2015). Safety lessons: Shifting paradigms and new directions for patient safety research. *Journal of Health Services Research & Policy, 20*(1 suppl), 1–8. https://doi.org/10.1177/1355819614558340

Marriott, R., Reibel, T., Gliddon, J., Griffin, D., Coffin, J., Eades, A., Robinson, M., Bowen, A., Kendall, S., Martin, T., Monterosso, L., Stanley, F., & Walker, R. (2020). Aboriginal research methods and researcher reflections on working two-ways to investigate culturally secure birthing for Aboriginal women. *Australian Aboriginal Studies, 1*, 36–53.

McCullough, K., Whitehead, L., Bayes, S., Williams, A., & Cope, V. (2020). The delivery of primary health care in remote communities: A grounded theory study of the perspective of nurses. *International Journal of Nursing Studies, 102*, 103474. https://doi.org/10.1016/j.ijnurstu.2019.103474

Monsen, K., Kelechi, T., McRae, M., Mathiason, M., & Martin, K. (2018). Nursing theory, terminology, and big data: Data-driven discovery of novel patterns in archival randomized clinical trial data. *Nursing Research*, *67*(2), 122–32. https://doi.org/10.1097/NNR.0000000000000269

Mwakanyanga, E., & Tarimo, E. (2018). Intensive care nurses' knowledge and practice on endotracheal suctioning of the intubated patient: A quantitative cross-sectional observational study. *PLoS One*, *13*(8), e0201743. https://doi.org/10.1371/journal.pone.0201743

Nairn, S. (2019). Research paradigms and the politics of nursing knowledge: A reflective discussion. *Nursing Philosophy*, 17 July. https://onlinelibrary.wiley.com/doi/abs/10.1111/nup.12260

Nursing and Midwifery Board of Australia. (2016). *Registered Nurse Standards for Practice*. 1 June 2016.

Polit, D., & Beck, C. (2017). *Nursing Research: Generating and Assessing Evidence for Nursing Practice* (10th edn). Philadelphia, PA: Lippincott.

Regan, K. M., Carol, C., & Vorderer, L. (2018). Paradigm shifts in inpatient psychiatric care of children: Approaching child- and family-centered care. *Journal of Child and Adolescent Psychiatric Nursing*, 26 July. https://doi.org/10.1111/jcap.12193

Richardson-Tench, M. (2008). The scrub nurse: Basking in reflected glory. *Journal of Advanced Perioperative Care*, *3*(4), 125–31.

Roberts, F. E., & Goodhand, K. (2018). Scottish healthcare student's perceptions of an interprofessional ward simulation: An exploratory, descriptive study. *Nursing & Health Sciences*, *20*(1), 107–15. https://doi.org/10.1111/nhs.12393

Ruiz, L. M. (2020). Multidisciplinary team attitudes to an advanced nurse practitioner service in an emergency department. *Emergency Nurse: The Journal of the RCN Accident and Emergency Nursing Association*, *28*(1), 33–42. https://doi.org/10.7748/en.2018.e1793

Rutberg, S., & Bouikidis, C. (2018). Focusing on the fundamentals: A simplistic differentiation between qualitative and quantitative research. *Nephrology Nursing Journal*, *45*(2), 209–12.

Sand, A.-S., Grimsgaard, S., & Pettersen, I. (2020). Patient and public involvement in health research: A Nordic perspective. *Scandinavian Journal of Public Health*, *48*(1), 119–21. https://doi.org/10.1177/1403494819863522

Slemon, A., Bungay, V., Jenkins, E., & Brown, H. (2018). Power and resistance: Nursing students' experiences in mental health practicums. *Advances in Nursing Science*, *41*(4), 359–76. https://doi.org/10.1097/ANS.0000000000000221

Takkal, A., Horrox, K., & Rubio-Garrido, A. (2018). The issue of space in a prison art therapy group: A reflection through Martin Heidegger's conceptual frame. *International Journal of Art Therapy*, *23*(3), 136–42. https://doi.org/10.1080/17454832.2017.1384031

Ziegler, S. (2005). *Theory-Directed Nursing Practice* (2nd edn). New York, NY: Springer Publishing Company.

FURTHER READING

Green, H. E. (2014). Use of theoretical and conceptual frameworks in qualitative research. *Nurse Researcher*, *21*(6), 34–8.

Richardson-Tench, M. (2012). Power, discourse, subjectivity: A Foucauldian application to operating room nursing practice. *ACORN Journal*, *25*(3), 36–7.

SEARCHING AND REVIEWING THE LITERATURE

Chapter learning objectives

The material presented in this chapter will assist you to:

1 identify the purpose of searching and reviewing the literature
2 provide examples of different types of literature reviews
3 identify relevant literature sources
4 conduct a focused search of the literature using a structured search strategy
5 outline the components of a literature review
6 develop an efficient system for cataloguing references.

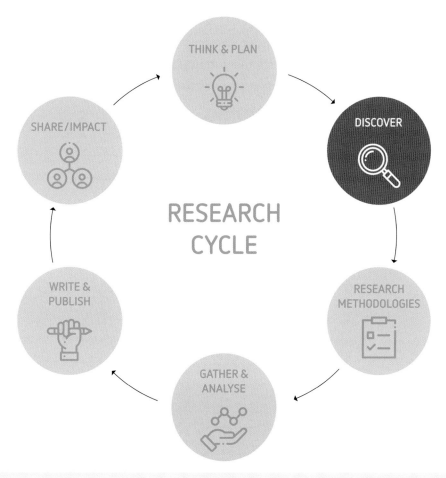

Research cycle

The primary focus of this chapter is the process of searching and reviewing the literature, a component of discovering what is known about a topic, which is highlighted in the research framework diagram above.

Introduction

There is a plethora of scholarly literature related to nursing, midwifery and allied health, available from numerous sources that are either discipline-specific or from other health-related disciplines. From an academic perspective, **literature** encompasses not just credible research papers, but includes any other relevant material found in books, journal articles, seminar and conference proceedings, unpublished theses, media, government reports and personal communication between researchers.

The number of journals and articles published each year continues to grow. In 2014 it was reported that 2.5 million articles were being published by more than 28 000 active scholarly peer-reviewed English-language journals each year (Ware & Mabe, 2015). In the most recent STM report (Johnson, Watkinson & Mabe, 2018), the number of publications has increased to 3 million articles, with the number of scholarly peer-reviewed English-language journals reported at 33 100, indicating a growth of 5% to 6% per year. With the multitude of resources currently available, many in digital format, searching and reviewing the literature can be time-consuming and daunting, posing a challenge for even the most experienced researcher. It is therefore essential for clinicians to develop their skills in searching and reviewing the literature.

A **literature review** encompasses a review, critical analysis and synthesis of published sources of literature on a particular topic. It is an integral part of the research cycle (see **Figure 2.1**), a continuous quest to learn more and to help gather evidence about a particular topic. A literature review should summarise findings that have emerged from

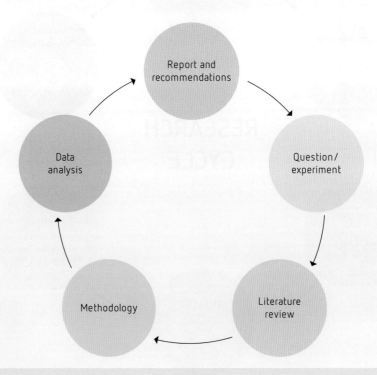

▶ **Figure 2.1** The research cycle

research evidence. A conclusion about the accuracy and completeness of the evidence should also be reached, essentially identifying what is known and where the gaps currently exist (Ridley, 2012). The order in which these elements are completed might vary, but all parts are integral to **rigorous** reporting of research outcomes.

While completing a literature review is an integral part of the research process, it is also important to help find evidence to answer clinically relevant questions or to identify whether recommendations in the literature are **evidence-based** and address clinical problems. Conducting a structured literature review also helps to manage the overwhelming amount of information available (George, Ferguson & Pearce, 2014).

The purpose of a literature review

There are a number of reasons for undertaking a literature review. The initial purpose is to demonstrate a comprehensive understanding of the literature by describing, summarising and evaluating the evidence that has been sourced. The most common purposes for undertaking a literature review are to present a critical review of the background of the topic under discussion and to establish a justification for further research. It is not the aim to answer the question posed or find all the evidence published (Ridley, 2012). Familiarity with the body of research is developed, which provides a context for the research project.

A literature review is required in three different contexts:

1 to determine what has been written about a particular topic or problem
2 to prepare a review of the literature as part of a preliminary stage in a large research project, such as a thesis proposal
3 to prepare a literature review as a component of a research project or research grant application (Knopf, 2006; Lau & Kuziemsky, 2016).

Why review the literature?

Conducting a literature review will assist in:

- identifying topics or questions that require further investigation
- defining the research problem
- planning the design and methodology of a study
- establishing a link between what is being proposed and what has already been investigated
- integrating findings of a study with an existing body of knowledge
- providing exposure to the approaches used by researchers who have previously investigated the research problem
- reviewing the type of design previously selected (e.g. experimental, phenomenological or grounded theory approach)
- avoiding replicating studies that have already been conducted
- identifying the limitations of the research
- identifying the problems or difficulties previous researchers have encountered so they can be avoided
- combining research findings to support evidence-based practice.
  Additional factors are presented in Figure 2.2.

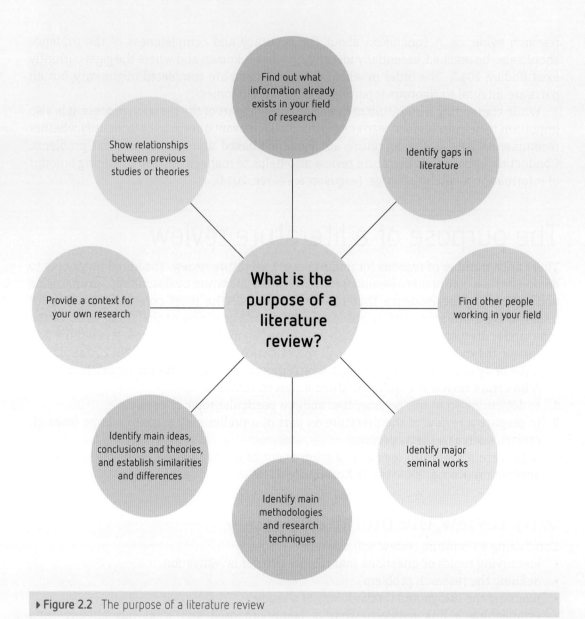

▶ **Figure 2.2**   The purpose of a literature review

Types of literature reviews

If a literature review is required to support a study, then the type of review that has been chosen to address the topic should be clearly stated. An overview of the literature may be required to provide background or context and/or to demonstrate the key published studies on a particular topic. This type of literature review is commonly seen in undergraduate work and in applications for research grants where word limitations require conciseness. A more comprehensive literature review would indicate greater depth in searching and analysing and is common in research reports, as well as in honours- and masters-level research (Ridley, 2012).

An **integrated literature review** combines diverse methodologies to formulate a conclusion, but cannot necessarily be confirmed on a hierarchy scale of evidence. These reviews are, however, of particular use to nurses and midwives as they include context, holistic care components and more subjective elements of their practice (Whittemore & Knafl, 2005).

Scoping reviews are a relatively new approach to synthesising evidence, providing an alternative to literature reviews and systematic reviews. Although the purpose of a scoping review is to provide an indication of the volume and the type of studies available on a particular topic, as well as provide an overview of the literature, a rigorous and transparent method in the appraisal of the literature is required to ensure the results are trustworthy (Munn et al., 2018).

As described by Munn and colleagues (2018, p. 2), scoping reviews are used:

- to identify the types of available evidence in a given field
- to clarify key concepts/definitions in the literature
- to examine how research is conducted on a certain topic or field
- to identify key characteristics or factors related to a **concept**
- as a precursor to a systematic review
- to identify and analyse knowledge gaps.

Protocols and implementation for a systematic review have been discussed in Chapter 1. It is important to note that if the intention is to publish a **systematic review**, it is important to check the protocol requirements in the guidelines published by the research institutes, such as the Joanna Briggs Institute. A systematic review is conducted within a rigid framework, includes a clearly formulated question and appraisal of the quality of the studies and interprets the results using a systematic process (Tawfik et al., 2019).

ACTIVITY

Access the following articles and identify the different search strategies that have been used to support the literature review. Discuss these findings with your colleagues.

- Reardon, M., Abrahams, R., Thyer, L., & Simpson, P. (2020). Prevalence of burnout in paramedics: A systematic review of prevalence studies. *Emergency Medicine Australasia, 32*(2), 182–9. https://doi.org/10.1111/1742-6723.13478
- Coleman, R., Hartz, D., & Dahlen, H. (2020). The experiences of Aboriginal and Torres Strait Islander Bachelor of Midwifery students: An integrative literature review. *Women and Birth.* https://doi.org/10.1016/j.wombi.2020.02.008
- Thornton, R., Nicholson, P., & Harms, L. (2019). Scoping review of memory making in bereavement care for parents after the death of a newborn. *Journal of Obstetric, Gynecologic and Neonatal Nursing, 48*(3), 351–60. https://doi.org/10.1016/j.jogn.2019.02.001

Characteristics of a well-conducted literature review

A well-conducted literature review:

- clearly articulates the search strategy used for locating previous research
- details inclusion and exclusion criteria (the reasons why some studies were included or excluded in the review)

- demonstrates the relationship between the author's study and other research already conducted (Denney & Tewksbury, 2013; Paltridge & Starfield, 2007)
- tells the reader a story (provides a road map) about what has been studied in the past and evaluates the literature rather than just reporting each study separately (Denney & Tewksbury, 2013; Kamler & Thomson, 2006)
- contains the author's voice and critique; the author demonstrates a command of the literature (Galvan, 2009)
- demonstrates synthesis, appraisal and application of the literature (Holbrook et al., 2007)
- highlights trends, themes and gaps in the literature (Denney & Tewksbury, 2013; Pyrczak & Bruce, 2017)
- cites seminal or landmark studies and explains why certain studies are important (Galvan, 2009)
- justifies the rationale for the researcher's study to be conducted (Denney & Tewksbury, 2013; Moule & Goodman, 2009)
- consists mainly of primary sources (Krainovich-Miller, 2006; Ridley, 2012)
- expresses opinions about the quality and importance of the cited research (Pyrczak & Bruce, 2017)
- provides a framework for establishing the importance of the study to be conducted as well as a benchmark for comparing the results with other findings (Creswell, 2009)
- is presented in the form of an essay, not an annotated list (Pyrczak & Bruce, 2017)
- reflects the cumulative significance of the body of research rather than the relevance of each study's findings (Polit & Beck, 2009).

Characteristics of a poor literature review

Poorly written literature reviews often present with the following characteristics:
- digression from the topic without a clear focus
- a focus on the limitations and criticism of previous research
- a simple summary (e.g. sample size, method, results) without a critical analysis and critique of previous research findings
- failure to critique studies that are unfavourable to the writer's view or area of research (Polgar & Thomas, 2008)
- exclusion of seminal studies
- failure to include current research.

Primary and secondary literature sources

Depending on the originality of the literature, sources are categorised as either primary or secondary, with both published in refereed journals and websites. **Primary sources** include original theories or findings written by the person or persons involved at the time of the inquiry. **Secondary sources** are the theories or studies to which an author refers. Secondary sources have the limitation of being filtered through the writer's own attitudes and biases, but sometimes the original is not available.

Although a secondary source may provide a different interpretation of the original material, it may only convey the essence of the work and is not the work itself (Parahoo, 2006). While it may be acceptable to use secondary sources for undergraduate assignments, they are best avoided in postgraduate studies. A clue to identifying a secondary source is a reference 'cited by ...'. Examples of secondary sources include textbooks, magazine articles, encyclopedias and internet sites aimed at dispersing public health information or commercial ventures to the public.

Another distinction is between scholarly and unscholarly work. Scholarly works are usually the more valuable sources for research purposes. They include works such as theoretical papers; reports of research methodologies, procedures or instruments; reports of research results; review papers, books written by authorities and works of art, drawings and posters.

Further considerations are systematic reviews and evidence-based practice (EBP) guides, as the implications of the hierarchy of evidence can have a profound effect on the resultant findings.

Common sources of literature

Journals

Professional journals are the most valuable resource for researchers. They have varying degrees of scope for their various audiences. The scope ranges from broad-interest journals such as the *Australian Journal of Advanced Nursing*, *International Journal of Nursing Practice* and *Nursing Inquiry* to more specific specialty journals such as the *Australian and New Zealand Journal of Mental Health Nursing*, or concept-specific journals such as the *Journal of Transcultural Nursing*. Journals can be discipline-specific to nursing, such as *Collegian* or *Contemporary Nurse*, or they can be multidisciplinary, such as the *Australian Journal of Rural Health*.

Some journals, such as *Clinical Nursing Research, Nursing Research* and *Western Journal of Nursing Research*, are dedicated to publishing research. Other journals, such as *Qualitative Health Research*, have a particular methodological focus.

Frequently, knowledge from different disciplines is featured in discipline-specific journals, such as *Critical Care Medicine, Journal of Infection and Public Health, Health Psychology* or *Journal of Physiotherapy*, which could be useful sources of material for all healthcare professionals.

Journals can be international, such as *Clinical Nursing Research*, which accepts papers from any country; or they can have a national focus, such as *Collegian* and *Contemporary Nurse*, which publish only Australian research.

Electronic journals are journals published only on the internet, such as *Online Journal of Issues in Nursing*. Given the high cost of publishing journals using traditional printing methods, electronic journals are becoming increasingly popular.

FOR EXAMPLE

PUBLICATION RANKINGS

Publications are often subject to formal or informal rankings according to the impact within a given research field. Therefore, it is worth considering journal rankings before deciding where to publish, as some journals carry more prestige than others in the academic world. The journal ranking list does change over time, so it is worth seeking help from librarians for the most up-to-date and relevant version. Another resource includes the updated Excellence in Research for Australia (ERA) list, compiled by the Australian Research Council (ARC, 2019), which can be accessed from https://www.arc.gov.au/excellence-research-australia > ERA > ERA Reports.

A journal **impact factor** is a measure of the frequency with which the average article in a journal has been cited in a particular year. It is calculated by dividing the number of citations in the journal citation report by the total number of articles published in the two previous years. These measures can be accessed through the Web of Science Journal Citation Report, usually retrieved through a university or hospital library.

For example, a journal that publishes original research relevant to nursing, midwifery and other health-related professions, *International Journal of Nursing Studies*, has a higher impact factor (3.57) than *Nurse Education Today*, a journal that publishes nursing, midwifery and interprofessional healthcare education (2.442).

ACTIVITY

Access the Web of Science Journal Citation Report and identify the impact factor for the journals listed below. Discuss the outcome and identify the top-ranked journal with a colleague.

- *Physiotherapy Theory and Practice*
- *Australasian Journal of Paramedicine*
- *Nursing Inquiry*
- *Journal of Midwifery & Women's Health*
- *BMC Public Health*

Books

Textbooks are not usually considered reliable sources of contemporary research, even if they are research texts, primarily because of the time lag of up to five years between when the research project is written up, when it is published in a journal and when it is then cited in a book. Nevertheless, books can be valuable sources of literature and ideas (Ridley, 2012), particularly for undergraduate assignments.

For example, when searching for books related to bereavement, loss and grief (limited to books only and dates from 2014 to 2019), 27 books were included in the search. (See Figure 2.3.)

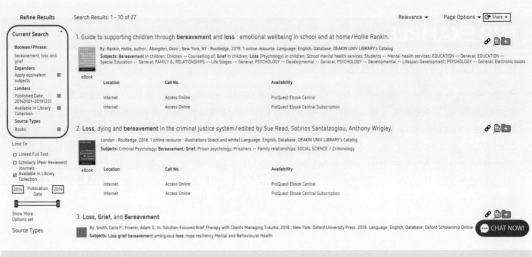

▸ **Figure 2.3**   Library search for textbooks

Conference proceedings

Conference papers and proceedings are also useful and may be listed as references (Ridley, 2012). These documents are usually harder to access, but with the growth of electronic media, such papers and proceedings are often available on the internet. Check if the papers presented have been **peer reviewed** to strengthen the credibility in the findings or submissions. Using similar keywords, peer-reviewed conference abstracts can be accessed via the web or databases. Most conferences abstracts include a word count (maximum word count), an introduction/background, results and conclusion section. See Figure 2.4.

Bereavement, Loss and Grief

P019
Memory-Making in Neonatal
End-of-Life Care

Rebecca Thornton[1,2], Lou Harms[1],
Pat Nicholson[1,2]
[1]*University of Melbourne, Melbourne, VIC, Australia*
[2]*Deakin University, Melbourne, VIC, Australia*

Background: The loss of a child in the first hours or days of life is a profoundly distressing event for parents. Provision of appropriate psycho-social care for bereaved parents is critical. Current perinatal and neonatal palliative care guidelines recommend supporting parents to create memories with their baby. However, little is currently known about the impact of these activities on parents' experience of loss.

Method: This study utilized a grounded theory approach. Eighteen bereaved parents participated in in-depth interviews to explore memory-making interventions in the context of end-of-life care in the Neonatal Intensive Care Unit.

Results: Three key themes emerged which have the potential to guide memory-making interventions in neonatal end-of-life care. Firstly, participants expressed the need to parent their baby, both before and after the baby's death. Secondly, mementos were important to parents, not only as a way of remembering the baby but also as evidence of the baby's brief life. Finally, parents wanted guidance and support from staff to make the most of the time they have with their baby.

Conclusion: Understanding how parents experience memory making interventions is critical in ensuring neonatal health practitioners provide appropriate support for bereaved families, ultimately improving the quality of care.

▶ **Figure 2.4**   Conference Abstract

Source: Thornton, R., Harms, L., & Nicholson, P. (2018). Memory-making in neonatal end-of-life care. *Journal of Pain and Symptom Management*, 56(6). https://doi.org/10.1016/j.jpainsymman.2018.10.281

Reports

Reports by governments and other institutions are another useful source of information. The Australian Bureau of Statistics (visit https://www.abs.gov.au/) makes available a large number of statistical reports. For example, information about the number of births in Australia can be accessed (as shown in Figure 2.5).

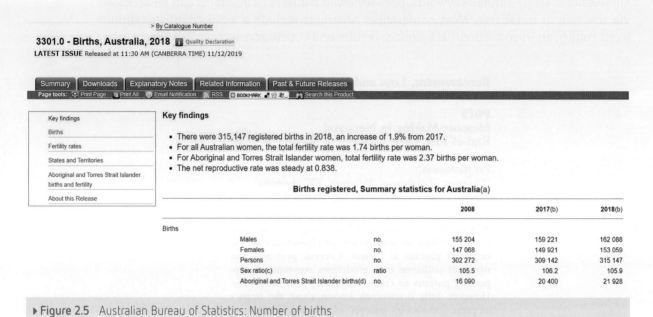

> Figure 2.5   Australian Bureau of Statistics: Number of births

Source: Australian Bureau of Statistics (Reference period: December 2019) 3301.0 - Births, Australia, 2018
https://www.abs.gov.au/AUSSTATS/abs@.nsf/mf/3301.0, ABS Website, accessed 30 November 2020.

Theses

A thorough search of the literature will include a search for relevant theses, although it is not necessary for undergraduate assignments to include this type of literature.

University libraries often hold hard copies of theses by students who completed their studies at the institution. An abstract provides details about the research project and the thesis can be downloaded if available through open access. (See the example in Figure 2.6.) A Google search may indicate where other Australian theses can be accessed, for example the National Library of Australia's Trove service (visit http://trove.nla.gov.au).

Grey literature

Grey literature is sometimes overlooked when completing a literature review as it is not found in peer-reviewed journals; however, the importance of grey literature is increasing. Grey literature includes government and scientific reports, and other literature that is not controlled by commercial publishers (George, Ferguson & Pearce, 2014; Ridley, 2012).

Memory-making in neonatal end-of-life care

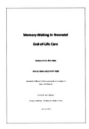

Download

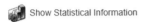

Memory-Making in Neonatal End-of-Life Care (2.238Mb)

Show Statistical Information

Author

Thornton, Rebecca Kate

Date

2019

Affiliation

Social Work

Metadata

Show full item record

Document Type

PhD thesis

Access Status

Open Access

URI

http://hdl.handle.net/11343/224196

Description

© 2019 Dr. Rebecca Kate Thornton

Abstract

Experiencing the death of an infant places parents at risk of prolonged and profound grief, therefore providing appropriate psychosocial support for parents is crucial. Current perinatal palliative care guidelines recommend memory-making activities, such as collecting or creating mementos and spending time caring for the infant, as an important aspect of bereavement care. However, evidence to support such interventions is scant. This study used the grounded theory method described by Corbin and Strauss (2015) to explore bereaved parents' experiences of memory-making in neonatal end-of-life care. Eighteen bereaved parents participated in extensive semi-structured interviews. The core psychosocial process underpinning parents' experience of memory-making was identified as "Affirmed Parenthood". This core category was supported by three key themes; "Being a parent", "Creating evidence" and "Being guided". "Being a parent" included spending time with the baby before and after death, touching and holding the baby, and providing physical care. "Creating evidence" captured parents' efforts to collect or create tangible evidence of their baby's life through photographs and other mementos, and by involving others with their baby to ensure that people outside the immediate family would have memories of their child. Finally, "Being guided" represented parents' need to be supported and encouraged throughout the process of memory-making. Where all three key themes were addressed in bereavement care, parents experienced affirmation of the significance of their baby's life, affirmation of the significance of their loss, and affirmation of their role as the baby's parents.

Keywords

neonatal; perinatal; bereavement; grief; memory; loss; death; parent

▶ **Figure 2.6** Doctoral thesis (unpublished)

Source: Thornton, R. (2019). Memory-making in neonatal end-of-life care. Unpublished doctoral dissertation. The University of Melbourne. https://minerva-access.unimelb.edu.au/handle/11343/224196

Examples include the National Safety and Quality Health Service Standards. These standards were developed by the Australian Commission on Safety and Quality in Health Care, with the aim of protecting the public from harm and improving the quality of health service provision. This publication can be found at https://www.safetyandquality.gov.au > Publications and resources (see Figure 2.7).

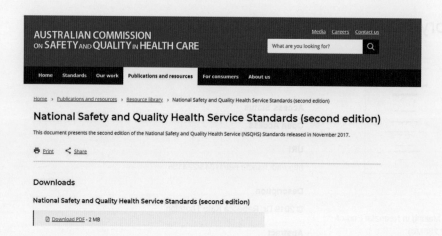

▶ **Figure 2.7** Australian Commission on Safety and Quality in Health Care: National Safety and Quality Health Service Standards

Source: Australian Commission on Safety and Quality in Health Care. https://www.safetyandquality.gov.au/publications-and-resources/resource-library/national-safety-and-quality-health-service-standards-second-edition

---

ACTIVITY

Go to CINAHL and find the following article: Murphy, J. (2010). Using mobile devices for research: Smartphones, databases, and libraries. *Online*, 34(3), pp. 14–18.
Read about how personal electronic devices can be used to aid and update research strategies.

Identifying relevant and credible literature

Relevant and credible literature concerning clinical issues needs to be contemporary. It can be sourced from peer-reviewed journals, most of which are found on electronic sites available through a library. The key database for nursing and allied health journals is **CINAHL Complete** (Cumulative Index to Nursing and Allied Health Literature). Other databases relevant to nursing and midwifery include MEDLINE, PsycINFO and PubMed. There are a number of key databases that are more specific for allied health professions; for example, PEDro for physiotherapy and ProQuest's Linguistics + Language Behaviour Abstracts (LLBA) for speech and audiology. Informit Health subset, an Australian online library database, is a valuable database for students and researchers when searching for Australian literature. Equally important are the EBP libraries, such as **Cochrane Australia** and Joanna Briggs Institute.

Sometimes a hand search through journals specific to a topic is required, which is driven by the subject under investigation. Take, for example, John Fields' 2007 thesis 'Caring to death'. To collate the data required for this **discursive analysis**, professional bodies, legal proceedings and newspaper accounts were sourced. But if the pharmacological management of type 2 diabetes was being explored, a general search via Google would not be used to source information as many of the sites or articles would lack credible evidence. The vast majority of the literature search would centre on recent **peer-reviewed journal articles**.

The challenge facing researchers today, however, is not to dismiss all websites or texts but to be rigorous in identifying relevant and credible sources of information (Ridley, 2012). The following example demonstrates how different types of literature have been used to support a change in clinical practice.

FOR EXAMPLE

LEVELS OF EVIDENCE TO SUPPORT EVIDENCE-BASED PRACTICES

Hand hygiene is regarded as one of the most important means of reducing the spread of infections. In fact, in 1847 Ignaz Semmelweis observed a higher mortality rate in women post-delivery when a medical student was involved with the birth when compared with a midwife. When asked to wash their hands prior to performing clinical procedures, a two per cent reduction in patient mortality was observed (Best & Neuhauser, 2004). Although hand-scrubbing techniques implemented at the start of the 20th century included the use of a brush, studies published in the 1980s discouraged this technique as the use of a disposable sponge was shown to be just as effective in reducing bacterial counts on the hands of personnel (WHO, 2009). In a recent systematic review, Liu and Mehigan (2017) found that despite the implementation of guidelines for completing a surgical scrub, poor compliance was found among staff. Participants across the studies preferred to use an alcohol-based hand-rubbing technique compared to the brush-based protocol as it resulted in less skin damage. It was suggested by Liu and Mehigan that the implementation of hand-rubbing protocols could be effective in increasing compliance and prevent surgical site infections.

Peer-reviewed journal article

Grey literature

Systematic review

Selecting relevant literature

When searching for literature, a number of articles may be eliminated by reading the abstract. It is best to do this at the literature search stage to avoid wasting time. Not all entries in an index have an abstract, so it then becomes necessary to review the article itself by skimming through the introduction and conclusion. If only research articles are to be included in the review, articles that are in non-research journals can be immediately eliminated.

Other considerations concerning the quality of the article is the date when the study was carried out and the type of journal in which it appears. A journal article may be referred to as a peer-reviewed or refereed article. The system of peer review requires the journal editor to send the article without any form of identification to at least two reviewers who have expertise in the field. These reviewers then critique the article using similar methods to those detailed in Figure 2.8. The editor then sends the reviews to the author who makes any required revisions and then resubmits their article to be considered for publication. This process is followed until the reviewers and editor are satisfied with the work or the author withdraws the paper. Thus, the peer-review system helps to maintain a standard of excellence in research scholarship (see Kearney & Freda, 2005).

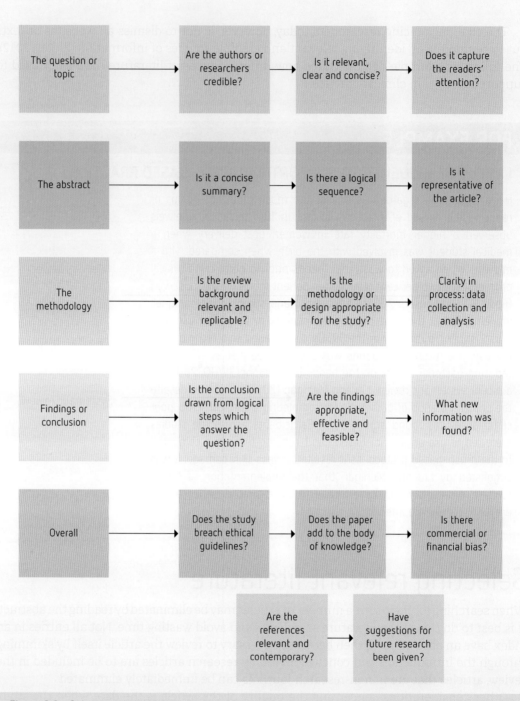

▶ Figure 2.8   Critiquing an article

Conducting the literature search

When embarking on a literature review the type of research methodology will direct the search for contemporary evidence. Quantitative research requires a literature search to be completed at the beginning of the project. If it is a long project, say a year or more, a literature search will also be conducted at the end of the project to ensure the latest information is included in the final report. If it is a very long project, such as a major thesis, a top-up search is completed at least every six months. This is easily achieved using electronic media, with many journals providing the option of receiving alerts concerning any updates for specific topics.

Qualitative research requires a different approach to timing the **review of the literature**. The purpose and timing of the literature review will vary based on the type of study being conducted. A thorough literature review may be discouraged prior to data collection; this is to avoid becoming immersed in the literature to support an impartial and unbiased standpoint on the topic. For example, in a grounded theory study a formal review of the literature is delayed to prevent the researcher from imposing existing knowledge or theories during the process or outcomes of the study (Birks & Mills, 2011; Bryant & Charmaz, 2019). Reviewing the literature before undertaking the study can influence the researcher's openness, which may result in important observations going unnoticed. A review of the literature may be completed as the study progresses to identify what has already been done by other researchers, or once the study has been completed, depending on the design of the study.

Undertaking a literature review

As mentioned previously, a literature review involves a critical analysis of the literature, focused on a particular research topic. There are a number of steps involved, as shown in Figure 2.9 and discussed in the following sections.

Step 1: Select the type of literature review

There are different types of literature reviews, each with its own purpose and method. It is therefore important to select the one that best suits the purpose of the literature review before commencing with the literature search. Two main types of reviews include traditional and systematic reviews.

Traditional literature reviews:
- provide an overview of the discipline area
- support an argument or discussion
- critically analyse the available literature on the topic
- provide a summary of the evidence.

Systematic reviews:
- critique and synthesise all the available evidence for a focused question
- include the production of a transparent and reproducible process that summarises the results of well-designed studies.

Step 2: Plan the literature search

In light of the ever-improving access to information, it is worth remembering that a literature review forms part of an ongoing discussion as opposed to a definitive work. The findings are important and add to the body of knowledge, and as such the reviewer's pathway while compiling the literature review is important and should be included in the

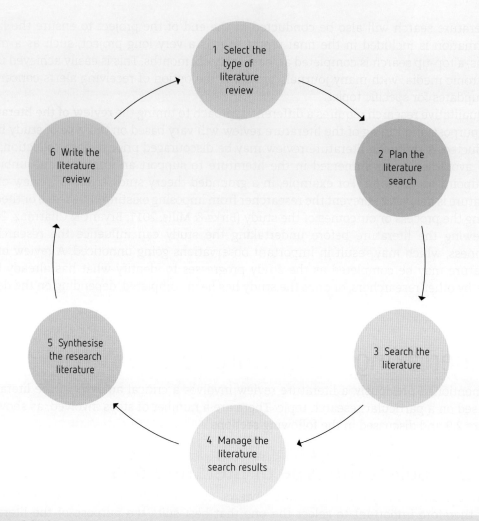

▶ Figure 2.9   Six steps to producing a literature review

Source: Nippers, I., & Sutton, A. (2014). Oxygen therapy: professional compliance with national guidelines. *British Journal of Nursing, 23*(7), 382–6.

literature review. Therefore, an organised and systematic method of searching the literature and keeping records is a key component of an efficient review. This includes refining the research question and identifying the scope of the literature review.

Step 3: Search the literature

Using a keyword search in the databases generates evidence if there is a match between the keywords entered and what is found in the abstract or title of the article. One of the challenges when undertaking a search is to include all synonyms (e.g. teens; teenager; youth; adolescents) in the search to avoid missing articles relevant to the topic. Therefore, before searching databases a search strategy needs to be developed to assist in formulating the topic into a research question, providing a prompt in developing search concepts and key search terms. If the key search terms are not appropriately framed this will lead to a search outcome that could include hundreds of non-usable abstracts and irrelevant information.

When formulating a research question the PICOT (patient, intervention, comparison, outcome, time) format can be used as a guide for conducting an efficient, thorough and focused search (Riva et al., 2012). It is a tool that can be used for further refining the research topic into concepts or components, making it easier to find relevant articles.

FOR EXAMPLE

PICOT QUESTION

You are interested in exploring whether handwashing among healthcare workers reduces healthcare-acquired infections. Using the PICOT model, this would be written as:

P – healthcare workers

I – handwashing

C – no comparison group as it would be unethical for healthcare workers not to perform handwashing in clinical practice

O – hospital-acquired infection

T – time is not relevant to this question and is not included in the literature search.

Therefore, the search question would be: 'Does handwashing among healthcare workers reduce hospital-acquired infection?' Key search terms would include 'healthcare workers', 'handwashing' and 'hospital-acquired infection'.

In a similar manner, PIE is better suited as a way to focus when exploring a qualitative research question.

P – patient/population/problem

I – interest area

E – evaluation/effect.

Concept mapping is another method of identifying search keywords. Once the topic has been summarised, in three or less sentences, the main concepts are broken down into keywords, including alternative words (synonyms). The main concepts and alternative search terms are then listed in a table, which becomes part of the search planner for the literature search. When the keywords have been developed, alternative spelling should be checked, including British and American spelling, for example, anaesthetist (British) and anesthetist (American). An additional column can be included in the table so that all limits for the search are recorded. An example of a basic search planner is provided below.

	Alternative search terms			Limits (e.g. population, age group, gender, language, date range, publication type)
Concept 1	Teenager	Adolescent	Youth	
Concept 2	Aboriginal	Indigenous Australian	Torres Strait Islander	
Concept 3	Mental health	Wellbeing	Quality of life	

A systematic log of the recorded database searches should be recorded as it should be reported in the literature review. A more detailed search planner example has been completed for the question: 'Does handwashing among healthcare workers reduce hospital-acquired infection?'

	Concept 1	AND →	Concept 2
List all key words / terms as stated in your topic description above	hospital-acquired infection / hospital-acquired infection		handwashing / hand washing
	OR ↓		OR ↓
List search terms using truncation (*) and wildcards	infection*		handwash* hand wash*
	OR ↓		OR ↓
List synonyms, alternate spelling, language	cross infection OR nosocomial infection		hand hygiene OR hand disinfection

Your search strategies for each database should be recorded. The following template demonstrates how the literature search can be recorded.

Date	Database	Search strategy	Result: Numbers of hits
		• Keywords, variants, * or ? • Linking words – AND, OR, NOT • Limiters used to narrow search, date range, peer reviewed and scholarly	• Relevant • Full text found? If not … follow through with Find It @[university] InterLibrary Loan, Google Scholar • Export to EndNote • Create an alert to receive updates

Inclusion of medical subject headings (MeSH)

Each article citation is associated with a set of MeSH terms that describe the content of the citation. These are based on article content, specifically developed to create a targeted search and retrieve more relevant articles required for the topic under consideration. A list of similar search terms can be accessed through CINAHL or MeSH, depending on the database. Headings and subheadings are then added to the list of current search terms, which are used to refine the literature search. CINAHL headings or MeSH tutorials are available on the databases for users who are unfamiliar with developing alternative search terms (Richter & Austin, 2012).

Step 4: Manage the literature search results

When first setting out to review the literature, it may be difficult to decide how much to search. Although the depth of the search will depend on experience, searching skills and financial resources, it is important to search enough to ensure that all relevant information is accessed. It should not result in so much information that there is the danger of becoming overwhelmed by the task of trawling through the evidence. Another factor to be considered is the amount of time required to complete a thorough search, something that is often underestimated.

It is important that when reading the literature, it is focused, with an analytical approach adopted, rather than blindly accepting what the author has written. The extent of reading the literature depends, in part, on how much information is available on the topic or research question. If the literature is limited, it may be necessary to read related material. Conversely, if there is a great deal of available information, it may be necessary to narrow the topic.

It is best to begin with the most current references and work backwards until no new information is accessed. If the topic is contemporary, such as HIV/AIDS (which was unheard of before 1980), there will be limited literature from the early 1980s. Changes in health trends, such as the incidence of pertussis (whooping cough), should also be noted. If limits are included in the search information about the pre-vaccine years, which is relevant to the topic, relevant information may be excluded from the search results. Generally, 10 years is a reasonable period to include in the search. It should be noted that important **seminal** works, which are highly original papers from which further study has flowed, should be included. These original papers can usually be obtained from other references and may well be older than the 10-year limit set in the search.

It may be necessary to narrow either the scope of the literature review or the topic reviewed. If too much literature is accessed, the topic may be too complex, so it will be necessary to narrow it down to make it more manageable. Non-research material that does not belong in a review of literature may be included in the search results; in this case research papers would be included and non-research material excluded. However, non-research material can be used for background reading information. So, as can be seen, it is important to identify the boundaries of the search and, when useful, use inclusion and exclusion criteria.

FOR EXAMPLE

INCLUSION AND EXCLUSION CRITERIA

The criteria for determining acute pain management of children presenting to the emergency department.

Inclusion criteria	Exclusion criteria
Paediatric patients	Adult patients
Emergency department presentation	Non-emergency presentation
Pain management intervention	Not pain management related / chronic condition management

The purpose of the literature review is another factor influencing the extent of the search. It is unlikely that a student undertaking a small undergraduate assignment is expected to include every article ever written on a topic. An important feature of completing a literature review is that wide reading on the topic is encouraged, with the inclusion of relevant material to support the argument presented.

With regards to the number of references that should be included in an assignment, it will depend on the type of assignment required for the unit. A typical assignment, one that requires an introduction, body and conclusion, will have most of the references included in the body of the assignment, which accounts for about 75% of the word count. For example, in a 2000-word essay, students will have 1500 words for the body. Each main point that is made should average around 200 to 400 words in total, which should be supported by two or three references. Therefore, one peer-reviewed reference should be used for roughly every 200 words. Although, this will depend on the discipline and the task. At the other end of the spectrum, a PhD thesis will require an extremely thorough review of the literature.

Search tips

Boolean operators and limiters

Searching with **Boolean operators** – AND, OR and NOT – will either create a very broad or very narrow search (Ridley, 2012). By joining similar terms or concepts (e.g. Indigenous Australians OR Aboriginal), either term will appear in the results. By joining different concepts (e.g. type 2 diabetes AND insulin administration) a more focused search with both terms will appear. The use of NOT excludes a term or concept and produces a more focused search (e.g. diabetes NOT juvenile). Common **limiters** are the availability of full text, publication date, publication type and language. **Expanders** are usually set as the default but these can be used to limit the search; for example, to full text only or English language only.

Phrase searching

Phrase searching uses inverted commas around two or more words as a command for the database that the words should be searched together in that order. For example "cognitive therapy". The search of a database or search engine will retrieve only that set of words when they appear next to each other and in the same order. To search by phrase simply put quotation marks, "…" around the words included in the search; for example, "climate change".

Truncation and wildcards

There are a few tips and tricks that can be used to get the most out of the database. Truncation and wildcard symbols can be used where there are unknown characters, multiple spellings or various word endings. The truncation symbol is usually the asterisk (*) and can be used to find variant endings and expand the results (Ridley, 2012); for example, nurs* will include nurse, nurses and nursing in the search. A wildcard symbol (?) can be used to replace a single character in a word that may include different spelling; for example, organi?ation will include organisation and organization in the search (George, Ferguson & Pearce, 2014).

All of the online search tips above are summarised in Table 2.1.

> **TIP**
>
> Neither the wildcard nor the truncation symbol can be used as the first character in a search term.

▶ Table 2.1 Online search tips

Search tip descriptors	Example
Boolean operator Boolean operators are a means of combining search terms to broaden or narrow the search results: • AND: narrows a search by telling the database that <u>all</u> keywords must be found in an article for it to be included in the search results • OR: broadens a search telling the database that any of the search terms can be present in the search results • NOT: used to narrow the search by eliminating all terms that follow the search term	• AND: joint pain AND quality of life • OR: Aboriginal OR Indigenous Australians OR Torres Strait Islander • NOT: Aids NOT hearing aids
Phrase searching Terms are searched in the exact order specified within quotation marks	"surgical patient" "body alignment"
Truncation Word variations or alternative spellings are searched by adding a truncation symbol to the end of terms Common symbol use is *	Nurs* will include nurse, nurses and nursing
Wildcards Wildcards are used to substitute a symbol for a single letter (character) of a word Common symbol used is ?	Search for variant spelling (American and British) Organi?ation will include organi**s**ation and organi**z**ation

All databases organise information about each article or book into specific fields; for example, author, abstract, date and so on. These fields can be used to build a more precise search. **Figure 2.10** shows how the specific fields can be used in the **MEDLINE** database.

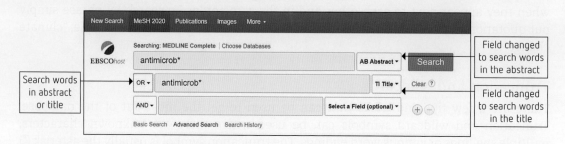

▶ **Figure 2.10** Example of MEDLINE specific fields

The following example outlines the benefits of using Boolean operators and limiters, combining or excluding keywords to produce a more focused result, with inappropriate hits excluded.

FOR EXAMPLE

USE OF BOOLEAN OPERATORS AND LIMITERS

The following search was performed on the MEDLINE Complete database using Boolean operators and limiters, as well as truncation, to narrow the search result for antimicrobial stewardship. This example can be replicated using a different topic.

Search #	Search terms/phrases	Limiters/expanders/ Boolean/ phrase included in the search	Number of hits
S1	AB antimicob* OR TI antimicrob*	Sources with antimicrobial (and variations of the word) in the abstract or title field	159 727
S2	AB "antibiot* resist*" OR TI "antibiot* resist*"	Sources with antibiotic resistance (and variations of the word) in the abstract or title field	62 229
S3	AB "antimicrob* stewardship" OR TI "antimicrob* stewardship"	Sources with antimicrobial stewardship (and variations of the word) in the abstract or title field	3 052
S4	AB antibacter* OR TI antibacter*	Sources with antibacterial (and variations of the word) in the abstract or title field	75 339

Search #	Search terms/phrases	Limiters/expanders/ Boolean/ phrase included in the search	Number of hits
S5	AB antibiotic* OR TI antibiotic*	Sources with antibiotic (and variations of the word) in the abstract or title field	327 704
S6	AB ("patient care" or "patient safety" or "patient outcome*") OR TI ("patient care" or "patient safety" or "patient outcome*")	Sources with the exact order specified within the quotation marks in the abstract or title field	131 316
S7	MH ("Patient Care" OR "Patient Care Team" OR MH "Patient-Centred Care"	Sources with the exact order specified within the quotation marks in the main heading field	1 003 138
S8	S6 OR S7	Sources from search number 6 or 7	1 107 905
S9	AB ((surgical OR surgery OR operat* OR procedure* OR peri-operative OR perioperative)) OR TI ((surgical OR surgery OR operat* OR procedure* OR peri-operative OR perioperative))	Sources with surgical or surgery or operation (and variations of the word) or peri-operative or perioperative in the abstract or title field	3 150 860
S10	MH ("operating rooms" OR "surgical procedures, operative+") OR MH "operating room nursing"	Sources with operating rooms or surgical procedures/operative (and variations of the word) or peri-operative room nursing in the main heading field	3 119 683
S11	MH ("operating rooms" OR "surgical procedures, operative"+") OR (S9 OR S10)	Sources with operating rooms or surgical procedures/operative (and variations of the word) or sources from search number 9 or 10	18 936
S12	MM "Antimicrobial stewardship"	Sources with the exact order specified within the quotation marks in the major heading field	954
S13	S1 OR S2 OR S3 OR S4 OR S5 OR S12	Sources from search number 1 or 2 or 3 or 4 or 5 or 12	488 652
S14	S8 AND S11 AND S13	Sources from search number 8 and 11 and 13	66

AB = abstract field; TI = title field; MH = exact subject heading; MM = exact major heading.

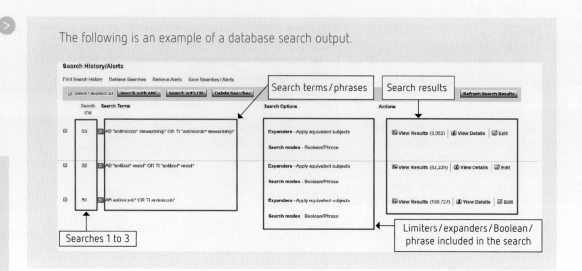

The following is an example of a database search output.

It is important when conducting a literature search to seek support from librarians and to take advantage of library tutorials, as both are imperative in developing good literature search techniques necessary for undertaking any research.

Step 5: Synthesise the research literature

After assessing the search output, it may be necessary to narrow the topic even further or redirect it slightly. The first stage is to superficially read all the material once or twice. This will provide a better sense of the important issues with regards to the topic and the methodologies of previous research, and will help to identify major points.

Reading a research article

In order to become familiar with the body of research on a particular topic, it is necessary to read research articles; therefore, it is helpful to understand the structure of this source of information. Research articles usually follow a logical standard order.

1   Title: should condense the article content in a few words which will capture the attention of readers.
2   **Abstract**: summarises details about the study.
3   Introduction: details the problem being researched and highlights the scope and significance of the study.
4   Identification of theoretical framework and statement of relationship to the current study: previous research, included in the literature review section, provides a summary of research relevant to the questions being explored. If it is a quantitative design, specific hypotheses and variables will be formally or informally identified. This section usually answers the questions 'What?' and 'Why?' If it is a qualitative study, hypotheses and variables will not be stated; rather, the project will be introduced in exploratory terms and the theory underlying the choice of methods may be described. It is at this point that **ethics approval** is noted where applicable.
5   Methodology section: outlines the design of the study, the population, the subjects recruited or participants involved, and the methodology used to answer the research question, including methods of data collection and analysis.

6   Results section: where the findings of the study will be presented.
7   Discussion section: includes a discussion of the significance of the findings and how they relate to previous findings as well as the theoretical framework.
8   Conclusions and recommendations: for implementing the findings.
9   References: provided at the end of the paper.
10 Acknowledgements: includes mention of any financial or commercial incentive for the research and persons or organisations who assisted in the study.

Language of research articles

In reading research articles, new researchers often experience problems with the scholarly language, particularly research terminology and statistics. It can seem as though the writer has difficulty communicating in plain language, particularly if a formal style of writing has been used. Such usage is a convention that has developed over many years, so when dealing with research terminology that is difficult, the best way to handle this problem is to read the paper and make notes of the words that need further clarification. Referring to the glossary provided in a research textbook is important so that familiarity with these terms develops. Sometimes a paper requires several readings as it usually gets easier with each reading. It often helps to do this as a group exercise. It is really no different from being dropped into the middle of a nursing specialty, such as critical care, and having to learn the jargon.

Having decided what material should be included in the review, deciding how to capture this information is the next step required. Before reading any material, it should be decided which method will be used. The pre-technology approach is to take notes by hand of key ideas from each article. This is time-consuming and has the additional disadvantage that the notes are a self-interpretation of the material and are therefore subject to bias. On the positive side, this method is relatively cheap and can be effective, provided not much information is required from the source. An alternative to handwriting is to photocopy or print a hard copy of the article, though this can be expensive and is not environmentally friendly.

An easier option is to save an electronic copy of the article via an electronic source of a journal that has what is called 'full text' capability. Software programs such as **EndNote** enable the cataloguing of bibliographic information electronically (as well as any notes made about each article) and have the advantage of being able to capture data from remote databases.

> **TIP**
>
> A very useful resource for students when learning how to read a research article is the textbook *How to Read a Paper: The Basics of Evidence-Based Medicine*, written by Trisha Greenhalgh (2014).

Documenting key ideas from the reading

Since it is impossible to work with a considerable number of articles, it is necessary to identify the key passages so that they can be referred to again. There are several ways of doing this. Whichever method is used, it is important to be able to link the source and the idea so that the idea can be attributed to its rightful source and thus avoid **plagiarism**. Plagiarism in its simplest form is taking someone else's work or ideas without acknowledging the source. This can expose the writer to academic censure.

One strategy for documenting findings from the articles includes the use of a summary table. Documenting the details in the table assists with organising how the articles will be organised in the literature review, as well as how the findings will be presented. An example of using a summary table has been presented in Table 2.2. Following that, Table 2.3 summarises the common options for cataloguing literature.

▸ Table 2.2   Summary table

Author/year	Study design	Sample/setting	Main findings	Strengths/limitations

Cooke et al., 2005	Randomised controlled trial	• Adult surgical care unit
		• Types of surgery:
		  – orthopaedics
		  – skin
		  – breast
		  – general
		  – urology
		• Patients = 180; 60 per group, 30F/30M
		• No loss to follow-up
		• Intervention – music via headphones
		• Placebo – headphones only
		• Control – standard care
		• State-Trait Anxiety Inventory (STAI) completed pre/post op
			Mean STAI scores significantly reduced in intervention group compared with placebo and control groups	• Methodologically sound for randomisation
				• No significant differences between groups at baseline
				• Assigning music may affect potential of music to help patient relax
				• Different types of procedures performed which would affect individuals
				• Detailed presentation of data provided with discussion and tables/charts

▸ Table 2.3   Methods of cataloguing literature

Method	Strengths	Limitations
EndNote	• Specifically designed for this purpose • Citations can be directly linked to Word documents and in a specific style • Once notes are made on an article, the hard copy of the article is no longer needed • Citation details (including abstracts) of each article are easily downloaded from electronic databases (e.g. CINAHL)	• The need to back up libraries • The need for ongoing familiarity with updates of software
Photocopy of articles	• Useful when there are few studies to critique • Notes on an idea can be easily highlighted and can be subject – and/or author-categorised	• Requires physical space for storage (e.g. filing cabinet) • Not easily transported • Must continually access original article when citing in the text
Summarising articles onto cards or A4 paper	• Can be subject- and/or author-categorised • Easily stored	• Cards or paper can be easily damaged or lost • Time-consuming to create • Not easily transported when used for large studies
Summarising articles into electronic database (e.g. Word, Excel)	• All notes on articles are in the one location, allowing easy comparison	• Not designed for this purpose • Time-consuming

FOR EXAMPLE

USING ENDNOTE

EndNote allows you to organise your references by creating groups and manually adding references to the group using a 'drag and drop' method. This method can be used to sort articles for inclusion or exclusion.

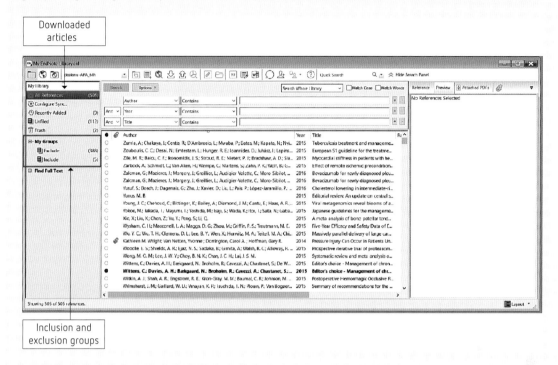

Although there are a number of quick reference guides and YouTube videos on 'how to use Endnote' (e.g. https://endnote.com/wp-content/uploads/m/pdf/en-online-qrc.pdf), most university libraries provide a comprehensive guide with the *most* up-to-date information on how to set up EndNote and the key functionality of the program.

Step 6: Writing the literature review

An outline or plan detailing the format of the literature review should be developed, including the type of structure of the review. For example, the review could be organised chronologically, conceptually or methodologically. This is usually guided by the detail included in the summary table.

The literature review should be coherent with the literature, organised into logical categories around the research question. The following tips should be remembered when writing.

1 Introduction: present an overview of the literature review and clearly identify the significance and importance of the review.

2 Critically analyse the relevant literature: present the literature/studies around the research topic/questions and the implications of each one, highlighting any gaps, inconsistencies or conflicting viewpoints.

3 Conclusion: summarise important points and give a brief explanation of how the information answers the original research question/topic. State whether more research is needed if the outcome of the literature review was inconclusive.

To develop an integrated argument from multiple sources, the arguments need to be linked together. The model of how this should be done has been provided in the following example. (The different colours in each sentence relate to the information provided in the boxes.)

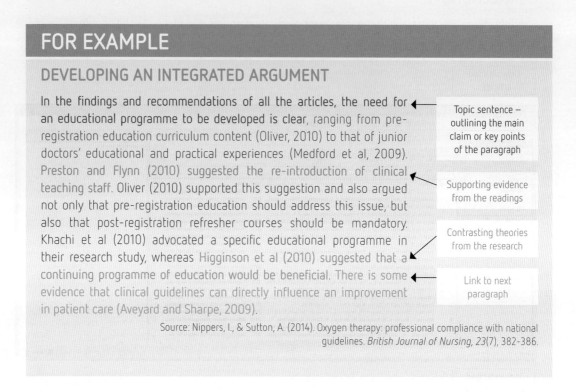

FOR EXAMPLE

DEVELOPING AN INTEGRATED ARGUMENT

In the findings and recommendations of all the articles, the need for an educational programme to be developed is clear, ranging from pre-registration education curriculum content (Oliver, 2010) to that of junior doctors' educational and practical experiences (Medford et al, 2009). Preston and Flynn (2010) suggested the re-introduction of clinical teaching staff. Oliver (2010) supported this suggestion and also argued not only that pre-registration education should address this issue, but also that post-registration refresher courses should be mandatory. Khachi et al (2010) advocated a specific educational programme in their research study, whereas Higginson et al (2010) suggested that a continuing programme of education would be beneficial. There is some evidence that clinical guidelines can directly influence an improvement in patient care (Aveyard and Sharpe, 2009).

Topic sentence – outlining the main claim or key points of the paragraph

Supporting evidence from the readings

Contrasting theories from the research

Link to next paragraph

Source: Nippers, I., & Sutton, A. (2014). Oxygen therapy: professional compliance with national guidelines. *British Journal of Nursing, 23*(7), 382-386.

References and bibliography

Ethics

It is necessary to reiterate the importance of acknowledging authorship, and ensuring that those who read the literature review can track down the original studies that have been acknowledged. There are various reference styles, such as the American Psychological Association (APA) and Harvard, and the appropriate one to use will be dictated by the university or the publishing company.

A list of the references used to support the literature review should be arranged alphabetically or numerically at the end of the work. The reference source should also be placed in-text supporting the concept, research finding or statement that acknowledges the author's original work. Bibliographies list the readings that supported the background of a topic and are not cited in-text; however, these are seldom used in health research or inquiry. As for referencing, a particular style may need to be adhered to if using a scholarly format. If there are any doubts about variances between reference and bibliography, follow the guidelines of the publication, faculty or subject, or discuss with a lecturer/supervisor. In the example provided in **Figure 2.11**, details about in-text-referencing can be viewed.

References included in the literature review are listed at the end of the paper in the reference list. Each entry should at least include information about the author(s), publication date, title and publisher. Depending on the type of source, additional information may be required. Examples from two types of sources, an article and a book, are provided in **Figure 2.12**.

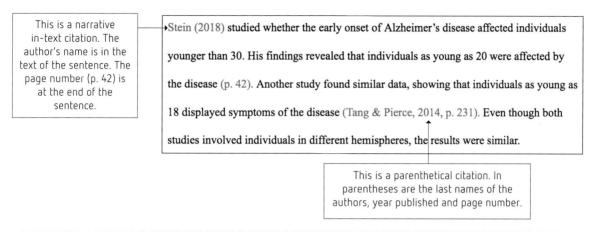

This is a narrative in-text citation. The author's name is in the text of the sentence. The page number (p. 42) is at the end of the sentence.

Stein (2018) studied whether the early onset of Alzheimer's disease affected individuals younger than 30. His findings revealed that individuals as young as 20 were affected by the disease (p. 42). Another study found similar data, showing that individuals as young as 18 displayed symptoms of the disease (Tang & Pierce, 2014, p. 231). Even though both studies involved individuals in different hemispheres, the results were similar.

This is a parenthetical citation. In parentheses are the last names of the authors, year published and page number.

▸ **Figure 2.11** Example of in-text referencing

Source: Citation Machine. (n.d.). https://www.citationmachine.net/APA

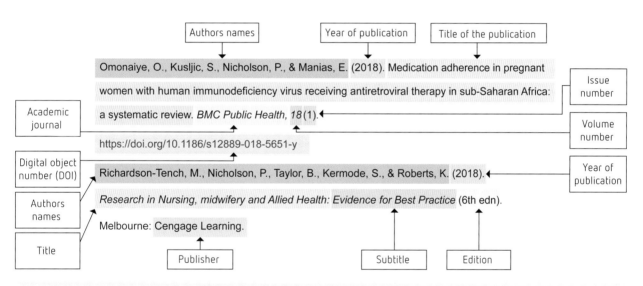

Authors names — Year of publication — Title of the publication

Omonaiye, O., Kusljic, S., Nicholson, P., & Manias, E. (2018). Medication adherence in pregnant women with human immunodeficiency virus receiving antiretroviral therapy in sub-Saharan Africa: a systematic review. *BMC Public Health, 18*(1).

https://doi.org/10.1186/s12889-018-5651-y

Richardson-Tench, M., Nicholson, P., Taylor, B., Kermode, S., & Roberts, K. (2018).

Research in Nursing, midwifery and Allied Health: Evidence for Best Practice (6th edn).

Melbourne: Cengage Learning.

Academic journal

Issue number — Volume number — Year of publication

Digital object number (DOI) — Authors names — Title

Publisher — Subtitle — Edition

▸ **Figure 2.12** Example of a reference list

Students may be required to complete an **annotated bibliography** as an exercise in formulating a literature review. This requires students to identify a number of key publications, and in their own words demonstrate their understanding of the content and meaning of the articles. The annotations usually include the full reference, with an approximately 200-word description. It may be necessary, for example, to explain or critique the populations and methods used, how findings were interpreted, the reliability of the findings and the strengths and limitation of the text. Annotations can be added to a personal reference library, and are useful as they are often superior to notes made on the article, which may be biased or too brief when returning to the works later.

FOR EXAMPLE

AN ANNOTATED BIBLIOGRAPHY

(1) Trevor, C.O., Lansford, B. and Black, J.W., 2004, 'Employee turnover and job performance: monitoring the influences of salary growth and promotion', Journal of Armchair Psychology, vol 113, no.1, pp. 56-64.

(2) In this article Trevor et al. review the influences of pay and job opportunities in respect to job performance, turnover rates and employee motivation. **(3)** The authors use data gained through organisational surveys of blue-chip companies in Vancouver, Canada to try to identify the main causes of employee turnover and whether it is linked to salary growth. **(4)** Their research focuses on assessing a range of pay structures such as pay for performance and organisational reward schemes. **(5)** The article is useful to my research topic, as Trevor et al. suggest that there are numerous reasons for employee turnover and variances in employee motivation and performance. **(6)** The main limitation of the article is that the survey sample was restricted to mid-level management, **(7)** thus the authors indicate that further, more extensive, research needs to be undertaken to develop a more in-depth understanding of employee turnover and job performance. **(8)** This article will not form the basis of my research; however it will be useful supplementary information for my research on pay structures.

Key

(1) Citation

(2) Introduction

(3) Aims and Research methods

(4) Scope

(5) Usefulness (to your research/ to a particular topic

(6) Limitations

(7) Conclusions

(8) Reflection (explain how thi work illuminates your topic or how it will fit in with your research)

Source: University of New South Wales Sydney. (n.d.). Annotated Bibliography. Sydney: UNSW. https://student.unsw.edu.au/annotated-bibliography

Putting it all together

The reasons for reviewing the literature were detailed at the beginning of this chapter. A structured step-by-step approach to completing a comprehensive literature review has also been presented.

The process of reviewing the literature may seem at first to be a chore that is difficult and complex. However, as students begin the process they will find that the time and energy invested will bring rewards in terms of generating new ideas. Students will also feel a sense of accomplishment when they have become conversant with the process of conducting a literature review. It is important to understand that undertaking a literature review is a key element in many undergraduate and postgraduate courses, as well as being an essential step in the research process. A suggested literature review workflow is shown in Figure 2.13.

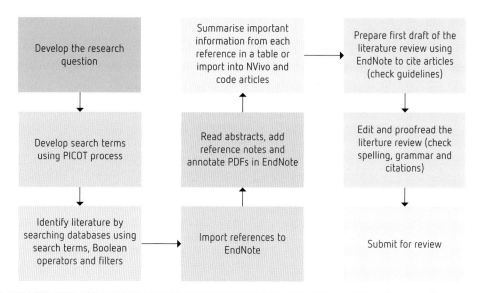

▶ **Figure 2.13**   Literature review workflow

Note: NVivo is a qualitative data analysis computer software package used to helps researchers organise, analyse and find insights in qualitative data; for example, when analysing interviews.

TIP   The following are 10 simple rules for writing a literature review (Golash-Boza, 2015; Pautasso, 2013).

1   Define the research topic and the audience.
2   Search the literature using a structured process.
3   Make notes about emerging themes while reading the articles.
4   Select the type of literature review required.
5   Keep the review focused.
6   Be critical and consistent.
7   Develop a logical structure.
8   Keep up to date and include relevant older studies.
9   Proofread all work before submitting the literature review.
10   Support ideas with references to avoid plagiarism.

SUMMARY

In this chapter, the purpose of conducting a literature search and literature review has been detailed. A summary of the literature review (see **Figure 2.14**) follows after this chapter summary.

1	Identify the purpose of searching and reviewing the literature	• A literature review:
		  – summarises and evaluates a body of evidence about a specific topic
		  – exposes research previously completed
		  – helps plan the design and methodology of a study
		  – integrates evidence relating to a topic

2	Provide examples of different types of literature reviews	• An integrated literature review provides a summary of the evidence, which gives an overview of the topic • A systematic review is a transparent and reproducible process that includes a critique of all available evidence
3	Identify relevant literature sources	• Journal articles may be eliminated by reading the abstract for relevancy • Articles in non-research journals can be removed from the review • The date a study was completed and the type of journal in which it appears are important factors to consider • Journal articles that are peer reviewed provide an indication of the quality review process prior to publication
4	Conduct a focused search of the literature using a structured search strategy	• A structured approach to searching the literature includes using keywords according to the PICOT format • Using MeSH creates a targeted search • Boolean operators and limiters are used when searching the literature to either narrow or broaden the topic
5	Outline the components of a literature review	• Each article follows a similar logical structure, with the abstract providing an overview of the study • Becoming familiar with research terms includes making notes in the articles and referring to the glossary included in the textbook
6	Develop an efficient system for cataloguing references	• Using a summary table to document key ideas from the readings identifies key themes and details how articles should be presented in the literature review • A reference system (e.g. EndNote) assists with linking ideas from the literature with the source, avoiding plagiarism and keeping a record of the search

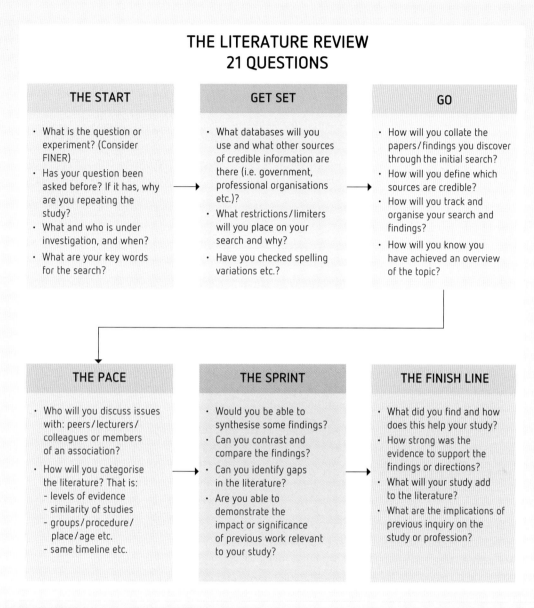

THE LITERATURE REVIEW
21 QUESTIONS

THE START

- What is the question or experiment? (Consider FINER)
- Has your question been asked before? If it has, why are you repeating the study?
- What and who is under investigation, and when?
- What are your key words for the search?

GET SET

- What databases will you use and what other sources of credible information are there (i.e. government, professional organisations etc.)?
- What restrictions/limiters will you place on your search and why?
- Have you checked spelling variations etc.?

GO

- How will you collate the papers/findings you discover through the initial search?
- How will you define which sources are credible?
- How will you track and organise your search and findings?
- How will you know you have achieved an overview of the topic?

THE PACE

- Who will you discuss issues with: peers/lecturers/colleagues or members of an association?
- How will you categorise the literature? That is:
  - levels of evidence
  - similarity of studies
  - groups/procedure/ place/age etc.
  - same timeline etc.

THE SPRINT

- Would you be able to synthesise some findings?
- Can you contrast and compare the findings?
- Can you identify gaps in the literature?
- Are you able to demonstrate the impact or significance of previous work relevant to your study?

THE FINISH LINE

- What did you find and how does this help your study?
- How strong was the evidence to support the findings or directions?
- What will your study add to the literature?
- What are the implications of previous inquiry on the study or profession?

▸ **Figure 2.14** Summary of the literature review

Source: Brown, S. (2002). Systematic review of nursing management of urinary tract infections in the cognitively impaired elderly client in residential care: Is there a hole in holistic care? *International Journal of Nursing Practice, 8*: 2–7.

REVIEW QUESTIONS

1 Explain the purpose of reviewing the literature before commencing a research project.
2 Describe the process of refining a literature search.
3 Identify sources of literature relevant to completing a literature review.
4 Discuss two methods of documenting key ideas identified in the literature.

CHALLENGING REVIEW QUESTIONS

1   During a literature search for relevant articles, over 10 000 articles' results have been sourced for the search terms you have used. Explain how this search can be refined using Boolean operators and limiters to help refine the search.
2   Explain the difference between completing a systematic review of the literature and a literature review that is conducted for an undergraduate assignment.
3   When undertaking a literature search, explain how the key ideas are recorded from the research and how this can assist with developing a systematic approach to completing a literature review.

CASE STUDY 1

Mathew, a third-year undergraduate social work student, is interested in finding out more about binge drinking among adolescents. In particular, he would like to learn more about the effects of alcohol consumption on teenagers' social interaction. Mathew has uncovered a lot of information and needs to refine the search. How would you go about assisting him?
1   Define Mathew's search.
2   Identify the keywords.
3   Locate relevant and credible papers.
4   Develop a system for managing his findings.

CASE STUDY 2

Heidi is a registered nurse who recently graduated with a first-class honours degree in nursing. She has been accepted into a PhD degree through a local university that has professional and academic links with a large tertiary referral hospital. A major research focus of the institution includes the health and quality of life for patients with dementia, a national health priority in Australia.
    As a fellow student, how should you advise Heidi in relation to each of the following?
1   Identify relevant and credible sources of literature.
2   Select relevant databases for conducting a literature search.
3   Set up an efficient system for keeping track of sources accessed.
4   Extract the relevant information from the literature.

REFERENCES

Australian Research Council. (2019). *State of Australian University Research 2018–19: ERA National Report.* Canberra: Australian Government.

Best, M., & Neuhauser, D. (2004). Ignaz Semmelweis and the birth of infection control. *Quality and Safety in Health Care, 13*(3), 233–4. https://doi.org/10.1136/qshc.2004.010918

Birks, M., & Mills, J. (2011). *Grounded Theory: A Practical Guide.* Los Angeles, CA: SAGE.

Brown, S. (2002). Systematic review of nursing management of urinary tract infections in the cognitively impaired elderly client in residential care: Is there a hole in holistic care? *International Journal of Nursing Practice*, *8*, 2–7.

Bryant, A., & Charmaz, K. (2019). *The SAGE Handbook of Current Developments in Grounded Theory*. London: SAGE.

Creswell, J. (2009). *Research Design: Qualitative, Quantitative, and Mixed Methods Approaches* (3rd edn). London: SAGE.

Cummings, S., Browner, W., & Hulley, S. (2007). Conceiving the research question. In S. Hulley, S. Cummings, W. Browner, D. Grady & T. Newman, *Designing Clinical Research* (3rd edn, pp. 17–26). Philadelphia, PA: Lippincott.

Denney, A. S., & Tewksbury, R. (2013). How to write a literature review. *Journal of Criminal Justice Education*, *24*(2), 218–34.

Fields, J. G. (2007). Caring to death: A discursive analysis of nurses who murder patients. PhD, Discipline of Nursing, University of Adelaide.

Galvan, J. (2009). *Writing Literature Reviews: A Guide for Students of the Social and Behavioral Sciences* (4th edn). Los Angeles, CA: Pyrczak Publishing.

George, G. S., Ferguson, L. A., & Pearce, P. F. (2014). Finding a needle in the haystack: Performing an in-depth literature search to answer a clinical question. *Nursing: Research and Reviews*, *4*, 65–76.

Golash-Boza, T. (2015). Writing a literature review: Six steps to get you from start to finish. https://www.wiley.com/network/researchers/preparing-your-article/writing-a-literature-review-six-steps-to-get-you-from-start-to-finish

Holbrook, A., Bourke, S., Fairbairn, H., & Lovat, T. (2007). Examiner comment on the literature review in PhD theses. *Studies in Higher Education*, *32*(3), 337–56.

Hulley, S. B., Cummings, S. R., Browner, W. S., Grady, D., & Newman, T. B. (2013). *Designing Clinical Research* (4th edn). Philadelphia: Lippincott Williams & Wilkins.

Johnson, R., Watkinson, A., & Mabe, M. (2018). *The STM Report: An Overview of Scientific and Scholarly Publishing* (5th edn). The Hague, Netherlands: International Association of Scientific, Technical and Medical Publishers. https://www.stm-assoc.org/2018_10_04_STM_Report_2018.pdf

Kamler, B., & Thomson, P. (2006). *Helping Doctoral Students Write: Pedagogies for Supervision*. London: Routledge.

Kearney, M., & Freda, M. (2005). Nurse editors' views on the peer review process. *Research in Nursing and Health*, *28*(6), 444–52.

Knopf, J. W. (2006). Doing a literature review. *PSOnline*. http://isites.harvard.edu/fs/docs/icb.topic1038752.files/Doing_a_Literature_Review.pdf

Krainovich-Miller, B. (2006). Literature review. In G. LoBiondo-Wood & J. Haber (eds), *Nursing Research: Methods and Critical Appraisal for Evidence-Based Practice*. St Louis, MO: Mosby.

Lau, F. Y. Y., & Kuziemsky, C. (2016). *Handbook of eHealth Evaluation: An Evidence-Based Approach*. University of Victoria. British Columbia: University of Victoria.

Liu, L. Q., & Mehigan, S. (2017). The effects of surgical hand scrubbing protocols on skin integrity and surgical site infection rates: A systematic review. *ACORN: The Journal of Perioperative Nursing in Australia*, *30*(2), 21–30.

Moule, P., & Goodman, M. (2009). *Nursing Research: An Introduction*. Los Angeles, CA: SAGE.

Munn, Z., Peters, M. D. J., Stern, C., Tufanaru, C., McArthur, A., & Aromataris, E. (2018). Systematic review or scoping review? Guidance for authors when choosing between a systematic or scoping review approach. *BMC Medical Research Methodology*. https://doi.org/10.1186/s12874-018-0611-x

Murphy, J. (2010). Using mobile devices for research: Smartphones, databases, and libraries. *Online*, *34*(3), 14–18.

Nippers, I., & Sutton, A. (2014). Oxygen therapy: Professional compliance with national guidelines. *British Journal of Nursing*, *23*(7), 382–6.

Paltridge, B., & Starfield, S. (2007). *Thesis and Dissertation Writing in a Second Language*. London: Routledge.

Parahoo, K. (2006). *Nursing Research: Principles, Process and Issues* (2nd edn). Basingstoke, UK: Palgrave Macmillan.

Pautasso, M. (2013). Ten simple rules for writing a literature review. *PLoS Computational Biology*, *9*(7), 1–4.

Polgar, S., & Thomas, S. (2008). *Introduction to Research in the Health Sciences* (5th edn). Edinburgh: Churchill Livingstone.

Polit, D., & Beck, C. (2009). *Essentials of nursing research* (7th edn). Philadelphia, PA: Lippincott.

Pyrczak, F., & Bruce, R. (2017). *Writing Empirical Research Reports: A Basic Guide for Students of the Social and Behavioral Sciences* (7th edn). Glendale, CA: Pyrczak Publishing.

Richter, R. R., & Austin, T. M. (2012). Using MeSH (Medical Subject Headings) to enhance PubMed search strategies for evidence-based practice in physical therapy. *Physical Therapy*, *92*(1), 124–32.

Ridley, D. (2012). *The Literature Review: A Step-by-step Guide for Students* (2nd edn). Los Angeles: SAGE.

Riva, J. J., Malik, K. M., Burnie, S. J., Endicott, A. R., & Busse, J. W. (2012). What is your research question? An introduction to the PICOT format for clinicians. *Journal of the Canadian Chiropractic Association, 56*(3), 167–71.

Tawfik, G. M., Dila, K. A. S., Mohamed, M. Y. F., Tam, D. N. H., Kien, N. D., Ahmed, A. M., & Huy, N. T. (2019). A step by step guide for conducting a systematic review and meta-analysis with simulation data. *Tropical Medicine and Health*, 1. https://doi.org/10.1186/s41182-019-0165-6

Ware, M., & Mabe, M. (2015). *The STM Report. An Overview of Scientific and Scholarly Journal Publishing* (4th ed). The Hague, Netherlands: International Association of Scientific, Technical and Medical Publishers.

Whittemore, R., & Knafl, K. (2005). The integrative review: Updated methodology. *Journal of Advanced Nursing, 52*(5), 546–53.

World Health Organization. (2009). WHO guidelines on hand hygiene in health care. First global patient safety challenge clean care is safer care. Geneva, Switzerland.

FURTHER READING

Cochrane Library, http://www.cochranelibrary.com/

Cronin, P., Ryan, F., & Coughlan, M. (2008). Undertaking a literature review: A step-by-step approach. *British Journal of Nursing, 17*(1), 17.

Evans, D., David G., Gruba, P., & Zobel, J. (2014). *How to Write a Better Thesis*. New York, NY: Springer.

Greenhalgh, T. (2014). *How to Read a Paper: The Basics of Evidence-Based Medicine*. Chichester, West Sussex, UK: John Wiley & Sons Inc.

Joanna Briggs Institute, https://jbi.global/

Lloyd Sealey Library. (2017). How to: Write a literature review: Writing a literature review. http://guides.lib.jjay.cuny.edu/c.php?g=322839&p=2162061

Macquarie University. (2012). Writing an article critique – postgraduate program in higher education. http://www.youtube.com/watch?v=u2cu6vsnoEM&feature=related

3 CRITICAL APPRAISAL OF RESEARCH EVIDENCE

Chapter learning objectives

The material presented in this chapter will assist you to:

1 provide a rationale for undertaking a critique of research evidence
2 explain how critically appraising the literature examines the value, trustworthiness and relevance of research evidence
3 analyse and evaluate the quality of research articles using critical appraisal criteria
4 list the necessary elements for critiquing a quantitative research article
5 list the necessary elements for critiquing a qualitative research article.

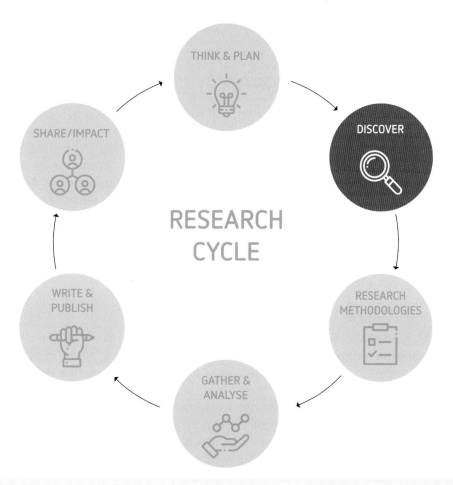

Research cycle

The focus of this chapter is on the critical appraisal of research evidence, the discovery component of the research frameworks diagram as highlighted above.

Introduction

Critically appraising research evidence is necessary to inform decisions about implementing the best available evidence in clinical practice, with the overall goal of improving patient outcomes (Dale, Hallas & Spratling, 2019). With the significant shift in healthcare professionals' use of evidence from scientific research in their clinical practice, being able to critically appraise research evidence is one of the most valuable skills a clinician should possess (Melnyk & Fineout-Overholt, 2019).

Findings from research articles that support the implementation of evidence-based practice lead to improved quality and patient safety, reduced variation in practices and reduced healthcare costs (Melnyk & Fineout-Overholt, 2015; Melnyk et al., 2012). It also promotes an attitude of inquiry among healthcare professionals, which leads them to become consumers of research and informed about safe patient care. Although critically appraising research articles may be a daunting experience, it is a fundamental skill for clinicians to be able to integrate the evidence with their own clinical experience and their patients' values when making decisions about patient care (Al-Jundi & Sakka, 2017).

This chapter provides an overview of the **critical appraisal** of research articles and outlines a systematic, logical order of the process, leading the reviewer to conclusions about the **trustworthiness**, value and relevance of the research evidence.

Why undertake research critiques?

There are a number of reasons why a critique of research evidence is necessary, one being that students may be required to critique a research article as part of an assignment. The aim of a student critique is to promote learning and to develop critical thinking skills. Undertaking a critique enables students to discriminate what to include in a review of the literature, to interpret results in light of previous research findings and to determine the suitability of including the article in a research proposal or report. The focus for a healthcare professional when undertaking a critique of a research project is to make an informed decision about the value of the research to their practice, in particular, evaluating the literature for its validity, impact and applicability (Gosall & Gosall, 2015).

Implications for practice

EBP

Gosall and Gosall (2015) suggest that critical appraisal of research allows clinicians to exclude studies that are poorly designed and will not lead to improved clinical outcomes. In other words, the aim of critical appraisal is to identify the quality of a research article, requiring the clinician to make a decision about which research evidence would have a clinically significant impact on their patient. It is important to note that improved outcomes will only be achieved when conclusions from critically appraised studies are applied to practice, and patient outcomes are monitored (Gosall & Gosall, 2015).

Developing critical appraisal skills requires using good judgement about the importance and credibility of the research results and deciding whether they will inform clinical practice.

There are three foundational factors to consider when appraising a research article – validity, reliability and relevance, as outlined below.

1   *Are the study results valid?* (**Validity**) This refers to whether the results were unbiased by critically evaluating the study's methodology and conclusions (Critical Appraisal Skills Programme [CASP], 2018), therefore determining whether the study was conducted properly. Bias can be introduced when conducting research, so it is important to recognise potential bias when reading articles that report research findings (Galdas, 2017; Melnyk & Fineout-Overholt, 2011).

2   *What are the results?* (**Reliability**) This involves reviewing the results and considering whether the study's results are clinically important. For example, were the results for the experimental group significantly better than the control group? Another important task is to determine the uncertainty about the results that have been reported. These are usually reported as *p* values and **confidence intervals**.

3   *Are the results relevant?* (**Applicability**) If the evidence is judged to be valid and important, the next step is to determine how the study can be applied to clinical practice, in particular taking into consideration the **population** characteristics or clinical setting, and determining how these differ to the clinicians' workplace. Critical appraisal skills provide a framework whereby these factors are examined in a transparent way, assisting the reviewer to make a judgement about the quality of the evidence (CASP, 2018).

A successful critique of a research paper is one that achieves a balance between the methodological flaws of the study and the relevance of the findings (Hannes, 2011). The following sections provide comprehensive guidance to assist healthcare professionals in undertaking a critique of quantitative and qualitative research articles.

Analysing and evaluating research using critique criteria

Assuming the appropriate material has been retrieved following a literature search (see Chapter 2), the process of critiquing research evidence includes skim reading the article for a general understanding of the study and evaluating which sources are most relevant to the research question. Reading the abstract is a quick way of obtaining information about the purpose, method, main findings and conclusions (Al-Jundi & Sakka, 2017). The articles should then be read in more detail several times while asking questions about the quality of the research using a critical appraisal tool. Following a thorough review of the article, the material is developed into a structured, logical argument.

When critiquing a research article, general questions about the quality of the research are considered, with more specific questions about parts of the research, in particular the recruitment and allocation of participants, collection of data, the results and how these have been reported. Each of these will be reviewed in turn in this chapter. In assessing the overall quality of the research, it is important to determine whether the results are statistically significant; that is, the results are not attributed to chance. There may, for example, be studies that did not achieve statistically significant results but the outcome of the study is considered to be clinically significant (Rajaretnam, 2015), and may be relevant for inclusion in a literature review section of a research proposal.

Most journals require authors to use the introduction, method, results and discussion (IMRAD) method (Teodosiu, 2019; Wu, 2011), which the National Standards Institute of the United States has adopted as the industry standard (Day, 1998; Day & Gastel, 2012). According to Day, IMRAD provides a framework that guides the author to address several questions essential to understanding a scientific study when it is published. It also increases the probability of the article being accepted for publication (Day & Gastel, 2012). When critiquing a study, it should be remembered that some journals have formats that do not necessarily conform to the IMRAD standard.

Using a critical appraisal tool assists with evaluating the evidence using structured questions or a checklist (Buccheri & Sharifi, 2017). There are several standard critical appraisal tools and checklists available to assist clinicians with evaluating the quality of published research articles. Standard critical appraisal tools and checklists, including those designed by the Critical Appraisal Skills Programme (CASP, 2018), CONSORT (2010), Joanna Briggs Institute (2020), Centre for Evidence-Based Medicine (n.d.) and Greenhalgh (2019), have been developed to assist clinicians when making informed decisions about the quality of research evidence. Many of these programs include tools for appraising various study designs, such as randomised controlled trials, systematic reviews and qualitative and qualitative studies. Although there is little consensus regarding the most appropriate tool for allied health research (Glenny, 2005; Katrak et al., 2004;), it is recommended that clinicians use the CASP tool for research studies and the AGREE II tool when appraising clinical guidelines (Dale, Hallas & Spratling, 2019).

A framework for critiquing health research, one that includes a list of questions for critiquing both qualitative and quantitative research, was developed to assist undergraduate students develop critical appraisal skills (Caldwell, Henshaw & Taylor, 2011). Dale, Hallas and Spratling (2019) describe undertaking a critical appraisal using an updated checklist adapted from Caldwell, Henshaw and Taylor (2011) and Dale (2005), as shown in Figure 3.1. Details about what should be included are listed in the checklist and should be used to guide students when learning how to critically appraise an article.

Critiquing a quantitative research article

The following is an example of a critical review of a randomised controlled trial article using the critical appraisal skills programme (CASP) randomised controlled trial standard checklist (CASP, 2019a).

Excerpts from the published research article, 'A novel multi-component online intervention to improve the mental health of university students: Randomised controlled trial of the Uni Virtual Clinic' by Farrer and colleagues (2019) are used in the following sections as examples of how to undertake a critical appraisal of clinical research.

There are three broad issues that should be considered when appraising a research article.

1   Is the basic study design valid for a randomised controlled trial? (Section A)
2   Was the study methodologically sound? (Section B)
3   What were the results? (Section C)
4   Will the results help locally? (Section D) (CASP, 2019a).

The CASP tool includes 11 questions that guide appraising an article in a systematic way. A number of prompts, designed as a reminder of why the questions are important, are includes with each question (CASP, 2019a).

Abstract
- Does the abstract discuss the purpose, methods, sample, results, and conclusions with implications for practice?

Background
- Is the purpose justified by the literature?
- Are only the most relevant, primary, and up-to-date sources included?
- Does the review address all the concepts proposed in the study?

Theoretical framework
- Does the theoretical or conceptual framework or philosophical background relate to the concepts or phenomena of study and the methods used in the study?

Statement of problem and purpose
- Are the problem and purpose clearly stated?
- Are the key variables or concepts identified and defined, if applicable?
- Is the problem significant to improve outcomes for children and their families?
- Are the definitions clear?
- Is (are) the hypothesis(es) and/or the research question(s) clearly stated?

Methodology
- Is the design appropriate for the study's purpose?
- Is the sampling method appropriate and the sample size adequate? Does it include a description of the sample inclusion and exclusion criteria? For qualitative studies, is the selection of participants described and the sampling method identified?
- Is the study approved by an institutional review board (i.e., IRB)?
- Is the mechanism for obtaining assent from any child over 7 years of age described?
- Is the setting clearly described?
- Is there a rationale for selection of the instrument(s)?
- Has the validity and reliability for the instrument(s) been established? if not, are the methods for doing so described?
- Are the limitations for the instrument(s) given? Has (have) the instrument(s) been ploted?
- Is the process for administration of the instrument(s) given?
- Are the data collection methods appropriate for the study? For quantitative studies, is the data collection method valid and reliable? For qualitative studies, is the data collection method auditable?
- Are data analysis methods described and appropriate? Are the statistical methods used consistent with the study design? For quantitative studies, is the data analysis method valid and reliable? For qualitative studies, is the data analysis method credible and comfirmable?

Results
- Are the data presented objectively and factually?

Discussion/conclusions
- Are the findings explained with regard to their significance?
- Is the relationship between the findings and the conceptual or theoretical framework or philosophical background discussed?
- Is the relationship between the findings and previous relevant research explained?
- For quantitative studies, are the results generalizable? For qualitative studies, are the results transferable?
- Are the conclusions linked to the study objectives?
- Do the conclusions flow from the data and the analysis?
- Are the limitations of the study presented?

▶ **Figure 3.1** Questions for critical appraisal of a research study

Source: Reprinted from *Journal of Pediatric Health Care*, 33/3, Juanita Conkin Dale, Donna Hallas and Regena Spratling, Critiquing research evidence for use in practice: revisited, 183–6., Copyright 2019, with permission from Elsevier.

Section A: Is the basic study design valid for a randomised controlled trial?

1   Did the study address a clearly focused research question? Yes ☑ No ☐ Can't tell ☐
Consider: Was the study designed to assess the outcomes of an intervention?
Is the research question 'focused' in terms of:
- Population studied
- Intervention given
- Comparator chosen
- Outcomes measured?

Source: The Critical Appraisal Skills Programme (CASP), www.casp-uk.net

FOR EXAMPLE

IS THE BASIC STUDY DESIGN VALID FOR A RANDOMISED CONTROLLED TRIAL?

The trial by Farrer and colleagues (2019) addresses a clearly focused issue and included the *population* (undergraduate and postgraduate students from a mid-sized university), details about the *intervention* (participants allocated to the intervention condition received a weekly email and a text message via mobile phone encouraging them to engage with the Uni Virtual Clinic [UVC]), *control* (participants allocated to the control condition did not receive any program content or contact with researchers during the 6-week intervention period) and *outcome* (mixed models analysis demonstrated that use of the UVC was associated with small significant reductions in social anxiety and small improvements in academic self-efficacy; most of the participants reported satisfaction with the UVC).

TIP

A method of generating a random allocation sequence using either a random-numbers table or a computer software program is used to divide participants into each experimental condition in order to reduce any bias.

2   Was the assignment of participants to interventions randomised?
Yes ☑ No ☐ Can't tell ☐
Consider:
- How was randomisation carried out? Was the method appropriate?
- Was randomisation sufficient to eliminate systemic bias?
- Was the allocation sequence concealed from investigators and participants?

Source: The Critical Appraisal Skills Programme (CASP), www.casp-uk.net

FOR EXAMPLE

WAS THE ASSIGNMENT OF PARTICIPANTS TO INTERVENTION RANDOMISED?

A researcher who was independent of the trial generated a sequence of random integers between the values of 1 and 2 at https://www.random. org/, and manually allocated participants to the trial conditions according to this sequence [randomisation of participants to the treatment arm].

Source: Farrer, L. M., Gulliver, A., Katruss, N., Fassnacht, D. B., Kyrios, M., & Batterham, P. J. (2019). A novel multi-component online intervention to improve the mental health of university students: Randomised controlled trial of the Uni Virtual Clinic. *Internet Interventions, 18*.

3   Were all participants who entered the study accounted for at its conclusion?
Yes ☑ No ☐ Can't tell ☐
Consider:
- Were losses to follow-up and exclusions after randomisation accounted for?
- Were participants analysed in the study groups to which they were randomised (intention-to-treat analysis)?
- Was the study stopped early? If so, what was the reason?

Source: The Critical Appraisal Skills Programme (CASP), www.casp-uk.net

FOR EXAMPLE

WERE ALL PARTICIPANTS WHO ENTERED THE STUDY ACCOUNTED FOR AT ITS CONCLUSION?

The primary and secondary outcome variables were analysed on an **intention to treat (ITT)** basis. [The flow of participants through the trial is depicted in a CONSORT diagram (p. 7).] … A total of 840 students clicked on the study invitation and were screened for eligibility. Of these, 259 (30.8%) consented and were eligible for the trial and 200 completed the baseline questionnaire and were randomised. The majority ($n = 144$, 72%) of participants completed the post-intervention questionnaire, and 47.5% ($n = 95$) completed the 3-month follow-up questionnaire.

Source: Farrer, L. M., Gulliver, A., Katruss, N., Fassnacht, D. B., Kyrios, M., & Batterham, P. J. (2019). A novel multi-component online intervention to improve the mental health of university students: Randomised controlled trial of the Uni Virtual Clinic. *Internet Interventions, 18.*

Section B: Was the study methodologically sound?

4   Were the participants 'blind' to intervention they were given? Yes ☐ No ☑ Can't tell ☐
Were the investigators 'blind' to the intervention they were giving to participants? Yes ☑ No ☐ Can't tell ☐
Were the people assessing/analysing outcome/s 'blinded'? Yes ☑ No ☐ Can't tell ☐

Source: The Critical Appraisal Skills Programme (CASP), www.casp-uk.net

FOR EXAMPLE

WERE THE PARTICIPANTS 'BLIND' TO INTERVENTION THEY WERE GIVEN?

The trial researchers [study personnel] were blinded to condition allocations [concealment of allocation of participants from the researchers involved in the trial]. During the 6 week intervention period, participants allocated to the intervention condition received a weekly e-mail and a text message via mobile phone, encouraging them to engage with the UVC. [It was not possible to conceal allocation from the participants (students).]

Source: Farrer, L. M., Gulliver, A., Katruss, N., Fassnacht, D. B., Kyrios, M., & Batterham, P. J. (2019). A novel multi-component online intervention to improve the mental health of university students: Randomised controlled trial of the Uni Virtual Clinic. *Internet Interventions, 18.*

5   Were the study groups similar at the start of the randomised controlled trial? Yes ☑ No ☐ Can't tell ☐
Consider:
- Were the baseline characteristics of each study group (e.g. age, sex, socio-economic group) clearly set out?
- Were there any differences between the study groups that could affect the outcome/s?

Source: The Critical Appraisal Skills Programme (CASP), www.casp-uk.net

FOR EXAMPLE

WERE THE GROUPS SIMILAR AT THE START OF THE RANDOMISED CONTROLLED TRIAL?

Table 1 presents the demographic and clinical characteristics of the sample at baseline. ...There were no significant differences between participants randomised to the intervention or control conditions on any baseline demographic or symptom variables.

Source: Farrer, L. M., Gulliver, A., Katruss, N., Fassnacht, D. B., Kyrios, M., & Batterham, P. J. (2019). A novel multi-component online intervention to improve the mental health of university students: Randomised controlled trial of the Uni Virtual Clinic. *Internet Interventions, 18*.

6   Apart from the experimental intervention, did each study group receive the same level of care (that is, were they treated equally)? Yes ☑ No ☐ Can't tell ☐
Consider:
- Was there a clearly defined study protocol?
- If any additional interventions were given (e.g. tests or treatments), were they similar between the study groups?
- Were the follow-up intervals the same for each study group?

Source: The Critical Appraisal Skills Programme (CASP).

FOR EXAMPLE

APART FROM THE EXPERIMENTAL INTERVENTION, DID EACH STUDY GROUP RECEIVE THE SAME LEVEL OF CARE?

Eligible participants were required to provide an e-mail address and mobile phone number, and were e-mailed a link to the baseline survey. ... All participants received an e-mail containing a link to the post-intervention survey 6 weeks after they completed the baseline survey, and a link to the follow-up survey was sent 3 months after the post-intervention survey.

Source: Farrer, L. M., Gulliver, A., Katruss, N., Fassnacht, D. B., Kyrios, M., & Batterham, P. J. (2019). A novel multi-component online intervention to improve the mental health of university students: Randomised controlled trial of the Uni Virtual Clinic. *Internet Interventions, 18*.

Section C: What are the results?

7   Were the effects of intervention reported comprehensively? Yes ☑ No ☐ Can't tell ☐
Consider:
- Was a power calculation undertaken?
- What outcomes were measured, and were they clearly specified?
- How were the results expressed? For binary outcomes, were relative and absolute effects reported?
- Were the results reported for each outcome in each study group at each follow-up interval?
- Was there any missing or incomplete data?

Source: The Critical Appraisal Skills Programme (CASP), www.casp-uk.net

- Was there differential drop-out between the study groups that could affect the results?
- Were potential sources of bias identified?
- Which statistical tests were used?
- Were p values reported?

FOR EXAMPLE

WERE THE EFFECTS OF INTERVENTION REPORTED COMPREHENSIVELY?

The purpose of this trial was to examine feasibility and the effectiveness of the intervention on depression symptoms, anxiety symptoms and a range of other symptom outcomes, as well as satisfaction with and usage of the intervention. [Baseline, post-intervention and 3-month follow-up surveys assessed depression, anxiety, self-efficacy, quality of life, adherence and satisfaction with the UVC intervention.]

PRIMARY OUTCOMES (DEPRESSION AND ANXIETY SYMPTOMS)

Participants in both conditions showed reductions in depression symptoms ($F = 43.02$, $p < 0.001$) and anxiety symptoms ($F = 25.49$, $p < 0.001$). … Between-group effect sizes at post-intervention were small for both depression ($d = -0.16$) and anxiety ($d = -0.16$). Similarly, small effect sizes were observed between conditions at 3 months.

Source: Farrer, L. M., Gulliver, A., Katruss, N., Fassnacht, D. B., Kyrios, M., & Batterham, P. J. (2019). A novel multi-component online intervention to improve the mental health of university students: Randomised controlled trial of the Uni Virtual Clinic. *Internet Interventions, 18.*

TIP
- ANOVA F-test: analysis of variance to analyse the differences among group means in a sample.
- $p < 0.001$: the probability that this result could have happened by chance is only 0.1%.
- Cohen's d: an appropriate effect size for the comparison between two means (i.e. two groups to see how different they are). $d = 0.2$ is considered a 'small' effect size, which means that if two groups' means don't differ by 0.2 standard deviations or more, the difference is trivial, even if it is statistically significant.

FOR EXAMPLE

WERE THE EFFECTS OF INTERVENTION REPORTED COMPREHENSIVELY?

Participants in the intervention condition showed significant reductions in social anxiety symptoms and significant improvement in academic self-efficacy over time compared to participants in the control condition. …

Participants in both conditions showed significant reductions in distress … and significant improvements in quality of life … over time.

INTERVENTION ADHERENCE AND USAGE

Of those in the UVC condition who returned a post-intervention survey, 75.8% ($n = 47$) accessed the UVC during the intervention period at least once. Most of these participants logged in to the program around once per week ($n = 30$, 63.8%) and 42.6% ($n = 20$) spent between 5 and 15 minutes using the program per visit.

SATISFACTION

Most participants who returned a post-intervention survey reported being satisfied with the intervention; 61.7% ($n = 29$) of participants were either 'very satisfied' or 'somewhat satisfied' following use of the UVC.

In terms of specific features of the program, 32.6% of participants ($n = 15$) reported that they liked the interactive symptoms quizzes the most, followed by the problem solver tool on the homepage ($n = 7$, 15.2%) and the self-help modules ($n = 6$, 13.0%).

Source: Farrer, L. M., Gulliver, A., Katruss, N., Fassnacht, D. B., Kyrios, M., & Batterham, P. J. (2019). A novel multi-component online intervention to improve the mental health of university students: Randomised controlled trial of the Uni Virtual Clinic. *Internet Interventions, 18*.

TIP

A 95% confidence interval is a range of values that you can be 95% certain contains the true mean of the population.

---

8 Was the precision of the estimate of the intervention or treatment effect reported?
Yes ☐ No ☐ Can't tell ☑
Consider:
- Were the confidence intervals (CIs) reported?

Source: The Critical Appraisal Skills Programme (CASP),

FOR EXAMPLE

WAS THE PRECISION OF THE ESTIMATE OF THE INTERVENTION OR TREATMENT EFFECT REPORTED?

Although *p* values have been reported, confidence intervals have not been reported in the article (Farrer et al., 2019).

---

9 Do the benefits of the experimental intervention outweigh the harms and costs?
Yes ☐ No ☐ Can't tell ☑
Consider:
- What was the size of the intervention or treatment effect?
- Were harms or unintended effects reported for each study group?
- Was a cost-effectiveness analysis undertaken? (Cost-effectiveness analysis allows a comparison to be made between different interventions used in the care of the same condition or problem.)

Source: The Critical Appraisal Skills Programme (CASP), www.casp-uk.net

FOR EXAMPLE

DO THE BENEFITS OF THE EXPERIMENTAL INTERVENTION OUTWEIGH THE HARMS AND COSTS?

The trial found no evidence for the effectiveness of the Uni Virtual Clinic in reducing symptoms of depression, anxiety or psychological distress, or improving quality of life or general self-efficacy, compared to a no-treatment control group. ... The trial demonstrated some utility in reducing social anxiety and improving academic self-efficacy among students, and was rated well in terms of satisfaction and usability. ... Interventions such as the UVC have the potential to reimagine the way mental health services are delivered in universities, which may reduce the prevalence of mental disorders in this high-risk population.

Source: Farrer, L. M., Gulliver, A., Katruss, N., Fassnacht, D. B., Kyrios, M., & Batterham, P. J. (2019). A novel multi-component online intervention to improve the mental health of university students: Randomised controlled trial of the Uni Virtual Clinic. *Internet Interventions, 18.*

Section D: Will the results help locally?

10 Can the results be applied to your local population/in your context? Yes ☐ No ☐ Can't tell ☐ [The answer to this question will vary depending on the clinician's area of practice.]
   Consider:
   - Are the study participants similar to the people in your care?
   - Would any differences between your population and the study participants alter the outcomes reported in the study?
   - Are the outcomes important to your population?
   - Are there any outcomes you would have wanted information on that have not been studied or reported?
   - Are there any limitations of the study that would affect your decision?

11 Would the experimental intervention provide greater value to the people in your care than any of the existing interventions? Yes ☐ No ☐ Can't tell ☐ [The answer to this question will vary depending on the clinician's area of practice.]
   Consider:
   - What resources are needed to introduce this intervention taking into account time, finances, and skills development or training needs?
   - Are you able to disinvest resources in one or more existing interventions in order to be able to re-invest in the new intervention?

Source: The Critical Appraisal Skills Programme (CASP), www.casp-uk.net

Ethical requirements

In quantitative research, it is important to critique the ways in which the ethical rights of the participants were safeguarded throughout the project. Check carefully to see that the report includes explanations regarding the ethical requirements.

EBP

Figure 3.2 presents questions for consideration regarding the ethical aspects of a study.

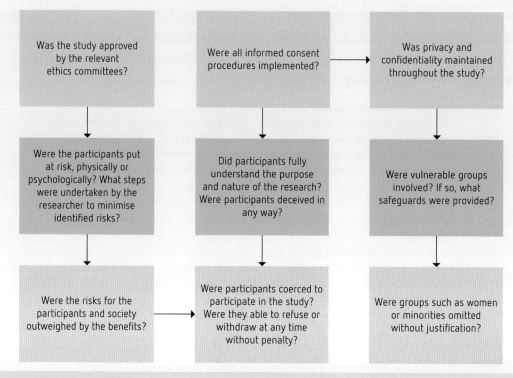

▶ **Figure 3.2** Questions for critiquing the ethical aspects of a study

Critiquing a qualitative research article

This section will emphasise some key questions when critiquing a qualitative research article, building on the questions raised in the previous section. An example of a critical review of a qualitative article is presented, and some explanation given as necessary, using a critical appraisal skills programme qualitative research checklist (CASP, 2019b).

There are close and direct connections between critiquing qualitative research and quantitative research processes, the format of a qualitative research proposal, the presentation of the results and the elements of a qualitative research article.

Qualitative research concentrates on people's experiences, attitudes and beliefs, and their perception of a situation. It is not the opposite of quantitative research and is not just a set of techniques for collecting descriptive data; it has a theoretical foundation. This is important because this foundation is essential if the knowledge generated from qualitative research is to be seen as legitimate. Qualitative research can address issues for the patient, such as the experience of living with chronic pain.

In the following example excerpts from the published research article, 'Creating evidence: Findings from a grounded theory of memory-making in neonatal bereavement care in Australia', by Thornton, Nicholson and Harms (2020), are used in the following sections as examples of how to undertake a critical appraisal of a qualitative research article.

Section A: Are the results of the study valid?

1 Was there a clear statement of the aims of the research? Yes ☑ No ☐ Can't tell ☐
Hint: Consider:
- What was the goal of the research?
- Why was it thought important?
- Why is it relevant?

Source: The Critical Appraisal Skills Programme (CASP), www.casp-uk.net

FOR EXAMPLE

WAS THERE A CLEAR STATEMENT OF THE AIMS OF THE RESEARCH?

The purpose of this study was to explore the significance of memory-making activities for parents experiencing the death of a neonate, and the impact that these activities have on parents' experience of bereavement.

Source: Thornton, R., Nicholson P., & Harms, L. (2020). Creating evidence: Findings from a grounded theory of memory-making in neonatal bereavement care in Australia. *Journal of Pediatric Nursing, 53*, 29 – 35.

2 Is a qualitative methodology appropriate? Yes ☑ No ☐ Can't tell ☐
Hint: Consider:
- Does the research seek to interpret or illuminate the actions and/or subjective experience of research participants?
- Is qualitative research the right methodology for addressing the research goal?

Source: The Critical Appraisal Skills Programme (CASP), www.casp-uk.net

FOR EXAMPLE

IS A QUALITATIVE METHODOLOGY APPROPRIATE?

This study was conducted using the **grounded theory** approach described by Corbin and Strauss … Although there is an increasing body of research exploring perinatal bereavement, little is known about bereavement interventions in the context of neonatal death.

Source: Thornton, R., Nicholson P., & Harms, L. (2020). Creating evidence: Findings from a grounded theory of memory-making in neonatal bereavement care in Australia. *Journal of Pediatric Nursing, 53*, 29 – 35.

3 Was the research design appropriate to address the aims of the research?
Yes ☑ No ☐ Can't tell ☐
Hint: Consider:
- Has the researcher has justified the research design (e.g. have they discussed how they decided which method to use)?

Source: The Critical Appraisal Skills Programme (CASP), www.casp-uk.net

FOR EXAMPLE

WAS THE RESEARCH DESIGN APPROPRIATE TO ADDRESS THE AIMS OF THE RESEARCH?

Although there is an increasing body of research exploring perinatal bereavement, little is known about bereavement interventions in the context of neonatal death. A grounded theory approach was selected to address this gap in the literature and enable the development of a substantive theory that could be used to guide practice.

4   Was the recruitment strategy appropriate to the aims of the research?
Yes ☑ No ☐ Can't tell ☐
Hint: Consider:
- Does the researcher explain how the participants were selected?
- Did they explain why the participants they selected were the most appropriate to provide access to the type of knowledge sought by the study?
- Were there any discussions around recruitment (e.g. why some people chose not to take part)?

Source: The Critical Appraisal Skills Programme (CASP), www.casp-uk.net

FOR EXAMPLE

WAS THE RECRUITMENT STRATEGY APPROPRIATE TO THE AIMS OF THE RESEARCH?

To be eligible to participate parents needed to have experienced the death of their infant in a neonatal unit in Australia, and to be able to communicate in English without an interpreter. The decision was made not to exclude parents on the basis of time elapsed since the loss, as limited evidence exists for such restrictions ... Eighteen bereaved parents were selected to participate in the study using theoretical sampling ... This cyclical approach to data collection and analysis enabled the researchers to make sampling decisions based on the emerging theory.

Source: Thornton, R., Nicholson P., & Harms, L. (2020). Creating evidence: Findings from a grounded theory of memory-making in neonatal bereavement care in Australia. *Journal of Pediatric Nursing, 53,* 29 – 35.

5   Was the data collected in a way that addressed the research issue?
Yes ☑ No ☐ Can't tell ☐
Hint: Consider:
- Was the setting for the data collection justified?
- Was it clear how data was collected (e.g. focus group, semi-structured interview etc.)?
- Has the researcher justified the methods chosen?

- Has the researcher made the methods explicit (e.g. for interview method, is there an indication of how interviews are conducted, or did they use a topic guide)?
- Were methods modified during the study? If so, has the researcher explained how and why?
- Is the form of data clear (e.g. tape recordings, video material, notes, etc.)?
- Has the researcher discussed saturation of data?

Source: The Critical Appraisal Skills Programme (CASP), www.casp-uk.net

FOR EXAMPLE

WAS THE DATA COLLECTED IN A WAY THAT ADDRESSED THE RESEARCH ISSUE?

Data were collected using extended digitally-recorded semi-structured interviews. Parents were offered a choice of in-person, telephone or Skype interviews … In keeping with the tenets of grounded theory, an initial interview guide was developed with several broad, open-ended questions. … The interview guide was updated after each interview, enabling exploration of emergent categories and subcategories … Sampling continued until no new categories or subcategories were emerging from subsequent interviews, and until the categories and subcategories were well developed in terms of their properties and dimensions, adding to the theoretical rigour of the emerging grounded theory.

Source: Thornton, R., Nicholson P., & Harms, L. (2020). Creating evidence: Findings from a grounded theory of memory-making in neonatal bereavement care in Australia. *Journal of Pediatric Nursing, 53*, 29 – 35.

6   Has the relationship between researcher and participants been adequately considered?
Yes ☑ No ☐ Can't tell ☐
Hint: Consider:
- Did the researcher critically examine their own role, potential bias and influence during (a) formulation of the research questions and (b) data collection, including sample recruitment and choice of location?
- How did the researcher respond to events during the study and did they consider the implications of any changes in the research design?

Source: The Critical Appraisal Skills Programme (CASP), www.casp-uk.net

FOR EXAMPLE

HAS THE RELATIONSHIP BETWEEN RESEARCHER AND PARTICIPANTS BEEN ADEQUATELY CONSIDERED?

Bereaved parents were informed of the study via community-based not for profit perinatal bereavement services (for example, SANDS and Red Nose). Each organisation posted news items either in their regular newsletters or via open Facebook groups, enabling parents to contact the researchers to express interest in participating. [Parents were not contacted directly by the researcher.]

Source: Thornton, R., Nicholson P., & Harms, L. (2020). Creating evidence: Findings from a grounded theory of memory-making in neonatal bereavement care in Australia. *Journal of Pediatric Nursing, 53*, 29 – 35.

Section B: What are the results?

7 Have ethical issues been taken into consideration? Yes ☑ No ☐ Can't tell ☐
Hint: Consider:
- Were there sufficient details of how the research was explained to participants for the reader to assess whether ethical standards were maintained?
- Did the researcher discuss issues raised by the study (e.g. issues around informed consent or confidentiality or how they have handled the effects of the study on the participants during and after the study)?
- Was approval sought from the ethics committee?

Source: The Critical Appraisal Skills Programme (CASP), www.casp-uk.net

FOR EXAMPLE

HAVE ETHICAL ISSUES BEEN TAKEN INTO CONSIDERATION?

Prior to commencing data collection, ethics approval was obtained from the University Human Ethics Sub-Committee. Due to the emotive nature of the topic, minimising the distress of participants was a key concern. Strategies included standard provisions for the protection of **privacy** and ensuring informed consent, as well as a specific distress protocol and the provision of support for parents throughout the research process … participants were encouraged to debrief at the end of the interview and were offered a follow-up phone call the next day.

Source: Thornton, R., Nicholson P., & Harms, L. (2020). Creating evidence: Findings from a grounded theory of memory-making in neonatal bereavement care in Australia. *Journal of Pediatric Nursing, 53,* 29–35.

8 Was the data analysis sufficiently rigorous? Yes ☑ No ☐ Can't tell ☐
Hint: Consider:
- Is there an in-depth description of the analysis process?
- Is thematic analysis used? If so, is it clear how the categories/themes were derived from the data?
- Did the researcher explain how the data presented was selected from the original sample to demonstrate the analysis process?
- Is sufficient data presented to support the findings?
- To what extent are contradictory data taken into account?
- Did the researcher critically examine their own role, potential bias and influence during analysis and selection of data for presentation?

Source: The Critical Appraisal Skills Programme (CASP), www.casp-uk.net

FOR EXAMPLE

WAS THE DATA ANALYSIS SUFFICIENTLY RIGOROUS?

In the current study, this [data analysis] was achieved through line-by-line coding, with each line or phrase from the transcript being given one or more conceptual labels or codes … In this study, the use of an evolving interview guide enabled researchers to check emerging concepts with new participants, while extensive memos were recorded regarding all sampling and theoretical decisions........ NVivo 11 (QRS International) was used to code interviews at each level of analysis and to facilitate constant comparison throughout data analysis.

Source: Thornton, R., Nicholson P., & Harms, L. (2020). Creating evidence: Findings from a grounded theory of memory-making in neonatal bereavement care in Australia. *Journal of Pediatric Nursing, 53*, 29–35.

9 Is there a clear statement of findings? Yes ☑ No ☐ Can't tell ☐

Hint: Consider whether:
- Are the findings explicit?
- Is there adequate discussion of the evidence both for and against the researcher's arguments?
- Did the researcher discuss the credibility of their findings (e.g. triangulation, respondent validation, more than one analyst)?
- Are the findings discussed in relation to the original research question?

Source: The Critical Appraisal Skills Programme (CASP), www.casp-uk.net

FOR EXAMPLE

IS THERE A CLEAR STATEMENT OF FINDINGS?

This study resulted in the development of a grounded theory titled 'affirmed parenthood'. The core category affirmed parenthood was supported by three key categories; 'Being a parent', 'Being guided' and 'Creating Evidence'. 'Being a parent' included spending time with the baby before and after death, holding or touching the baby, and providing physical care. 'Being guided' represented parents' need to be supported and encouraged throughout the process of memory-making. Finally, 'Creating evidence' captured parents' efforts to collect or create tangible evidence of their baby's life through photographs and other mementos, and by involving others with their baby to ensure that people outside the immediate family would have memories of their child.

Source: Thornton, R., Nicholson P., & Harms, L. (2020). Creating evidence: Findings from a grounded theory of memory-making in neonatal bereavement care in Australia. *Journal of Pediatric Nursing, 53*, 29–35.

Section C: Will the results help locally?

10 How valuable is the research? Yes ☑ No ☐ Can't tell ☐

Hint: Consider:
- Did the researcher discuss the contribution the study makes to existing knowledge or understanding (e.g. did they consider the findings in relation to current practice or policy, or relevant research-based literature)?
- Did they identify new areas where research is necessary?
- Have the researchers discussed whether or how the findings can be transferred to other populations or considered other ways the research may be used?

Source: The Critical Appraisal Skills Programme (CASP), www.casp-uk.net

FOR EXAMPLE

HOW VALUABLE IS THE RESEARCH?

The grounded theory of 'affirmed parenthood' was underpinned by three categories: being a parent, being guided and creating evidence. 'Creating evidence' was achieved by parents through bereavement photography, through the collection or creation of mementos, and through involving others during and after the neonatal unit stay. This evidence helped to affirm the baby's existence, to affirm the role of the parents, and to affirm the grief that parents experienced. These findings are well aligned with the current literature surrounding perinatal bereavement care, and support the use of memory-making interventions in neonatal end of life care. This research contributes to understandings of the significance and impact of memory-making activities for parents experiencing the loss of an infant in the neonatal unit.

Source: Thornton, R., Nicholson P., & Harms, L. (2020). Creating evidence: Findings from a grounded theory of memory-making in neonatal bereavement care in Australia. *Journal of Pediatric Nursing, 53,* 29–35.

SUMMARY

This chapter discussed the critical appraisal of research and outlined how to critique both quantitative and qualitative research articles.

1	Provide a rationale for undertaking a critique of research evidence	• Undertaking a critique of research evidence:
		  – promotes learning and develops critical thinking skills as a requirement of an assignment
		  – enables students to discriminate what should be included in a literature review
		  – determines the suitability of the evidence for a literature review in a research proposal or article

2	Explain how critically appraising the literature examines the value, trustworthiness and relevance of research evidence	• To judge the trustworthiness, value and relevance in a particular context • To make an informed decision about the value of the research to clinical practice

3	Analyse and evaluate the quality of research articles using critical appraisal criteria	• Standard critical appraisal tools and checklists include those designed by the Critical Appraisal Skills Programme (CASP, 2018), CONSORT (2010) and Joanna Briggs (2020)
		• When critiquing a research article the following questions need to be answered:
		  – What is the clinical question that needs to be answered?
		  – What is the study design and is it appropriate?
		  – Who are the subjects and how were they recruited into the study?
		  – What is being measured and how was this done?
		  – What measures have been taken to reduce bias and confounding factors?
		  – Who funded the study and are there any competing interests? Has this been reported?

4	List the necessary elements for critiquing a quantitative research article	• Elements in a critique of a quantitative article to check for:
		  – title describes the article
		  – abstract summarises the article
		  – introduction makes the purpose clear
		  – problem is properly introduced
		  – purpose of the study is explained
		  – research question(s) are clearly presented
		  – theoretical framework informs the research
		  – literature review is relevant, comprehensive and includes recent research
		  – methods section details how the research questions were addressed or the hypotheses were tested
		  – analysis is consistent with the study questions and research design
		  – results are clearly presented and statistics clearly explained
		  – discussion explains the results in relation to the theoretical framework, research questions and significance to nursing
		  – limitations are presented and their implications discussed
		  – conclusion includes recommendations for nursing practice, future research and policymakers
		  – level and quality of the evidence
		  – the study is or is not applicable to clinical practice

| 5 | List the necessary elements for critiquing a qualitative research article | • | Elements in a critique of a qualitative article to check for:
– title and research summary/abstract summarises the article
– elements of the literature review are relevant, comprehensive and include recent research
– theoretical assumptions about the chosen methodology are detailed
– ethical requirements have been addressed
– data analysis and interpretation processes detailed
– comprehensive discussion of findings, insights and examples presented
– recommendations for practice included
– final conclusions are congruent with the overall method and process of the research |

REVIEW QUESTIONS

1 Explain the three foundational factors when appraising a research article.
2 Explain the process of critiquing a research article.
3 Explain why it is important for clinicians to be able to critically review research articles.
4 Identify the differences when critiquing quantitative and qualitative research articles.
5 Describe the process for critiquing the ethical components of a research article.

CHALLENGING REVIEW QUESTIONS

1 You have been asked to review the literature and make recommendations about evidence-based practice in relation to sustainability and recycling in the healthcare setting. Explain how you will approach reporting on the current evidence and recommendations for clinical practice.
2 Explain how critiquing research articles is linked to evidence-based practice.
3 Explain how engagement in research activities can be promoted in clinical settings.

CASE STUDY 1

Prisha is an undergraduate nursing student beginning third year. Prisha is considering her options for a graduate position after she completes her course. As a student nurse, Prisha is aware that stress and burnout are important considerations for hospital nurses and would like to ensure she is fully prepared.

Prisha has found a research paper that she found to be interesting, one published by Kim (2019) that employed a descriptive cross-sectional design when examining emotional labour strategies, stress from emotional labour and burnout in nurses.

Kim, J-S. (2019). Emotional labor strategies, stress, and burnout among hospital nurses: A path analysis. *Journal of Nursing Scholarship*, *52*(1), 105–12. https:// doi:10.1111/ jnu.12532

1 Why is it important to critically appraise the research evidence Prisha is about to read?
2 How do the concepts of validity, reliability and applicability relate to the critical appraisal of the research evidence Prisha is reviewing in relation to her future?
3 There are a variety of tools available to critically appraise research evidence. Can you help Prisha by suggesting an appropriate tool she could use to critically appraise the Kim (2019) research article?

CASE STUDY 2

Shellie is a final-year midwifery student whose capstone research unit requires her to undertake a literature review on a topic of interest. Shellie has always been interested in the benefits of alternative healthcare. After working with a midwife who used reflexology in her practice, she decides to explore the effectiveness of reflexology in pregnancy, labour and birth. After determining her search terms and inclusion criteria, Shellie undertakes a database search and identifies 110 articles for initial review. After reviewing each article's abstract, Shellie identifies 25 primary research articles that appear suitable for inclusion. The articles report and discuss the findings from qualitative, quantitative and mixed-methods research studies. Shellie then undertakes a critical appraisal of each article to determine the quality of quality of the research and suitability for inclusion in her literature review.

1   What are the three key issues to think about when critiquing a research paper?
2   Why is the use of critical appraisal tools recommended for appraising the quality of research literature?
3   What ethical requirements should Shellie critique as part of her appraisal process?
4   As part of her critique process, Shellie designs a summary table to compare each of the articles for suitability for inclusion in her literature review. What headings would you suggest she include?

REFERENCES

Al-Jundi, A., & Sakka, S. (2017). Critical appraisal of clinical research. *Journal of Clinical & Diagnostic Research, 11*(5). https://doi.org/10.7860/JCDR/2017/26047.9942

Buccheri, R. K., & Sharifi, C. (2017). Critical appraisal tools and reporting guidelines for evidence-based practice. *Worldviews on Evidence-Based Nursing, 14*(6), 463–72. https://doi.org/10.1111/wvn.12258

Caldwell, K., Henshaw, L., & Taylor, G. (2011). Developing a framework for critiquing health research: An early evaluation. *Nurse Education Today, 31*(8), e1–7.

Centre for Evidence-Based Medicine. (n.d.). The Centre for Evidence-Based Medicine. https://www.cebm.net/

CONSORT. (2010). CONSORT transparent reporting of trials. http://www.consort-statement.org/

Critical Appraisal Skills Programme (CASP). (2019a). CASP Randomised Controlled Trial Standard Checklist. https://casp-uk.b-cdn.net/wp-content/uploads/2020/10/CASP_RCT_Checklist_PDF_Fillable_Form.pdf

Critical Appraisal Skills Programme (CASP). (2019b). CASP Qualitative Research Checklist. https://casp-uk.b-cdn.net/wp-content/uploads/2018/03/CASP-Qualitative-Checklist-2018_fillable_form.pdf.

Critical Appraisal Skills Programme (CASP). (2020). CASP Checklists Critical Appraisal Skills Programme. https://casp-uk.net/casp-tools-checklists/

Dale, J. C. (2005). Critiquing research for use in practice. *Journal of Pediatric Health Care, 19*, 183–6.

Dale, J. C., Hallas, D., & Spratling, R. (2019). Critiquing research evidence for use in practice: Revisited. *Journal of Pediatric Health Care, 33*(3), 342–6. https://doi.org/10.1016/j.pedhc.2019.01.005

Day, R. (1998). *How to Write and Publish a Scientific Paper* (5th edn). Cambridge, UK: Cambridge University Press.

Day, R. A., & Gastel, B. (2012). *How to Write and Publish a Scientific Paper* (7th edn). Cambridge, UK: Cambridge University Press.

Farrer, L. M., Gulliver, A., Katruss, N., Fassnacht, D. B., Kyrios, M., & Batterham, P. J. (2019). A novel multi-component online intervention to improve the mental health of university students: Randomised controlled trial of the Uni Virtual Clinic. *Internet Interventions, 18*.

Galdas, P. (2017). Revisiting bias in qualitative research: Reflections on its relationship with funding and impact. *International Journal of Qualitative Methods, 16*, 1–2. https://doi.org/10.1177/1609406917748992

Glenny, A.-M. (2005). No 'gold standard' critical appraisal tool for allied health research. *Evidence-Based Dentistry, 6*(4), 100–1.

Gosall, N., & Gosall, G. (2015). *The Doctor's Guide to Critical Appraisal* (4th edn). Knutsford, UK: Pastest.

Greenhalgh, T. (2019). *How to Read a Paper: The Basics of Evidence-Based Medicine and Healthcare* (6th edn). Oxford: Wiley Blackwell.

Hannes, K. (2011). Critical appraisal of qualitative research. In: J. Noyes, A. Booth, K. Hannes, A. Harden, J. Harris, S. Lewin, C. Lockwood (eds). *Supplementary guidance for inclusion of qualitative research in Cochrane systematic reviews of interventions. Version 1.* Cochrane Collaboration Qualitative Methods Group. http://cqrmg.cochrane.org/supplemental-handbook-guidance

Joanna Briggs Institute (JBI). (2020). Joanna Briggs Institute Critical appraisal tools. https://jbi.global/critical-appraisal-tools

Katrak, P., Bialocerkowski, A. E., Massy-Westropp, N., Kumar, V. S., & Grimmer, K. A. (2004). A systematic review of the content of critical appraisal tools. *BMC Medical Research Methodology*, 4, 22.

Melnyk, B. M., & Fineout-Overholt, E. (eds). (2019). *Evidence-Based Practice in Nursing and Healthcare: A Guide to Best Practice* (4th edn). Philadelphia, PA: Wolters Kluwer.

Melnyk, B. M., & Fineout-Overholt, E. (2015). *Evidence-Based Practice in Nursing and Healthcare: A Guide to Best Practice*. Philadelphia, PA: Wolters Kluwer Health.

Melnyk, B. M., & Fineout-Overholt, E. (2011). *Evidence-Based Practice in Nursing and Healthcare: A Guide to Best Practice*. Philadelphia, PA: Wolters Kluwer/Lippincott Williams & Wilkins.

Melnyk, B. M., Fineout-Overholt, E., Gallagher-Ford, L., & Kaplan, L. (2012). The state of evidence-based practice in US nurses: Critical implications for nurse leaders and educators. *Journal of Nursing Administration*, 42(9), 410–17.

Rajaretnam, T. (2015). *Statistics for Social Sciences*. SAGE.

Teodosiu, M. (2019.). Scientific writing and publishing with IMRAD. *Annals of Forest Research*, 62(2), 201–14. https://doi.org/10.15287/afr.2019.1759

Thornton, R., Nicholson, P., & Harms, L. (2020). Creating evidence: Findings from a grounded theory of memory-making in neonatal bereavement care in Australia. *Journal of Pediatric Nursing*, 53, 29–35.

Wu, J. (2011). Improving the writing of research papers: IMRAD and beyond. *Landscape Ecology*, 26, 1345–9. https://doi.org/10.1007/s10980-011-9674-3

FURTHER READING

Cooper, H. (2009). *Research Synthesis and Meta-Analysis: A Step-by-Step Approach* (4th edn). London: SAGE.

Crombie, I. (2008). *The Pocket Guide to Critical Appraisal* (2nd edn). Oxford, UK: Wiley.

Day, R., & Gastel, B. (2006). *How to Write and Publish a Scientific Paper* (6th edn). Westport, CT: Greenwood Press.

Fineout-Overholt, E., Melnyk, B. M., Stillwell, S., & Williamson, K. (2010). Evidence-based practice, step by step: Critical appraisal of the evidence part III. *American Journal of Nursing*, 110(11), 43–51. https://doi.org/10.1097/01.NAJ.0000390523.99066.b5

Greenhalgh, T. (2014). *How to Read a Paper. The Basics of Evidence-Based Medicine* (5th edn). Oxford, UK: Wiley.

Livingstone, W., van de Mortel, T., & Taylor, B. (2011). A path of perpetual resilience: Exploring the experience of a diabetes-related amputation through grounded theory. *Contemporary Nurse*, 39(1): 20.

Malloch, K., & Porter-O'Grady, T. (2010). *Introduction to Evidence-Based Practice in Nursing and Health Care*. Sudbury, MA: Jones and Bartlett.

Pain, E. (2016). How to review a paper. https://www.sciencemag.org/careers/2016/09/how-review-paper

Polgar, S., & Thomas, S. A. (2013). *Introduction to Research in the Health Sciences*. Edinburgh: Churchill Livingstone.

Ridley, D. (2012). *The Literature Review. A Step-by-Step Guide for Students* (2nd edn). Los Angeles, CA: SAGE.

Polit, D., & Beck, C. (2006). *Essentials of Nursing Research: Methods, Appraisal and Utilization* (6th edn). Philadelphia, PA: Lippincott.

Polit, D., & Beck, C. (2017). *Nursing Research: Generating and Assessing Evidence for Nursing Practice* (10th edn). Philadelphia, PA: Lippincott.

Pyrczak, F., & Bruce, R. (2007). *Writing Empirical Research Reports: A Basic Guide for Students of the Social and Behavioral Sciences* (6th edn). Glendale, CA: Pyrczak.

Schneider, Z. (2013). *Nursing and Midwifery Research: Methods and Appraisal for Evidence-Based Practice*. Chatswood, NSW: Mosby.

Truluck, C. A., & Leggett, T. (2016). Critical appraisal of health professions research. *Radiologic Technology*, 87(3), 355–8.

Chapter learning objectives

The material presented in this chapter will assist you to:
1   identify sources and strategies that can help you find research problems
2   understand the usefulness of literature in finding research problems
3   recognise how professional trends and research priorities influence the research area
4   state the criteria for selecting research problems
5   state a research problem or purpose and ask a specific research question
6   refine the question, formulate a hypothesis and identify variables in quantitative research
7   define an area and identify intentions in qualitative research.

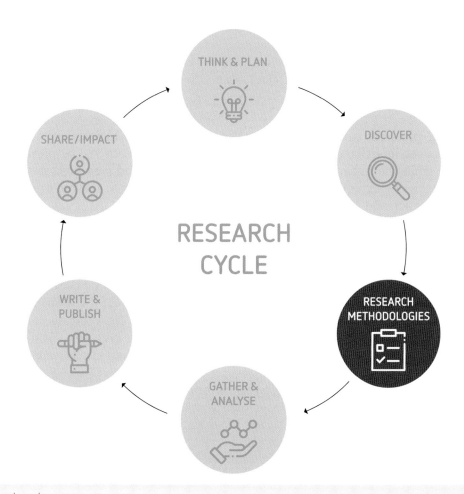

Research cycle

The primary focus of this chapter is formulating a research question for study. This fits with the discover stage

Introduction

This chapter describes how to formulate a research question, which includes identifying the people, literature, professional trends and research priorities that pertain to that question. In selecting **research problems**, you will see that you need to consider factors such as the preparedness of the researcher; the difficulty, feasibility and legitimacy of the problem; and adequate resources to fund the project. This chapter also describes the process for stating a problem in quantitative and qualitative research. It differentiates between hypotheses and **variables** identification in quantitative research, and the definition and intention clarification process of a **research area** in qualitative research.

Many research projects begin with a research question that asks about a problem or issue and therefore guides the study. It is the fundamental core of a research project. It focuses the study, determines the methodology and guides all stages of inquiry, analysis and reporting. A clearly stated research question is vital because it assists in the development of a clear research aim. Further, it allows for smooth progress through the project because it keeps the research interest in focus as it challenges, examines and analyses previous understandings while seeking new and/or amended knowledge.

ACTIVITY

Write a sentence about a problem you would like to research in your health discipline and ask two questions related to that research problem.

Research problems and research questions are different, although the terms are sometimes used interchangeably. Generally, the research problem will be presented as a statement, while the research question will be more specific and presented as a question. Sometimes the research questions are not listed in the research article but are implicit in the data collection and analysis methods.

FOR EXAMPLE

RESEARCH PROBLEMS

Lin and colleagues (2018) identified an issue in nurses not adhering to evidence-based wound care clinical practice guidelines (CPGs) in preventing surgical site infections (SSI). While not stated as a problem, the focus of the research was on the facilitators of and barriers to adherence of nurses to CPGs.

The qualitative study employed 'ethnographical data collection techniques' to collect using semi-structured interviews and focus groups. Hospital policy and procedure documents were also examined. Thematic analysis utilised inductive and deductive approaches revealing four themes: 'adhering to aseptic technique', 'knowledge and information seeking', 'documenting wound care and educating' and 'involving patients in wound care'. Facilitators and barriers were identified within each theme.

Marcusson-Rababi and colleagues (2019) identified a 'disparity in the burden of gynaecological cancer for Indigenous women compared with non-Indigenous women in Australia'. The problem was not clearly stated but the focus of the research was Indigenous women's lived experience of gynaecological cancer care services and factors that impact on the women's engagement with the care. Hospital-based care providers were also interviewed.

Data was collected by in-depth qualitative interview at approximately three months post initial referral. Interviews were thematically analysed resulting in four broad themes: 'navigating the system', 'communicating and decision making', 'coping with treatment demands' and 'feeling welcome and safe in the hospital'.

Beginners are often surprised to discover that finding the right research problem can be one of the most difficult parts of the research process. There is a boundless number of potential research problems in healthcare and it may be difficult to recognise a suitable research topic.

Despite the difficulty involved in choosing a problem, a good research project ultimately rests on the quality of the problem. This chapter presents sources of both quantitative and qualitative research problems and how to develop a research question.

Finding research problems: sources

It is very important to select the right problem in terms of its relevance, significance and feasibility. Spending adequate time doing so at the beginning of the process can pay dividends by preventing the waste of time and energy involved in selecting a problem that turns out to be unsatisfactory.

Sources

There are a number of sources of research problems. Critical observation of practice will lead to problem formation. Just analysing a conversation in handover may lead to ideas for research topics. This could be questions such as what factors encourage or discourage specific client outcomes (e.g. post-operative pain) and thinking about how you might measure the outcomes. You can listen to what your clients say or do not say during practice interactions.

In clinical practice, one often asks whether a particular approach is the best way to carry out an intervention.
- Why are procedures done a certain way?
- Are they based on scientific findings or on tradition or opinion? For example:
  - Are routine post-operative observations following surgery necessary?
  - How effective is acupuncture on post-operative pain?

Examine your own practice for observations or questions related to current practice. Look at what is happening and ask how it ought to be different. Questions could be asked about the nature and effects of phenomena and relationships in professional practice. Ideas for research topics that may be found in one's experience are often more relevant and interesting than those that are remote. There may be more enthusiasm for researching a problem that could have some impact on an individual's practice or practice setting or on what is frustrating at work.

TIP

Individual professional experience is a source of research problems.

TIP

A work manager, lecturer or supervisor may be a source of research problems. They usually will be able to help find a problem, discuss the implications of selecting that problem and give general ideas a more specific focus.

FOR EXAMPLE

GROUNDED THEORY

Smith, Leslie and Wynaden (2016) used a grounded theory study to explore the levels of support provided to perioperative nurses participating in multi-organ procurement surgery and the impact on their overall wellbeing. Participants were perioperative nurses who had previous participatory experience. Data was collected by semi-structured in-depth interviews and analysed by constant comparison. This study provided new insights into how nurses manage and cope with participating in organ procurement surgery and the support services needed.

Colleagues may be another source of help in finding a problem. Brainstorming with friends and colleagues about problems they have encountered may help to clarify research ideas. Joining a nursing blog may be a useful source of ideas. Talking to colleagues at work, at professional meetings and at conferences (particularly research conferences) is another source. Listening to speakers at conferences can provide a feeling for the issues of the moment, especially if the speakers are leaders. The informal part of a conference is fertile ground for the generation of new questions. Ideas and issues emanating from these situations can become research problems.

Once an area of interest is identified, talking to the expert clinicians in the field can lead to research problems that they have identified. Such problems will probably be topical, relevant and worthwhile.

Research literature

The professional literature is a rich source of problems. Once an area of interest has been identified, look at the relevant research periodicals. Reading a study will often suggest ideas about how it could have been improved and thus lead to ideas for further research.

EBP

EVIDENCE FOR BEST PRACTICE

SURGERY AND OUTCOMES

Lockwood, Kable and Hunter (2018) used a quasi-experimental design using an intervention and control group to measure a nurse-led evidence-based venous thromboembolism prevention program compared to usual care in hip and knee arthroplasty patients and associated clinical outcomes.

Adherence and compliance were measured for pre- and post-operative strategies, including nurse-led components. Data were collected by a purpose- developed audit form. Post-discharge patient adherence data were collected after discharge via a post-discharge questionnaire.

Results showed that the intervention group had a mean compliance score of 11.09, higher than the control group score of 7.10. Post-discharge compliance results were not significantly different.

The study showed that a nurse-led intervention achieved higher compliance with translating evidence-based guidelines into routine patient care for hip and knee arthroscopy patients.

Another source of inspiration can be the recommendations at the end of a research article. Garvey and colleagues (2018) identified the level of and factors associated with distress in 155 Indigenous Australian cancer survivors approximately six months post discharge. Their closing recommendation was that: 'Further research is required to identify the specific aetiologies of distress'.

This recommendation could lead the reader to plan a similar study that incorporates these recommendations into its design by identifying the main research problem and listing specific research questions to cover the identified areas.

Sometimes, when reading through the literature, certain research themes may emerge. For example, professional journals may feature research undertaken in specific areas, such as in oncology and perioperative nursing. Reading the articles carefully is recommended for identifying a research interest to pursue in these areas – especially if this would extend the research results already published.

The literature may also reveal a gap that needs to be filled. Boström and colleagues (2020), who examined registered nurses' experience of communicating with patients when practising person-centred-care (PCC) over the phone, were motivated because of the lack of research into this practice. They argued the need for research by acknowledging that how registered nurses (RNs) practice PCC in clinical work, especially at a distance by telephone, is still largely unknown (p. 2).

FOR EXAMPLE

IDENTIFYING A LACK OF RESEARCH

Walshe (2020) identified a lack of research on the way that district nurses provide palliative care to people at home. An ethnographical study was conducted by non-participant observation of district nurse–palliative care patient encounters and post-observation interviews. Two core themes were determined from the data: 'planning for the future' and 'caring in the moment'. Recommendation on further research on the disparity with what was done compared to what was said to be done was made.

In another example, Bridges and colleagues (2020) undertook a systematic review and synthesis of 61 qualitative studies and two systematic reviews describing older patients' experiences of care in acute hospital settings.

Falls by patients in hospitals and aged care facilities has engendered a plethora of research; in particular, research on education programs to prevent falls.

Stephenson and colleagues (2016) assessed falls prevention practices in Australian hospitals. The project utilised evidence-based audit criteria and implementation interventions in multiple acute hospital settings to demonstrate quality improvement in falls prevention practices. We can see that research such as this adds to the development of evidence-based practice (EBP), which is discussed further in this chapter.

The literature can also provide examples of studies that you may wish to *replicate*, which means to repeat a study using the same methodology. Replication is generally considered to be desirable to verify existing findings and increase their validity by carrying out identical research with a variety of subjects in different settings. Replication is most suited to quantitative research because test and retest is encouraged, based on objective epistemological assumptions. In contrast, qualitative research does not favour replication because its assumptions about knowledge are that it is relative and context dependent, so there is no point trying to exactly replicate research into a human experience. Even so, qualitative researchers may opt to adopt many different approaches in exploring the same or similar research interests and phenomena to achieve multiple layers of meaning that add to the richness of possibilities and insights.

There may be few quantitative studies published that replicate others, so the outcome is often many small, unrelated studies with a limited generalisability of results. In quantitative research, there is a need for more research that builds upon earlier research and addresses its limitations. Be aware, though, that originality is a requirement for research projects in many higher degrees. It is also important to realise that, in some cases, replication may not be necessary or advisable. This is especially true if you are taking a qualitative approach, which assumes that people are unique in their respective contexts and that absolute replication is not possible. In such cases, the research would still need to be original but not necessarily based on the research method used previously.

Influences on the research area: professional trends and research priorities

There are many aspects that may influence areas for research. One influence is trends within the profession, such as the change in scope of practice. Another is at the government level with the development of national health priorities. These two areas are discussed below.

Professional trends

Major events that affect the profession can be a source of research topics. Reading journals that deal with professional issues can give advance warning of trends and assist in selecting a topic. One such event was the worldwide introduction of EBP (Sackett et al., 1997). EBP lends itself well to research because it demands that the latest evidence from research be used in clinical practice situations. EBP will be discussed further in Chapter 13. Other professional trends surface in professional journals from time to time; research and scholarship ensures that they are thoroughly explored through critical debate and argumentation. Keep reading the journals of relevant disciplines to remain in touch with the trends.

Identified research priorities

EBP

At a national level, governments that relay directives to peak professional research bodies may set research priorities. The Australian Government may direct its health priorities to the National Health and Medical Research Council (NHMRC), and in the United Kingdom, the National Health Service (NHS) may inform the Medical Research Council of its research priorities. Given that the research priorities are government directives, it logically follows that funding is provided for research into these areas. Even though research may be at a far more modest level, be aware of national research priorities and adapt a manageable project for one's own research interests. In this way, even though large funding grants may not be obtained, the project can be published in professional journals that reflect the national research trends and priorities.

Criteria for selecting research problems

The researcher

The researcher must have the appropriate experience and skills to address the research problem; and frequently, research experience is related to qualifications. Beginning skills can be learned in undergraduate programs, although many such programs are now focusing on the preparation of research consumers rather than researchers. Advanced research skills are learned in research degrees – specifically, honours, research masters and doctoral degrees. In advanced degrees, you begin to understand some of the assumptions that underlie the use of certain qualitative methodologies, such as grounded theory, action research and postmodern influences on critical feminisms.

An inexperienced researcher should select a problem that can use a simple design and instruments in quantitative research, or a relatively uncomplicated methodology with congruent methods and processes in qualitative research. In either case, the project for a new researcher is likely to lead to easy analytical processes in which a high degree of success and enjoyment will be experienced. It is better to carry out a simple project well than to do a complex one poorly. Complicated designs requiring sophisticated measurement techniques and complex data analyses are best left to more experienced researchers, and obtuse methodologies with dense philosophies can wait until undertaking postgraduate research. If physical equipment is involved or specialist computer programs are necessary, consider the technical expertise required to run them.

To be able to research a problem effectively, adequate knowledge of the general area is needed. It is easier to research in an area of familiarity as knowledge of the terminology and major ideas are there. A physiotherapist would find it easiest to do research in physiotherapy from a theoretical base of physiotherapist knowledge. Familiarity with relevant theories and concepts will assist in planning research that is linked to theory. Knowledge of previous research in the area will also help to select an appropriate problem to research.

Researching an area of interest and choosing a problem for which there is a genuine desire for an answer will help maintain enthusiasm for the project during the difficult periods. The interest factor is more important in a longer project than in a shorter one because it is more difficult to sustain interest over a longer period.

The problem

The problem selected should fall within the general area specific to that discipline; for example, nursing or physiotherapy. Knowledge of what constitutes research in a discipline is required. Does this problem have a specific discipline focus or is it common across the multidisciplinary spectrum? A nurse will need to ascertain where the boundaries lie between nursing and medical research, and research in behavioural science. A rule of thumb is that

TIP

Ensure the research problem is relevant to the specific profession/ discipline. For example, links can be made with nursing's major domain concepts of person, health, environment and nursing.

having control over the decision making in that area of practice makes it a suitable subject for research. Research about client health is valid for many health disciplines.

Importance

Another consideration is the importance of the research problem. For a beginning researcher, it need not be a problem that addresses the most important questions in the field, but it must be a question worth answering. Professional journals pay attention to significance for specific disciplines, particularly in the areas of clinical application. Clinical nursing research, for example, requires authors to address the clinical significance of the research. Given the amount of time and effort that will be invested in a study, it is important to select a topic that will produce findings of benefit to some person or group, be it the client, healthcare worker, healthcare agency, community or society. Ask the following questions:

- Will the answer to the research question have the potential to lead to improvements in client health, community health or practice?
- Will it lead to changes in protocols or policies in your institution?
- Will the study lead to the development of knowledge?
- Will it test a theoretical proposition or explore a new area of knowledge?

Feasibility

Feasibility (i.e. whether the research can actually be carried out) also needs to be considered. By their very nature, some problems are difficult or even impossible to research. For quantitative research, choose variables that can be measured using the current technology. It would, for example, be impossible to assess neonates' attitudes to neonatal intensive care units, but data can be collected from their parents about their experiences. For qualitative research, state the question broadly enough to permit a broad explanation of the phenomenon to be explored and make sure it is aligned with the theoretical assumptions of how knowledge is produced through research.

FOR EXAMPLE

PHENOMENOLOGY

LeBlanc and colleagues (2018) used a phenomenological methodology in their study in which they explored the lived experience of intensive care nurses caring for patients with delirium. This meant that they used one-on-one interviews in a conversational style using open-ended questions.

Legitimacy

Legitimacy is a criterion that also needs to be considered. Just because a study can be carried out does not necessarily mean it should be. Nor should a research problem reflect a moral position. These areas involve religious beliefs, politics or ethics, so they are frequently value laden. For example, 'Should organ donation be compulsory?' is not a suitable research topic because it is trying to answer a moral question that is best answered by ethical debate. This does not mean that value-laden, subjective areas cannot be researched. Many qualitative approaches value subjectivity and the researcher within the research process. It is a matter of eliminating the 'should' aspect of the question. Such questions can be rephrased along these lines; for example, 'What is the lived experience of a parent donating a loved one's organs?'

Research questions that show the researcher is biased and trying to prove a point are also unsuitable. A research question such as: 'What is the connection between illegal refugees and violent crime?' indicates bias on the part of the researcher and is therefore unsuitable. But such questions can often be rephrased in a way that makes them suitable for research; for example, 'What perception of their own competence do graduates of University X hold?'

Ethical standards are another consideration. Do not proceed with any research project that involves harming or deceiving the subjects, coercing the subjects to participate or exposing them to risks out of proportion to the benefits of the research. If any research project does not comply with the ethical guidelines of the NHMRC and the relevant human research ethics committee(s), it will not be approved.

Ethics

Resources

Time

Make sure there is sufficient time to carry out the project. A research project often takes longer than expected so make sure that the project will not consume more time than is available. Also, consider the time available to spend working on the project and balance this with other work and personal commitments.

Nature of the project

A collaborative process between the researcher and the participants, such as action research, will take longer than something like a questionnaire.

Nature of the problem

Consider the nature of the problem being studied. A study of client progress through a lengthy treatment, for example, would not be feasible if there is only one semester to carry out the project. Also consider whether data would have to be collected at a specific time of year and if they do, how that fits in with other commitments.

Money

Every project has some cost attached. Some universities allocate money to students for research projects and may provide equipment such as computers and software. Hospitals may also have a research budget for focused clinical projects. However, it is unlikely that either will support the costs of expensive student projects. Clarify from the outset the amount of financial support that will be provided. If the amount available from the university, healthcare facility, one's own funds or funds from sponsors is insufficient, rethink the project and scale it down to a more realistic level, or choose another topic.

In deciding whether a project is affordable, consider its real costs, the budget available and the cost–benefit ratio. Before making a final decision, make a list of all projected expenses, including an adjustment for price rises. This might include:

- costs for obtaining literature:
  - photocopying, computer searches, books and journal subscriptions
  - permission to use other people's text(s) (i.e. copyright fees).
- costs for carrying out the project:
  - stationery and other consumables (e.g. printer cartridges)
  - pay for the participants in the project under conditions agreed to by an ethics committee
  - postage (including return postage for questionnaires) will be a major cost for postal surveys, as will printed questionnaires and self-addressed envelopes; however, the use of online surveys may mitigate these costs
  - digital recording equipment will be needed for field research that involves interviews, and you may need to rent or purchase equipment such as video cameras, computers or instruments if they are not available through your institution
  - hire of labour for data collection and management
  - transportation, accommodation and possibly living costs if travel is involved
  - communication costs such as telephone calls and internet access
- costs for the data-analysis stage: you may need to purchase computer software or hire specific services
- costs for the writing-up stage: you will need more stationery and consumables.

TIP

There is no such thing as free or no-cost research.

People

When beginning research in clinical settings, consider the people needed to help undertake the project. The availability of participants to study for the research is an important consideration. Clinical research is notorious for subjects and participants disappearing. It may not be possible to locate enough people who meet the criteria for participating in the study, particularly if the criteria are unusual. Potential participants may be geographically difficult to access, such as Indigenous Australians in remote areas, or participants might be hard to find, such as illegal drug users. Sometimes, people may already be involved in studies and will not have the time for involvement in two, or their participation in one study might preclude them from taking part in another.

Even if potential participants are eligible, they may be unwilling to help, especially if any discomfort is involved. Fear of unwanted consequences can make some people afraid of talking to a researcher about sensitive topics such as criminal behaviour or domestic violence, while others just do not trust a researcher. Elderly people may not be willing to sign a consent form because relatives have told them not to sign any documents.

There can also be procedural difficulties with accessing participants. If, for example, the participants will be children, parental or guardian consent will be required. In addition, approval from appropriate channels in your institution, such as your supervisor, the human research ethics committee and all the other required committees will be required

Another consideration is the gatekeepers who give or withhold permission to enter facilities for data collection. The authorities and medical staff in the clinical facilities to be involved must agree that the study can take place. Ensure permission is secured at the problem-formation stage, before undertaking the project.

Lastly, gaining administrative support is one of the highest priorities. If you are employed in a clinical facility, negotiation with authorities for use of the facilities or for time off to carry out the project will be needed.

ACTIVITY

Review the work carried out in the previous activities in this chapter to refine the research problem, question or purpose. Critically analyse decisions to see if the project is appropriate for the discipline, feasible, legitimate and able to be adequately resourced.

The research problem, purpose and question

It is normal for there to be a general statement of **research purpose** or aim of the study. This is usually found near the beginning of the study and sets out concisely, in broad terms, what the study hopes to accomplish; that is, its goals and aims. The purpose of this statement is to orient the reader to the study.

Bloxsome, Bayes and Ireson (2019) made clear that the aim of their study was 'to understand why Western Australian midwives choose to remain in the profession' (p. 209).

The more specific problem or question that the study seeks to answer can be stated either as a declarative statement or a question. Stating it as a question helps you to clarify exactly what it is that you want to find out.

Slomian and colleagues (2017) explored the extent to which a psychological distress episode in the year following birth could influence the needs of mothers during this period. Their objectives for the study were to (Slomian et al., 2017):

• explore the needs of mothers during this period
• compare these needs between mothers who did not have the feeling of living with a psychological disorder or a depression and mothers who lived with a psychological disorder or had the impression of living with a depression
• compare the needs expressed by the mothers with the perceptions of professionals and fathers about the mother's needs.

From these objectives, we are left in no doubt as to what the researchers are researching.

One way of structuring a research question to ensure that it is as comprehensive as possible is to divide it into a stem (the 'who, what, when, where or why' part of the question) and a topic (what the question is about). Begin by drafting the problem, question or purpose and making spontaneous responses to these questions. Clear and direct answers to the following simple questions will give the basis of posing a research problem, question or purpose:

• Who is involved in the research as participants?
• What is the area of interest?
• When is the research to be undertaken?
• Where is the research to be undertaken?
• Why is the research being undertaken?

Refining and formulating a hypothesis: identifying variables in quantitative research

The first step in formulating a research question is to either brainstorm topics or make a list of potential topics using the sources given earlier in this chapter. Figure 4.1 gives a brief outline of the process.

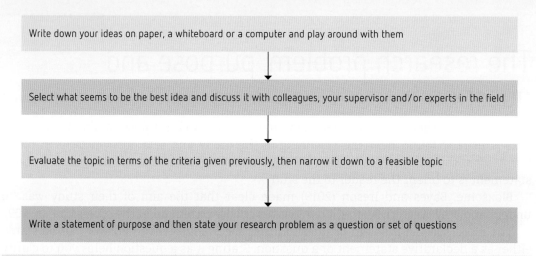

Write down your ideas on paper, a whiteboard or a computer and play around with them

Select what seems to be the best idea and discuss it with colleagues, your supervisor and/or experts in the field

Evaluate the topic in terms of the criteria given previously, then narrow it down to a feasible topic

Write a statement of purpose and then state your research problem as a question or set of questions

▶ **Figure 4.1**   The process: Refining and formulating the research question

During this process, reading the relevant literature to become an expert on the topic is important as this will help with the formation of relevant research questions.

Once the research problem and its consequent question (or questions) has been formulated, it is time to refine it. Frequently, the initial question is too broad and beyond the limits of a feasible study, making it necessary to narrow down the problem until there is a research question that can be undertaken. The narrowing process can relate to the topic or the setting for the research. The topic can be narrowed by removing its less important parts or, alternatively, narrowing the number of settings in which the study will be conducted or the types of participants included. It may be necessary to restrict the topic in several dimensions.

Suppose you would like to investigate if exercise improves mental health. To look at all forms of exercise and in different age groups would entail a large number of projects. To narrow this topic down, consider one exercise program such as an outdoor physical activity program with one age group such as adults or adolescents with clinical depression.

Stating a hypothesis and identifying variables

When undertaking quantitative research, first state the problem and then develop a hypothesis that will provide a working basis for investigation. Although stating a hypothesis might seem difficult at first, it is not; a hypothesis is simply a statement of what the researcher thinks is going to be the outcome of the investigation. Another definition of *hypothesis* is that it is 'the formal statement of the expected relationship or relationships between two or more variables in a specified population' (Gray, Grove & Sutherland, 2017, p. 7). We formulate hypotheses all the time, although we may not recognise them. We might say, 'Every time I forget my umbrella it rains'. This could be restated as a research hypothesis: 'On the days when I forget to take my umbrella, it is more likely to rain than on days when I remember to take it'.

In a quantitative research project, it is customary to formulate a formal research hypothesis that speculates about the relationship between two variables. To be a hypothesis, it must state a possible relationship and it must have at least two variables that enter into the relationship.

A variable, as its name suggests, is something that varies. In the example above, there are two variables:

1 whether I forget or remember my umbrella
2 whether it rains.

A variable that can be controlled by the researcher is called an **independent variable**. A variable that cannot be controlled by the researcher, or that is hypothesised to be affected by an independent variable, is a **dependent variable**. It is helpful to think of a dependent variable as an outcome variable. In the example above, even though the weather could be thought of as the dependent variable and remembering the umbrella as an independent variable, this is not strictly correct, as memory is not being manipulated. In instances where the researcher does not control the independent variable, it is more correct to speak of *research variables* than independent and dependent variables.

Research hypotheses can be stated as directional hypotheses, meaning that the researcher is speculating about the direction that the findings will take. To do this, the researcher must have some grounds for stating a direction. These grounds might consist of a theoretical prediction, previous research findings or a logical argument.

Even when a directional hypothesis is expressed, it is usually converted to a null hypothesis because in statistical analysis it is customary to try to demonstrate that the statement that there is no difference in the groups is rejected, rather than saying that there is a difference. This will be discussed further in Chapter 6.

If a hypothesis cannot be tested, it is not a hypothesis. Also, each hypothesis should deal with only one relationship and one set of variables, although a study may have more than one hypothesis being tested.

As discussed previously, variables are the parts of a hypothesis that vary and are defined in terms of the concept they measure. Variables also need to be stated in terms of how they are going to be measured, which is not always specified in the hypothesis itself. For example, if you were going to measure blood pressure, it would be stated whether it is measured with a sphygmomanometer or with a direct sensor in the blood vessel.

FOR EXAMPLE

STATING A HYPOTHESIS

Middleton and colleagues (2019) reported on the results of a randomised controlled trial that evaluated the effectiveness of an intervention to improve triage, treatment and transfer for patients with acute stroke admitted to the emergency department (ED).

> The details of the research are discussed in full in the research article. The researchers have made their research procedures as clear and transparent as possible to ensure that their research design and results are open to professional scrutiny and critique, to allow judgements relating to rigour.
>
> Many of these areas relating to quantitative research are described in Chapters 5 and 6.

So far, this chapter has described some general ideas for stating a research problem, question or purpose, and has shed some light on the process for doing so, with particular interest in developing a hypothesis and identifying variables in quantitative research. As there are many differences in quantitative and qualitative research assumptions, methods and processes, the next part of this chapter looks specifically at how to define an area and identify objectives in qualitative research.

Defining an area and identifying intentions in qualitative research

Qualitative research is based on particular assumptions about the nature of knowledge, such as the uncertain nature of 'truth' and claims to be 'truthful', how knowledge is generated and how it is judged to be **trustworthy** (see Chapter 1 for further information on the epistemological assumptions of qualitative research). In tune with its epistemological assumptions, qualitative researchers would not deign to state a hypothesis or even try to anticipate the variables in a question about human experience. Rather, the beginning of a qualitative project begins most often with defining a research area and identifying research objectives. The reason for stating that this is how a project 'begins most often' is that, given it varies so markedly through the various forms of qualitative interpretive and critical research, there is no hard and fast rule in qualitative research.

When defining an area for research, qualitative researchers typically begin with all the preliminaries mentioned in this chapter, including exploring sources and strategies such as people, literature, professional trends and research priorities. They also consider the criteria for selecting problems, such as researcher readiness, what problem to select and the money needed to make the project manageable. At the point of stating the problem, question or purpose of the study, they can diverge in various directions according to the qualitative approach they are taking.

If researchers are taking a qualitative interpretive approach – historical, grounded theory, ethnographic or phenomenological (see Chapter 7) – the beginning part of the project may look fairly standard in that there will be a clear statement of intent of the general area to be explored and the specific aims or objectives to be fulfilled.

FOR EXAMPLE

DEFINING AN AREA

Whitburn and colleagues (2017) utilised a qualitative study using an interpretive phenomenological analysis approach in their research in their study of women's experience of childbirth pain. The authors clearly stated that the study 'aimed to examine women's experiences within the perspectives of modern pain science'.

Harrison and colleagues (2019) employed a qualitative study using an interpretive phenomenological analysis approach. Their study questions were clearly stated:

- 'What are the attitudes of women diagnosed with gestational diabetes mellitus (GDM) towards physical activity during pregnancy?'
- 'What are the perceived barriers to and enablers of physical activity during pregnancy in women with GDM?'

Both of the above examples state broad intentions as an indication of what researchers are exploring. Unlike quantitative researchers, they do not state a hypothesis or list variables because the research areas are unexplored and qualitative researchers are open to what might emerge during the project. These two studies were also clinically focused and significant for EBP.

EBP

If researchers are taking a qualitative critical approach, such as action research, feminist research or critical ethnography (see Chapter 7), the beginning part of the project might vary markedly. Action research often requires research participants to work with the researcher as co-researchers, and the problem, question or purpose of the project emerges within group processes as the research evolves collaboratively. Once the thematic concern (issue) has been identified, the general objectives of the research are revisited within the research group. The following 'Evidence for best practice' feature shows you how the process evolves in an action research project and the significance for practice.

EVIDENCE FOR BEST PRACTICE

EBP

USING ACTION RESEARCH TO DEVELOP MIDWIVES' SKILLS TO SUPPORT WOMEN WITH PERINATAL MENTAL HEALTH NEEDS

AIM

The aim of this research was to identify and develop midwives' skills to support women with mental health needs during pregnancy.

SAMPLE

Participants comprised one mental health nurse and seven self-selected registered midwives working with pregnant women attending the selected hospital for antenatal care. The midwives were from hospital-based antenatal and community settings, caring for women during pregnancy, and varied in clinical experience and length of employment within the organisation.

RESULTS

Major findings were: (1) uncertainty about decision making in terms of when to refer women for specialised mental health care; (2) the need for education about open questions to identify women at risk of perinatal mental health issues; and (3) education about signs of perinatal mental health difficulties. Actions included the development of a perinatal mental health referral pathway.

This research, undertaken by Madden and colleagues (2017), is a significant example of research influencing practice.

In research influenced by postmodern ideas, there may be relatively little structure at the outset of the project. Researchers might state extremely broad intentions as a problem statement, and thereafter leave the direction and flow of the project open to what might eventuate for the participants and the researcher. As a result, a research problem, question or purpose could be located anywhere along a continuum from a highly structured and objective quantitative approach of stating a hypothesis and variables, through the less structured and subjective forms of problem definition and statement of intentions in qualitative interpretive and critical research, to the extreme relativist and subjective forms of free-form, open-ended research influenced by postmodern thinking.

SUMMARY

This chapter described the formulation of a research question.

1	Identify sources and strategies that can help you find research problems	• Your own work interests are a source of research problems • Critical observation of practice will lead to problem formation • Your colleagues, work manager, lecturer and/or supervisor expert clinicians in the field can be a source of research problems
2	Understand the usefulness of literature in finding research problems	• Professional literature is a rich source of problems • Reading a study often suggests ideas about how it could have been improved and thus leads to ideas for further research

3	Recognise how professional trends and research priorities influence the research area	• These can include:
		  – national research priorities
		  – major events that affect the profession

4	State the criteria for selecting research problems	• Select a problem that can use:
		  – a simple design and instruments in quantitative projects
		  – a relatively uncomplicated methodology with congruent methods and processes in qualitative research

5	State a research problem or purpose and ask a specific research question	• A clearly stated research question is essential • A research problem, question or purpose may be located anywhere along a continuum
6	Refine the question, formulate a hypothesis and identify variables in quantitative research	• The initial research question, problem or area may need to be refined because it is too broad and beyond the limits of a feasible study • Quantitative research requires a hypothesis; variables are the parts of a hypothesis that must be able to be measured
7	Define an area and identify intentions in qualitative research	• A qualitative project begins most often with defining a research area and identifying research intentions or objectives

REVIEW QUESTIONS

1 Differentiate between a research problem and a question.
2 Discuss why a statement of aim or purpose is necessary at the beginning of a project.
3 Describe how people, literature, professional trends and research priorities can help you to decide on a research problem/area.
4 Discuss why variables are not inherently dependent or independent.

CHALLENGING REVIEW QUESTIONS

1 Discuss why funds, however small, are needed for research.
2 Discuss how quantitative and qualitative research differs in stating research problems/questions/purposes.
3 Discuss why qualitative researchers do not state a hypothesis or try to anticipate the variables in a question about human experience.

CASE STUDY 1

Angela works as a physiotherapist in a multidisciplinary team in a large city hospital. For some time she has been considering undertaking postgraduate research with local university staff who oversee a teaching and research centre in her organisation. Angela has checked out her assumptions about what postgraduate research entails, and an academic working in the centre confirmed that she would be eligible to enter into a Master of Physiotherapy Studies.

The study itself is not a daunting prospect for Angela; however, deciding on how to research her chosen area is giving her some concern. She has noticed in her work that elderly women are often not listened to when they approach members of the health team and that they are seldom given adequate emotional support when they receive negative news about their health status. Therefore, in her research, Angela wants to 'give a voice' to elderly women and sensitise staff to their unique needs. She asks you for help in how to proceed. What will you advise her in relation to the following?

1 How can Angela decide on research, problem and resource criteria?
2 How can Angela pose this research interest as a hypothesis?
3 Identify the dependent and independent variables in the hypothesis.

CASE STUDY 2

Ravi is a paramedic who works in a regional area adjacent to a large National Park. The park attracts many bush walkers, cyclists and motorcycle riders and he has attended many trauma cases resulting from accidents associated with recreational bush walking, cycle, and motorcycle accidents.

Ravi is particularly interested in the management of long bone fractures as such patients are extremely difficult to extricate from a wilderness environment. Ravi is authorised to administer intravenous morphine to manage pain in patients with long bone fractures; however, he read a research article that demonstrated good outcomes using a combination of intravenous morphine and midazolam. Ravi would like to undertake research to determine if morphine alone or the morphine/midazolam combination would provide superior outcomes in patients with long bone fracture.

1 Develop a research question for this study.
2 Develop a research hypothesis for this study.
3 Identify dependent and independent variables in this study.

REFERENCES

Bloxsome, D., Bayes, S., & Ireson, D. (2019). 'I love being a midwife; it's who I am': A Glaserian grounded theory study of why midwives stay in midwifery. *Journal of Clinical Nursing*, 29(1–2), 208–20. https://doi.org/10.1111/jocn.15078

Boström, E., Ali, L., Fors, A., Ekman, I., & Andersson, A. E. (2020). Registered nurses' experiences of communication with patients when practising person-centred care over the phone: A qualitative interview study. *BMC Nursing*, 19(1). https://doi.org/10.1186/s12912-020-00448-4

Bridges, J., Collins, P., Flatley, M., Hope, J., & Young, A. (2020). Older people's experiences in acute care settings: Systematic review and synthesis of qualitative studies. *International Journal of Nursing Studies*, 102, 103469. https://doi.org/10.1016/j.ijnurstu.2019.103469

Engberg, S., & Schlenk, E. (2007). Asking the right question. *Journal of Emergency Nursing*, *33*(6), 571–3.

Garvey, G., Cunningham, J., Janda, M., Yf He, V., & Valery, P. C. (2018). Psychological distress among Indigenous Australian cancer survivors. *Supportive Care in Cancer*, 26(6), 1737–46. https://doi.org/10.1007/s00520-017-3995-y

Gray, J. R., Grove, S. K., & Sutherland, S. (2017). *Burns and Grove's The Practice of Nursing Research: Appraisal, Synthesis, and Generation of Evidence* (8th edn). St Louis, MO: Elsevier.

Harrison, A. L., Taylor, N. F., Frawley, H. C., & Shields, N. (2019). Women with gestational diabetes mellitus want clear and practical messages from credible sources about physical activity during pregnancy: A qualitative study. *Journal of Physiotherapy*, 65(1), 37–42. https://doi.org/10.1016/j.jphys.2018.11.007

LeBlanc, A., Bourbonnais, F. F., Harrison, D., & Tousignant, K. (2018). The experience of intensive care nurses caring for patients with delirium: A phenomenological study. *Intensive and Critical Care Nursing*, 44(44), 92–8. https://doi.org/10.1016/j.iccn.2017.09.002

Lin, F., Gillespie, B. M., Chaboyer, W., Li, Y., Whitelock, K., Morley, N., Morrissey, S., O'Callaghan, F., & Marshall, A. P. (2018). Preventing surgical site infections: Facilitators and barriers to nurses' adherence to clinical practice guidelines – a qualitative study. *Journal of Clinical Nursing*, 28(9–10), 1643–52. https://doi.org/10.1111/jocn.14766

Lockwood, R., Kable, A., & Hunter, S. (2018). Evaluation of a nurse-led intervention to improve adherence to recommended guidelines for prevention of venous thromboembolism for hip and knee arthroplasty patients: A quasi-experimental study. *Journal of Clinical Nursing*, 27(5–6), e1048–60. https://doi.org/10.1111/jocn.14141

Madden, D., Sliney, A., O'Friel, A., McMackin, B., O'Callaghan, B., Casey, K., Courtney, L., Fleming, V., & Brady, V. (2017). Using action research to develop midwives' skills to support women with perinatal mental health needs. *Journal of Clinical Nursing*, 27(3–4), 561–71. https://doi.org/10.1111/jocn.13908

Marcusson-Rababi, B., Anderson, K., Whop, L. J., Butler, T., Whitson, N., & Garvey, G. (2019). Does gynaecological cancer care meet the needs of Indigenous Australian women? Qualitative interviews with patients and care providers. *BMC Health Services Research*, 19(1). https://doi.org/10.1186/s12913-019-4455-9

Middleton, S., Dale, S., Cheung, N. W., Cadilhac, D. A., Grimshaw, J. M., Levi, C., McInnes, E., Considine, J., McElduff, P., Gerraty, R., Craig, L. E., Schadewaldt, V., Fitzgerald, M., Quinn, C., Cadigan, G., Denisenko, S., Longworth, M., Ward, J., D'Este, C., … McElduff, B. (2019). Nurse-initiated acute stroke care in emergency departments. *Stroke*, 50(6), 1346–55. https://doi.org/10.1161/strokeaha.118.020701

Sackett, D. L., Richardson, W. S., Rosenbery, W., & Haynes, R. B. (1997). *Evidence-Based Medicine: How to Practice and Teach EBM*. New York, NY: Churchill Livingstone.

Slomian, J., Emonts, P., Vigneron, L., Acconcia, A., Glowacz, F., Reginster, J. Y., Oumourgh, M., & Bruyère, O. (2017). Identifying maternal needs following childbirth: A qualitative study among mothers, fathers and professionals. *BMC Pregnancy and Childbirth*, 17(1). https://doi.org/10.1186/s12884-017-1398-1

Smith, Z., Leslie, G., & Wynaden, D. (2016). Coping and caring: Support resources integral to perioperative nurses during the process of organ procurement surgery. *Journal of Clinical Nursing*, 26(21–22), 3305–17. https://doi.org/10.1111/jocn.13676

Stephenson, M., McArthur, A., Giles, K., Lockwood, C., Aromataris, E., & Pearson, A. (2016). Prevention of falls in acute hospital settings: A multi-site audit and best practice implementation project. *International Journal for Quality in Health Care*. Feb; *28*(1):92–8. doi: 10.1093/intqhc/mzv113. Epub 2015 Dec 17. PMID: 26678803.

Walshe, C. (2020). Aims, actions and advance care planning by district nurses providing palliative care: An ethnographic observational study. *British Journal of Community Nursing*, 25(6), 276–86. https://doi.org/10.12968/bjcn.2020.25.6.276

Whitburn, L. Y., Jones, L. E., Davey, M.-A., & Small, R. (2017). The meaning of labour pain: How the social environment and other contextual factors shape women's experiences. *BMC Pregnancy and Childbirth*, 17(1). https://doi.org/10.1186/s12884-017-1343-3

FURTHER READING

Andrew, E., Briffa, K., Waters, F., Lee, S., & Fary, R. (2019). Physiotherapists' views about providing physiotherapy services to people with severe and persistent mental illness: A mixed methods study. *Journal of Physiotherapy*, 65(4), 222–9. https://doi.org/10.1016/j.jphys.2019.08.001

Avruscio, G., Tocco-Tussardi, I., Bordignon, G., & Vindigni, V. (2017). Implementing clinical process management of vascular wounds in a tertiary facility: Impact evaluation of a performance improvement project. *Vascular Health and Risk Management*, Volume 13, 393–401. https://doi.org/10.2147/vhrm.s137099

Bolton, G., & Isaacs, A. (2018). Women's experiences of cancer-related cognitive impairment, its impact on daily life and care received for it following treatment for breast cancer. *Psychology, Health & Medicine*, 23(10), 1261–74. https://doi.org/10.1080/13548506.2018.1500023

Flanagan, B., Lord, B., Reed, R., & Crimmins, G. (2019). Listening to women's voices: The experience of giving birth with paramedic care in Queensland, Australia. *BMC Pregnancy and Childbirth*, 19(1). https://doi.org/10.1186/s12884-019-2613-z

Hunter, J., Ussher, J., Parton, C., Kellett, A., Smith, C., Delaney, G., & Oyston, E. (2018). Australian integrative oncology services: A mixed-method study exploring the views of cancer survivors. *BMC Complementary and Alternative Medicine*, 18(1). https://doi.org/10.1186/s12906-018-2209-6

McLeod, G. A., Annels, K., Cohen, J., Edwards, S., Hodgins, D., & Vaughan, B. (2017). Work related musculoskeletal injuries sustained by Australian osteopaths: Qualitative analysis of effects on practitioner health, clinical practice, and patient care. *Chiropractic & Manual Therapies*, 25(1). https://doi.org/10.1186/s12998-017-0158-7

Murray, S. J., & Tuqiri, K. A. (2020). The heart of caring: Understanding compassionate care through storytelling. *International Practice Development Journal*, 10(1), 1–13. https://doi.org/10.19043/ipdj.101.004

Walker, S., Bellhouse, C., Fairley, C. K., Bilardi, J. E., & Chow, E. P. F. (2016). Pharyngeal gonorrhoea: The willingness of Australian men who have sex with men to change current sexual practices to reduce their risk of transmission – a qualitative study. *PLoS ONE*, 11(12), e0164033. https://doi.org/10.1371/journal.pone.0164033

Ward, A., Eng, C., McCue, V., Stewart, R., Strain, K., McCormack, B., Dukhu, S., Thomas, J., & Bulley, C. (2018). What matters versus what's the matter – exploring perceptions of person-centred practice in nursing and physiotherapy social media communities: A qualitative study. *International Practice Development Journal*, 8(2), 1–18. https://doi.org/10.19043/ipdj.82.003

Woods, J. A., Newton, J. C., Thompson, S. C., Malacova, E., Ngo, H. T., Katzenellenbogen, J. M., Murray, K., Shahid, S., & Johnson, C. E. (2019). Indigenous compared with non-Indigenous Australian patients at entry to specialist palliative care: Cross-sectional findings from a multi-jurisdictional dataset. *PLoS ONE*, 14(5), e0215403. https://doi.org/10.1371/journal.pone.0215403

5 QUANTITATIVE RESEARCH METHODOLOGIES

Chapter learning objectives

The material presented in this chapter will assist you to:
1 identify the purpose of conducting quantitative research
2 identify the differences between major types of quantitative research designs
3 describe the difference between an independent and dependent variable
4 explain the importance of validity and reliability when conducting scientific research
5 explain the preparation required for, and the process of, data collection.

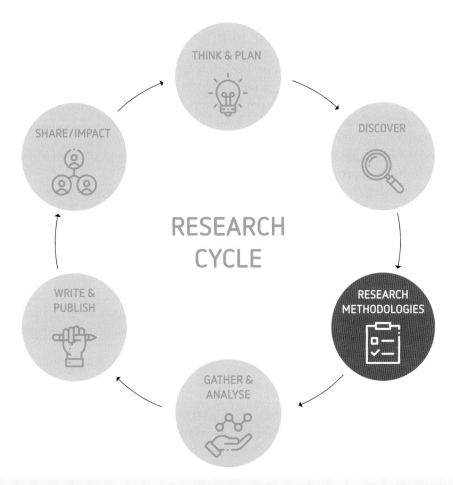

Research cycle

The primary focus of this chapter is understanding quantitative research methodologies, which is a key component of research methodologies when designing the project, as shown in the research cycle above.

Introduction

This chapter presents the key ideas and methods of quantitative methodologies. The methods are briefly discussed by way of introduction, including several major types of quantitative research designs, such as descriptive, analytical and experimental designs. It is recommended that students engage in further reading if a specific research method is used to address the hypothesis and answer the research questions when developing a research project.

What is a research design?

A research design refers to the logic or framework by which a project will answer a research question. It implies the organisation of the research components into a coherent and systematic plan to ensure the evidence obtained will address the research problem (Bryman, 2015). Therefore, the choice of design will depend on the research question, type of hypothesis being tested, purpose of the study, practical resources available, ethical considerations and the researcher's expertise. Selecting an appropriate research design is one of the most important decisions made when developing a research project. Researchers should be knowledgeable about various research designs before selecting a specific design to address their research question (Abutabenjeh & Jaradat, 2018).

There are a number of ethical issues that need to be considered as not all research designs are appropriate for answering a particular research question. For example, if a researcher wants to explore the impact of alcohol on fetal development, it would be inappropriate to consider a randomised controlled trial design. It is not ethical to potentially cause harm to an individual when conducting research (National Statement, 2007); therefore, a cohort design may be more appropriate in this situation.

There is increasing emphasis on the importance of incorporating new research findings into daily healthcare practice and improving patient safety. Therefore, it is important that all healthcare professionals participate in activities that improve patient outcomes and advance the profession by actively seeking opportunities to engage in evidence-based practice (Carter, et al. 2017). Evidence-based practice refers to finding the best possible evidence to inform clinical decisions. The hierarchical system of classifying evidence is the cornerstone of evidence-based practice (Burns, Rohrich & Chung, 2011; Rosen & Tsesis, 2016). Clinicians are therefore encouraged to find the highest level of evidence to answer clinical questions, improve the quality of care provided and achieve positive patient outcomes (Saunders & Vehvilainen-Julkunen, 2017).

There are several types of research designs, ranging from non-experimental research designs to controlled experimental research designs. A hierarchy of evidence, which ranks study types based on the rigour of the research method, was developed by Australia's National Health and Medical Research Council (NHMRC, 2009), and includes levels from I to IV, as shown in Figure 5.1. The highest level of evidence (Level I) includes evidence obtained from a rigorous systematic review of randomised controlled studies (Level II studies). Level II includes evidence obtained from well-designed randomised controlled trials, with three categories included in the next level.

Level III includes the following.

- Level III-1: pseudo-randomisation, where allocation of subjects may not be blinded.
- Level III-2: evidence obtained from comparative studies with concurrent controls, including non-randomised experimental trials, cohort studies, case-controlled studies and interrupted time series with a control group.
- Level III-3: evidence obtained from comparative studies with historical control, two or more single-arm studies, or interrupted time series without a parallel control group.

The final category, Level IV, includes evidence obtained from case series, either post-test or pretest post-test (NHMRC, 2009).

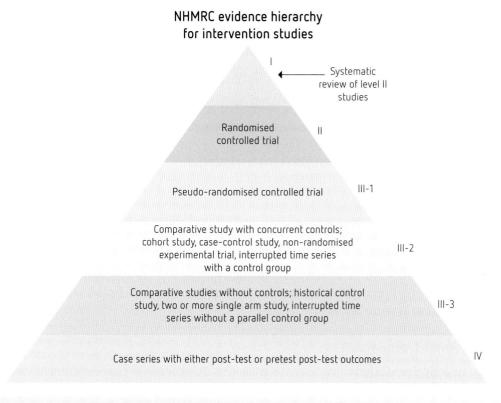

▶ **Figure 5.1** NHMRC hierarchy of evidence

Source: Adapted from National Health and Medical Research Council. (2009). NHMRC Levels of evidence and grades for recommendations for developers of clinical practice guidelines. https://www.nhmrc.gov.au/_files_nhmrc/file/guidelines/developers/nhmrc_levels_grades_evidence_120423.pdf

Major types of quantitative research designs

While there are many types of quantitative research designs, they are generally categorised as experimental and observational research (Grimes & Schulz, 2002). Traditional experiments include manipulation of a variable and random allocation of participants to either a control group, who receive standard treatment (i.e. medication), or an experimental group, who receive standard treatment plus exposure to an intervention (i.e. medication and a personalised exercise program). If done correctly, experimental designs provide evidence for 'cause and effect' and are therefore viewed as the gold standard for research (Sullivan, 2011).

Although observational research cannot draw the same conclusion as experimental designs, this type of research is not inferior or less important. Observational studies are further categorised into descriptive and analytical studies. Descriptive studies (e.g. case-series reports) do not include a comparison group. In this type of study, while the situation or phenomenon can be described, an association between variable cannot be examined. In contrast, analytical studies include a control group and examine the relationship between two or more variables (i.e. exposure versus non-exposure). Study designs that are either descriptive or analytical studies are detailed below.

- Analytical studies (include a control group):
  - cohort studies: populations are tracked from exposure to outcome (prospective)
  - case controlled studies: track backwards from outcome to exposure (retrospective)
  - cross-sectional studies: measure both exposure and outcome at a particular time point (i.e. snapshot).
- Descriptive studies (do not include a control or comparison group):
  - case report (one patient), case series (more than one patient) and case studies (one person, group or event)
  - cross-sectional studies (can also be descriptive).

An algorithm for classifying different research designs is displayed in Figure 5.2.

Observational studies

Descriptive designs

In quantitative research, a **descriptive design** is used to systematically describe the characteristics of a population, situation or area of interest. Descriptive design is defined as any study that is not truly experimental.

Simple descriptive designs

Simple descriptive designs are used to measure or observe a phenomenon of interest without manipulating the variables in the study (Melnyk & Fineout-Overholt, 2011). This type of design is sometimes referred to as 'correlational' or '**observational studies**', and provides information about the naturally occurring health status or other characteristics of a particular group. The researcher collects the necessary information using surveys, interviews or observation. Designs may also include a **cross-sectional study**, involving a one-time interaction with a group of people or following people over time, referred to as a **longitudinal study**.

FOR EXAMPLE

SIMPLE DESCRIPTIVE DESIGN

The Australian Census of Population and Housing, which is undertaken every five years, collects data on key characteristics of the Australian population. These data are used to identify how the population has changed and allow for future planning in Australia (Australian Bureau of Statistics, 2016).

In contrast, Hogh, Baernholdt and Clausen (2018) surveyed healthcare providers to investigate the impact of bullying on missed nursing care (described as insufficient time to provide the necessary care and the clinicians perception that the care provided was not enough to meet the needs of the client), in the aged care sector.

While the authors found that bullying was able to predict missed nursing care, the impact of bullying on the quality of care delivery was not identified. Using a descriptive design cannot determine degrees of difference between groups, relationships between variables or whether one variable causes another. It is a useful design with advantages that include being a quick and relatively inexpensive design which enables preliminary research data to be collected and used as a foundation for future studies.

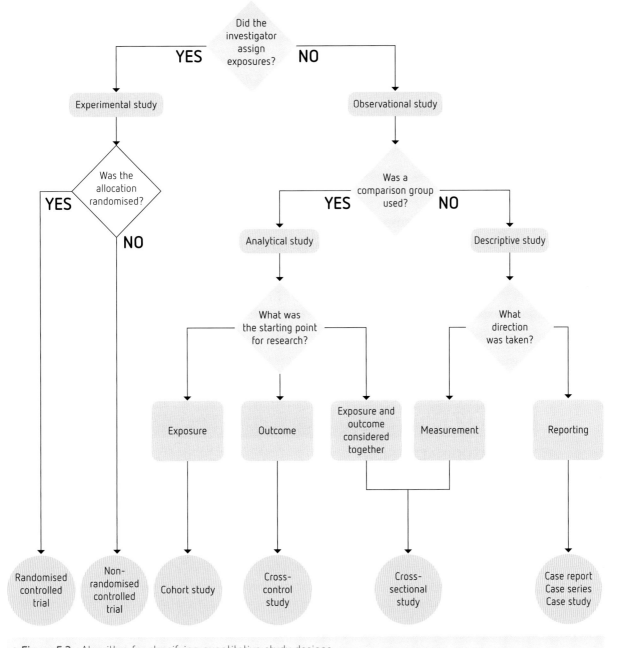

▶ **Figure 5.2**   Algorithm for classifying quantitative study designs

Source: Reprinted from *The Lancet*, vol. 359, David A Grimes and Kenneth F Schultz, An overview of clinical research: the lay of the land, p 57–61, copyright 2002, with permission from Elsevier.

Cross-sectional designs

Cross-sectional designs are snapshots, or cross-sections, of a population studied at a single point in time. They are sometimes referred to as one-shot designs because this type of design entails the collection of data of a population at a single point in time. Virtually all descriptive designs are cross-sectional, including those that are simple descriptive, comparative and correlational. Many experimental designs are also cross-sectional. The defining characteristic of a cross-sectional design is that there is only one snapshot of data taken.

FOR EXAMPLE

CROSS-SECTIONAL DESIGN

Savoia and colleagues (2020) explored the factors associated with access and use of personal protective equipment (PPE) during COVID-19 using a cross-sectional, online self-reporting survey. They found that receiving adequate information about the use of PPE was associated with correct donning and doffing procedures. While having adequate PPE supplies was identified in the study, the importance of adequate training and clear instructions about how to don and doff PPE were also highlighted.

Longitudinal designs

Longitudinal designs are observational research methods in which data are collected from the same group repeatedly at various points in time to see whether a phenomenon changes over time. This type of study may extend over several years, with some studies extending over many decades. Longitudinal designs can be used with correlational, experimental or quasi-experimental designs, with time-dependent patterns identified in the data. Many experimental designs in health research, such as clinical trials, are longitudinal because it is necessary to follow people through a full course of treatment, repeatedly gathering data, to determine whether any changes in their condition are occurring.

FOR EXAMPLE

LONGITUDINAL DESIGN

Evans and colleagues (2020) explored the immediate and aspirational employment plans and workforce choices of midwives prior to graduating from an Australian university. Reasons for staying in midwifery and perceptions around factors likely to influence job satisfaction were also explored. Almost 90 per cent of respondents either aspired to work in a continuity of care model or recognised that they would gain job satisfaction by providing continuity of care to women. Making a difference to the women in their care, working in models of care which enabled them to provide the necessary care and having the ability to make autonomous midwifery decisions were identified as factors that influenced job satisfaction. The authors concluded that aligning early graduate work experiences with continuity of care models may have a positive impact on the confidence and professional development of graduate midwives and lead to greater satisfaction and retention among midwives.

Comparative descriptive designs

A **comparative descriptive design** is one in which two or more groups are being compared using particular variables. This type of design generally has the same advantages and disadvantages as a simple descriptive design, but has the added advantage of enabling the comparison of groups. They produce weak evidence in comparison to experimental designed studies, although this design is slightly stronger than simple descriptive design; however, comparative descriptive designs are important in research because they are generally used to conduct an initial exploration of a research question when little is known about the topic.

FOR EXAMPLE

COMPARATIVE DESCRIPTIVE DESIGN

A comparative descriptive design was employed by Roulin and colleagues (2020) to describe and compare the nurses' and elderly patients' perceptions of caring attitudes and behaviours in an inpatient rehabilitation centre in Switzerland. While both nurses and patients considered comfort care as being important, nurses scored humanistic and clinical care as being most important, whereas the patients scored clinical aspects of caring as being more important. These results indicated the value of visible aspects of care delivery in rehabilitation departments.

Analytical designs

Correlational designs

A **correlational design** explores the relationships between two or more variables within one group but does not aim to determine cause and effect. It examines the direction of the relationship (positive or negative) and the strength of the relationship. Where pools of data already exist (e.g. patient medical records), this design can be implemented very quickly. Statistical analysis is conducted to determine whether there is a relationship between the variables and, if so, how strong it is and what direction it takes.

The advantage of a correlational design is that it is a relatively easy, fast and inexpensive way to obtain and process a lot of data that can be used to investigate relationships among variables. It is useful in exploratory research to determine relationships that can later be tested more explicitly by more exacting methodologies, such as an experimental design.

FOR EXAMPLE

CORRELATIONAL DESIGN

Bai and colleagues (2015) used a structured self-report questionnaire to investigate fatigue levels and fatigue predictors for patients undergoing haemodialysis using a cross-sectional correlation research design. Although a number of predictors of fatigue were identified (including age, marital status, employment status, physical activity and types of medications), depression was found to have the greatest impact on the patients' fatigue levels.

Cohort designs

A cohort design involves following two groups over time, including one group that has been exposed to a known risk factor and another unexposed group, to determine the occurrence of disease. The incidence of disease in the two groups is compared and the relative risk, or incidence rate, is calculated to determine whether there is an underlying link between exposure and the disease (Setia, 2016). Cohorts occur naturally, such as birth cohorts; for example, the *baby boomers* comprise people born between 1946 and 1960. Typically, a cohort is studied repeatedly at points of time over several years. As the study is conducted, outcomes from participants in each cohort are measured and relationships with specific characteristics are determined.

Another type of cohort is a one-off cohort. This is a unique group of people, all of whom were exposed to something unusual that may have affected their health. In Australia, studies have been conducted on military servicemen who were exposed to the atomic bomb tests at Maralinga and the servicemen exposed to Agent Orange during the Vietnam War.

In a **prospective study** subjects are followed over a period to determine whether their exposure status changes after baseline data information has been collected. Such data can be used to answer questions about the association between risk factors and disease outcomes (Setia, 2016). In contrast, a **retrospective study** involves identifying a cohort of individuals after they have developed the outcome of interest. This design is useful for unusual or occupational exposures whereby exposure status and the incidence of disease are determined retrospectively (Setia, 2016).

Other cohort studies are non-concurrent, meaning that the exposure occurred a long time ago, so researchers need to refer to data that may have been collected retrospectively and also collect new data.

FOR EXAMPLE

COHORT STUDY

The incidence of acute respiratory tract infection (ARTI) in exclusively breastfed infants was explored in a prospective cohort study, conducted at 116 midwifery centres in India. Data from the study confirmed the protective effective of exclusive breastfeeding against ARTI during the second and third months of life, with higher rates of ARTI found in infants who were not exclusively breastfed.

Source: Kuriakose, S., Kaimal, R., Cherian, V., & Peter, P. (2020). Comparison of incidence of acute respiratory infection in exclusively breastfed infants and not exclusively breastfed infants from 61 to 180 days of age: A prospective cohort study. *Journal of Family Medicine & Primary Care*, 9(6), 2823–2829. https://doi.org/10.4103/jfmpc.jfmpc_198_20

Time series designs

A time series design differs from a cohort study in that the participants are selected by the researcher and are not a naturally occurring group. In a time series design, the researcher makes several measurements, both before and after the treatment, which help to measure any variations in the data that are dependent on time.

Time series designs can help show that any changes that occur just after the implementation of the intervention are related to the treatment. Without the use of a control group, it is a weak design because it does not control for other events that may happen during the study. This design can become quasi-experimental with the use of a non-equivalent control group, or it can become experimental with the use of random assignment to control and experimental groups.

FOR EXAMPLE

TIME SERIES DESIGN

Chaboyer and colleagues (2010) undertook an observational time series study in two medical units to assess the effects of the implementation of improvement strategies on medication errors, patient falls and pressure ulcers.

Causal-comparative research designs

Causal-comparative research designs have certain characteristics of an experimental design, but do not fulfil the requirements of internal validity. For example, although quasi-experimental designs do not include random allocation of participants to control and **experimental groups** (Bryman, 2015), the intention of using this type of design is to estimate the effect of an intervention in the absence of randomisation (Miler, Smith & Pugatch, 2020). Healthcare research often includes quasi-experimental designs because random allocation in the clinical setting is often quite difficult.

Non-equivalent control group designs

This is the most common design of the quasi-experimental type. While this design does use a control group, it varies from the classic experimental design by using groups that have already been established, or are going to be established, but does not include randomisation of participants. The subjects are self-selected into the groups, or selected based on a criterion. Therefore, the non-equivalent control group design does not meet the criterion for random allocation to groups. One of the biggest problems with a non-equivalent control group design is that it cannot be absolutely determined whether the groups were equal to begin with because subjects are not randomly assigned to the groups. The collection of data about **extraneous variables**, including gender, age and educational levels, could establish whether the groups were equivalent on these variables. The inclusion of a pretest could also be included to establish whether the groups were initially equivalent in relation to the dependent variable.

Pre-experimental designs

A pre-experimental design does not use a **control group**; therefore, the evidence produced is not considered to be as strong as a randomised controlled trial. Even so, this type of design can still be useful, particularly where limited numbers of subjects prohibit the use of a control group. Pre-experimental designs include one-shot case studies and pretest post-test designs.

There are two types of non-equivalent control group designs:

1 *pretest post-test* has the advantage of establishing whether or not the groups were equivalent on the experimental variable before the treatment
2 *post-test only* is similar to the above design except that it only includes a post-test.

Without the pretest, it cannot be determined whether the groups were initially equal on the experimental variable; but, as noted earlier, not all studies are suited to a pretest.

Pretest post-test designs

In this design, a pretest and post-test are conducted involving only one group. This design is used where it is not possible to use a control group; for example, where there are too few subjects available.

This design features:
- random allocation of subjects to the control and experimental groups
- pretesting of both groups on the dependent variable
- administration of treatment to the experimental group but not the control group
- measurement of the dependent variable on a post-test.

The results of the experiment are established by a set of comparisons. The pretest measurements of both groups are compared to establish whether the groups were in fact initially equivalent. Pretest measurements will also establish a baseline measurement. The post-test measurements for both groups are compared with the pretest measurements to establish if there has been a change, and if so, the direction of the change. If the treatment has been successful, the experimental group should achieve a significantly different post-test measurement from the pretest measurement. A significantly different post-test measurement from the control group not receiving the treatment should also be achieved. The control group might also demonstrate a slight change in the same direction because of the placebo effect.

This is considered to be the best design because it controls for any changes during the course of the experiment.

The advantage of the pretest post-test design over the one-shot case study design is that it enables a comparison to be made of the measurement of the dependent variable after the experimental treatment with the results obtained before the treatment was implemented. This then allows some conclusions to be drawn about the size of the effect of the treatment.

FOR EXAMPLE

PRETEST POST-TEST DESIGN

Suppose a researcher wanted to test the effect of hyperbaric pressure on the size of pressure injuries. They would undertake a pretest measurement of the size of the pressure injury, then apply the hyperbaric pressure treatments. They would then measure the size of the pressure injury again. If the average size of pressure injury at the end of the program was lower, they might conclude that the hyperbaric pressure treatment had reduced the rate of pressure injuries. But the validity of the findings could be challenged on the grounds of history if, for example, other events, such as increased mobility of the patients, occur during the course of the study. The findings can also be challenged by the problem of maturation or changes in the subjects that occur spontaneously during the course of the experiment; for example, spontaneous remission of the pressure injury. This challenge could have been easily avoided by comparing the results with those of another group who had not been exposed to hyperbaric pressure but had shared all the other experiences of the experimental group; in other words, a control group.

An example of a pretest post-test design includes the study by White, Hemingway and Stephenson (2014) who evaluated the effectiveness of learning immediately after a workshop and the participants' view about the transferability of learning to clinical practice.

There are several threats to the validity of the findings in such a design. This type of design can be weakened by a testing effect where learning or skills are involved. There is no way of determining whether the process of pretesting influenced the results because there is no baseline measurement of the control group. There is also the problem of instrument decay, whereby changes in the assessing instrument can affect the results. This is more of a problem where physical instruments are used over a longer period, but it can be avoided by recalibrating the instruments against a known stable reference.

Post-test only control group design

This design is often used when a pretest is not possible or desirable. Two groups are involved, including a control group and experimental group:

- a post-test is administered to both groups
- a control group is used and subjects are randomly allocated to either of the two groups.

The advantage of this design is that it eliminates any testing effect and therefore may be used where the measurement is a test of learning or skill development.

A potential problem with this design is using it where the pretest post-test design should have been included in the design. If a control group is used with randomisation groups, it can be accepted that the groups were the same to begin with and that the results were due to the treatment. If the treatment was effective, there should be a significant difference between the two groups.

FOR EXAMPLE

POST-TEST DESIGN

Suppose a researcher wants to test the effect of a new dressing technique on wound healing and compare it with the effect of a traditional technique. If subjects are to be randomly allocated to control and experimental groups, each group should have the same type of dressing technique. This would mean that the nurses would probably have to do dressings using the two different techniques because of changing patient allocations, which would be confusing and difficult to manage. Similarly, randomly allocating the nurses to two different techniques on one ward would not work because of shifting patient allocations. Patients would mostly end up in both groups because continuity of nurse–patient allocation could not be guaranteed. For these reasons, the researcher would probably have to include two wards – an experimental and a control ward – and introduce the new technique into the experimental ward. This then becomes a non-equivalent control group design.

Kim and Lee (2020) used a quasi-experimental study with a non-equivalent control group design to explore the effects of medication error encouragement training (MEET) on medication confidence among nursing students. Both groups received theoretical training, with the experimental group receiving the MEET and the control group receiving traditional error-avoidance training. On completion of the training, the experimental group's confidence was significantly higher than those in the control group.

Solomon four-group design

This is a special type of experimental design that is used when the researcher is worried that the use of a pretest would affect the post-test readings. Two control groups and two experimental groups are included in this design. The pretest is administered to one control and experimental group only.

The results of an experiment with this design would be interpreted as follows. If the pretest did not have any effect, the two experimental groups should have the same result on the post-test. If the pretest did sensitise the subjects, the two experimental groups would have different results on the post-test. The comparison of the control with the experimental groups should be interpreted in the same way as for other experiments.

This is a powerful design to control for testing effect and intervening variables. One disadvantage of the design is the need to recruit more subjects into the study.

Factorial designs

Factorial designs involve measuring two or more independent variables on a dependent variable. For example, if the effects of both type and timing of back care on the development of pressure injuries was being measured, two different studies would be designed or a design that included two different independent variables or factors would be considered:

- the type of back care; for example, repositioning versus bed surface
- the frequency of back care; for example, four-hourly versus two-hourly.

This design would have four cells, to which subjects would be assigned randomly. More complex designs with more factors and levels are possible (see Table 5.1).

▸ Table 5.1   Independent variable example

	Four-hourly care	Two-hourly care
Repositioning	Group 1	Group 2
Bed surface	Group 3	Group 4

Thus, one group would have two-hourly back care using only repositioning, one would have two-hourly back care with a specific bed surface and so on. This type of study is referred to as a two-by-two factorial design because two factors and two levels of treatment are included in the study.

FOR EXAMPLE

FACTORIAL DESIGN

Rattray and colleagues (2011) used a factorial design to determine which professional, situational and patient characteristics predict nurses' judgements of patient acuity and the likelihood of referral for further review.

One-shot case studies

In a one-shot case study design, the effect of an event or phenomenon, or the administration of a substance or other treatment, is tested on a group after it has occurred. The conclusions are based on the general expectations of what the findings would have been if the experimental event had not occurred. Usually, this design is used for events that have happened without warning, or in a situation in which it is not possible to design a scientific experiment. In this design, subjects are frequently self-selected because they have been exposed to some experience or substance.

The advantage of this design is that investigation of phenomena is permitted to explore whether this may have had an effect on some characteristic of the participants. This type of design can provide information informing more sophisticated designs to measure the same effects, but it is considered a very weak design because the researcher has no control over the intervention and a control group is not included in the design of the study.

FOR EXAMPLE

ONE-SHOT SECTIONAL SURVEY

Mongkuo and Quantrell (2015) employed a cross-sectional pre-experimental one-shot care study design to explore the effects of excessive consumption of alcohol and other factors (such as enrolment status) and involvement in risky sexual behaviour among college student. Results reported from the study included the positive influence of alcohol on risky sexual behaviour, with females more like to engage in this type of behaviour. An interesting result from this study was that risky behaviour was found to increase with age, a finding that differed from previous research studies.

Single patient trial ($n = 1$) designs

It is possible to construct a counterbalanced design using a single participant. This is called a single patient trial or $n = 1$ design. The patient is their own control.

FOR EXAMPLE

SINGLE PATIENT TRIAL

If, for instance, a researcher is interested in which aromatherapy oil had the most beneficial effect on a patient's sleep patterns, they could measure the person's sleep pattern as a baseline and then introduce an aromatherapy oil for a week or more, and measure their sleep pattern again. This could be repeated introducing other aromatherapy oils to determine the most beneficial effects.

The advantage of this kind of design is that as well as being a useful guide to individual care for patients, it can also be carried out using individual patients in multiple settings and at different times on an ongoing basis. Data are aggregated to determine the outcome.

Experimental designs

Experimental designs are considered to be the most powerful quantitative research designs, producing the best evidence for cause-and-effect relationships between variables. The prime purpose of an experiment is to conclusively determine whether one variable has an effect on another variable.

Generally, the researcher sets up a situation in which one variable can be manipulated. This variable is called the independent treatment or causal variable. It is expected that the manipulation of the independent variable will have an effect on another variable, called the dependent outcome or effect variable. Any changes in the dependent variable are presumed to be caused by the independent variable – it is the presumed effect.

In health research, examples of independent variables include nursing interventions, educational programs, prescribing medication, types of wound dressings or exercise programs.

FOR EXAMPLE

TESTING A NEW DRESSING TECHNIQUE

The following research question is posed: 'Does dressing technique A (independent variable), when compared with dressing technique B (independent variable), cause a change to the rate of infection (dependent variable)?'

That is:

- independent variable = dressing technique A
- independent variable = dressing technique B
- dependent variable = rate of infection (i.e. dependent on the dressing technique)

Dressing technique A may result in no change to the rate of infection, but dressing technique B may cause a reduction in the rate of infection. The experimental design would prove that dressing technique B should be used in clinical practice.

Although the true experimental design is considered to be the gold-standard research design, the application of experimental designs to healthcare research has been limited for various reasons.

- Experimental research assumes that the relevant variables have been identified so that they can be controlled; therefore, it is important that variables associated with the study have been identified when selecting a design.
- There are many social variables of importance to health outcomes that cannot be manipulated.
- It is difficult to carry out experimental research in the clinical setting, where random assignment to groups and standardisation of research procedures may be impossible to achieve.

EBP

- The ethical questions concerning the best care of the patient must take precedence.

ACTIVITY

Explain which of the following research designs is appropriate for the research question: 'Is the prevalence of pressure injuries greater in patients who are overweight than in patients who have a normal BMI?'
- Simple descriptive design
- Comparative descriptive design
- Correlational design
- Experimental design

True experimental research designs

A true experimental design (randomised controlled trial [RCT]) enables researchers to draw valid conclusions from the research. Three major features are:
- the use of an equivalent control group to control for extraneous variables
- random assignment to experimental and control groups
- the ability to control and manipulate the independent variable.

True experimental research designs aim to reduce bias and include major features when testing the effectiveness of new treatments so that researchers can design their study to control for any potential sources of bias as much as possible. Well-planned and rigorously conducted RCTs remain the most robust research method for finding the real effect of an intervention. However, a biased study may harm a patient and result in a waste of valuable resources (Bhide, Shah & Acharya, 2018). A step-by-step guide to planning, conducting, analysing and reporting RCTs is provided in the article by Bhide, Shah and Acharya (2018).

ACTIVITY

1   Explain the three essential features of a true experiment.
2   Explain why placebos are used in clinical trials.

Use of a control group

A control group is one that is equivalent in every way to the experimental group, except for the experimental variable, which controls for extraneous variables and thus allows for comparisons to be made.

To eliminate factors such as spontaneous remission, a control group with no treatment is usually introduced in clinical therapeutic trials to enable the researcher to see what would happen without the treatment. At the end of the trial, the researcher would know whether any effect was due to the treatment or to spontaneous remission. The psychological effects of treatment can be avoided by the application of a placebo to a control group, and the information is masked from the participants to reduce or eliminate **bias**. Subjects are blind to the treatment if they do not know which drug they are receiving. If the person who administers the drug also does not know which drug is being given, the design is said to be a double-blind study to prevent observer bias.

Random assignment to groups

The random allocation of subjects to either the treatment or control groups ensures that they have an equal probability of being in either group. This eliminates any systemic bias in the groups that may affect the study variable. It warrants that any other variables are evenly distributed between the groups so that they should be comparable, except for the independent variable. The CONSORT flow diagram details the phases of an RCT involving two groups (including enrolment, intervention allocation, follow up and data analysis). A flow diagram from a randomised controlled study by Chawla and colleagues (2020) is displayed in Figure 5.3, detailing the number of patients assessed for eligibility, the number of patients randomised to each arm of the study and reasons for those who were excluded. The aim of this study was to evaluate the impact of soaking surgical mesh in 0.5% bupivacaine solution on post-operative pain after a laparoscopic ventral hernia repair. The study had 161 patients eligible to participate, with 47 patients excluded (reasons detailed in the flow diagram). The study allocated 58 patients to the intervention arm of the study (surgical mesh soaked in 0.5% bupivacaine solution) with 56 patients allocated to the control arm of the study (surgical mesh soaked in normal saline solution). After allocation, nine patients did not receive the allocated intervention (three in the intervention group and six in the control group) with no patients lost to follow up. Data from 105 patients were included in the data analysis, which showed a significant difference in early post-operative pain between the two groups (Chawla, et al. 2020).

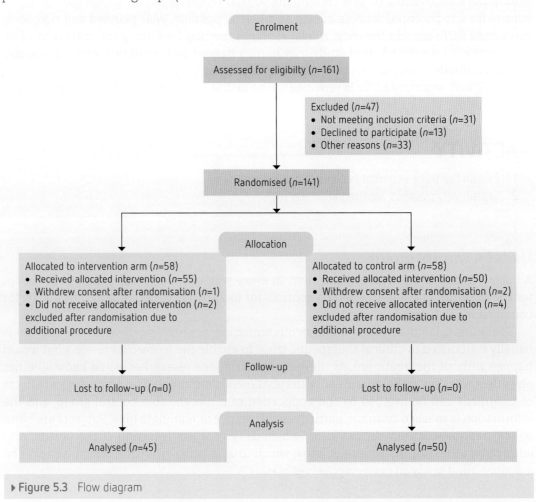

▶ **Figure 5.3** Flow diagram

Source: Chawla, T., Shahzad, N., Ahmad, K., & Ali, J. F. (2020). Post-operative pain after laparoscopic ventral hernia repair, the impact of mesh soakage with bupivacaine solution versus normal saline solution: A randomised controlled trial (HAPPIEST Trial). *Journal of Minimal Access Surgery, 16*(4), 328–34. https://doi.org/10.4103/jmas.JMAS_50_19

Manipulation of the independent variable

Manipulation of the independent variable should ensure that the levels are sufficient to produce different findings between the groups. If, for example, relaxation therapy is introduced as the independent variable, it should be conducted for a sufficient enough time to produce a significantly relaxed state in the participants.

Table 5.2 compares all the major research designs that have been discussed in this section.

▶ Table 5.2   Comparison of major research designs

	Simple descriptive	Comparative descriptive	Correlational	Experimental	Pre-experimental	Quasi-experimental
Describes participants	Yes	Yes	Yes	Yes	Yes	Yes
Compares groups	No	Yes	Yes	Yes	Yes	Yes
Investigates cause-and-effect relationships	No	No	No	Yes	No	Yes
Manipulates independent variable	No	No	No	Yes	No	Yes
Has a control group	No	No	No	Yes	No	Yes
Random assignment to groups	No	No	No	Yes	No	No

FOR EXAMPLE

RANDOMISED CONTROLLED TRIAL

An RCT designed by Marques and colleagues (2020) assessed the effects of respiratory physiotherapy compared with standard pharmacological care on symptoms and function in outpatients with lower respiratory tract infections (LRTI). Outpatients with LRTI were recruited and randomly allocated to the control (pharmacological) or experimental (pharmacological and respiratory physiotherapy) group. Adding respiratory physiotherapy to the pharmacological treatment of outpatients with LRTI resulted in greater recovery of symptoms and function parameters.

Validity and reliability in scientific research

Validity in research usually includes external and internal validity.

External validity

This term refers to the capacity for generalisation, or the extent to which the results apply to situations beyond the original (specific) study. It is not possible to include everyone from a population in health science research due to several factors, including a lack of time or funding. If the sample included in the study is representative of the population from which they have been selected, the results can be generalised to that population. For example, if the study included paediatric patients aged between 6 and 14 years old, presenting to the emergency department with a fractured arm, the results from the study can be generalised to all paediatric patients of that age group. If participants are not randomly sampled from the whole population, the results can only be applied to the population from which the sample was taken.

Internal validity

This term refers to the extent to which the design and data allow accurate conclusions to be made. This depends on the extent to which the measurement tool measures what it is supposed to measure. For example, if the effects of a new method of mouth care on the oral mucosa was being measured, a validated measuring tool should be used to ensure the data collected is measuring effects on mouth care.

Major threats to validity

There are various problems that can arise to threaten the internal validity of a study. *Mortality* or *attrition* refers to the loss of subjects from the study. Subjects may drop out from the experimental and/or control groups at different rates, leaving an imbalance in the number of subjects in the two groups. If this happens, comparisons of the groups may be invalid and the effect of the intervention may not be observed. *History* refers to events that were not a part of the study design but happened during the course of the study and may impact on the study results.

FOR EXAMPLE

THREATS TO INTERNAL VALIDITY

If a researcher was interested in exploring the effects of an educational program on attitudes towards the use of contraceptives, and during the study there was a major television campaign about contraception, this could affect the attitudes of the subjects to the extent that the results of the study could be attributed to the television campaign and not the educational campaign.

Maturation occurs during the course of the study and can change the subjects in ways that affect the results. This can be important in longitudinal studies and in studies in which children are involved, because of their physical, mental and social growth. The effect of maturation can be countered by using shorter intervals between observations.

The *testing effect*, whereby an initial test can affect the results of a second test, can present as a problem when testing learning or skills.

FOR EXAMPLE

TESTING EFFECT

Suppose that a study aims to test whether a diabetes educational program has an effect on blood glucose control. Before subjects are exposed to the program, a researcher will need to measure the levels of pre-program knowledge by a test. This test may stimulate subjects to learn more about diabetes, which subsequently interferes with the measurement of the effects of the educational program.

Selection effects occur after the non-random selection of subjects from the comparison groups. If subjects are not assigned randomly to the groups, the groups' characteristics may become unequal, which could make comparison invalid.

The *placebo effect* is due to an individual's belief that a treatment works regardless of whether it does or not. The placebo effect is evident when a patient recovers from pain after they are given a substance or treatment with no therapeutic value. The placebo effect can be controlled by administering to a control group an inert substance that looks exactly like the active drug. The recipients must be blinded to whether they are receiving a placebo or the active treatment.

Changing procedures and instrumentation are another threat to validity. If the measurement procedures change during the study, the results will change and the comparison will be invalid. The major method of dealing with this problem is to conduct a rigorous trial on a small group (a **pilot study**) to identify any problems and refine the procedure before embarking on the full experiment.

Another potential problem is *differences in instruments*. Instruments can measure differently and can affect the study results. Instruments should be calibrated so that a standard unit is measured in the same way and with the same degree of accuracy for each participant, thereby avoiding discrepancies in the data.

Differences in measurement refers to the fact that the use of several data collectors may mean different ways of measuring. Training data collectors to collect data and take measurements in the same way can control this effect. Interrater reliability can also be achieved by testing them until the set standard is achieved.

The **Hawthorne effect** suggests that people behave differently when they are aware that they are being observed. It is difficult to control for this variable without violating ethical principles, as it is unethical to watch people without their knowing it. The only way to surmount this problem is to use unobtrusive observation, such as participant observation, in which the researcher is part of the clinical team.

The *experimenter effect* refers to how the researcher may consciously or unconsciously affect the results of the experiment. For example, a researcher who is convinced of the value of a treatment may consciously or unconsciously promote the treatment to the recipient and cause artificially high ratings of the new treatment, augmenting the placebo effect. As a result, in trials of new drugs, the person dispensing the drug should also be blind to whether the client is receiving the placebo or the active treatment.

Some variables, known as **confounding variables**, are known to be statistically associated with the outcome but are not actually measured in the research study. For example, there

TIP

If during a study you want to measure body temperature, all thermometers should be calibrated to ensure the accuracy and similarity of the measurements. Any defective thermometers can then be eliminated giving you confidence in your equipment.

TIP

Matching subjects in your design can help to eliminate confounding effects.

may be an association between coffee drinking during pregnancy and low-birth-weight babies, but women who drink lots of coffee may also be more likely to smoke cigarettes, and cigarette smoking may be the real cause of low birth weight. These variables can also be identified and adjusted statistically by sophisticated statistical procedures such as multivariate analysis of variance (MANOVA) and multiple regression.

If the measured value of a variable differs from the true value of that variable, it is due to bias in the design. Bias has a number of typical sources, such as:

- sloppy measurement; for example, interviewer bias where interviewers unintentionally favour a particular view of an issue
- participant recall bias due to the effects of memory on reporting events
- reporting bias, which occurs when participants deliberately report the aspects of a phenomenon that are of most importance to them
- the poor selection of participants, which will result in a sample that has a biased concentration of some variable.

ACTIVITY

You are about to undertake a study of surgical patients in the hospital you work at to see whether the incidence of post-operative wound infections is higher among males than females. List three of the variables that might modify, confound or bias your findings in some way.

Reliability in scientific research

Reliability refers to the reproducibility of the results of a measurement technique. This means that, given the same circumstances, the technique will produce the same measurements. If multiple measurements of the same thing agree, then reliability is good. There are some useful measures of reliability that can be reported by researchers to demonstrate that their research findings are reliable.

Test-retest reliability

If two sets of measurements of the same thing are taken at different times and the measurements are compared to see how similar they are, this is an indication of test-retest reliability (stability). The strength of the reliability can be determined by calculating a correlation coefficient. The approach is useful for ensuring that measurement tools such as questionnaires are stable over time.

Interrater/observer reliability

Interrater/observer reliability refers to the consistency of measurements when different collectors or observers are involved. The strength of the reliability can be determined by calculating a correlation coefficient. It is an approach that is useful for ensuring that all observers conduct measurements with the same degree of precision.

FOR EXAMPLE

OBSERVER RELIABILITY

If a researcher was exploring whether nurses wearing tabards with 'drug round in progress – please do not disturb' embroidered on the front and back, during medication rounds it would be important to know that each of the observers is reliably scoring the activity during data collection.

Sampling

The two major methods of **sampling** use probability and non-probability samples. A **probability sample** resembles the population as closely as possible and is usually randomly selected. It is used to calculate the probability that the results can be generalised to the population. Probability samples include the simple random sample, stratified sample, cluster sampling and multistage sampling. To prevent sampling bias, the probability sample is chosen by objective techniques rather than by the subjective judgement of the researcher.

In a **non-probability sample**, subjective judgements contribute to the selection of the sample. The disadvantage of non-probability sampling is that the results cannot be generalised and conclusions cannot be made concerning the population about the sample from the findings. The types of non-probability sampling are the convenience sample, case-based sample, snowball sample and quota sample. Convenience samples are very common in clinical research, where there may not be enough people to consider probability sampling.

The size of the sample, to be determined before data are collected, must be sufficiently large to yield valid data or the study will lack internal validity. There are formulas available to assist in calculating the size of the sample so sufficient power to the results is calculated during the design of the study. The statistical power of a study includes determining the sample size required to detect an effect of a given size with a given degree of confidence.

Sample size and power calculations are appropriate mechanisms for determining sample size only when all data in the study are collected on the same **scale of measurement**.

Pilot study

A pilot study is a mini replica of a research project that is designed to test all aspects prior to commencement of the full study. It incorporates every part of the procedure of the main study and provides guidance for the larger study. It is important that a pilot study:
- be carried out in such a way as to be as close as possible to the larger study design
- be carried out in the setting in which the main study will be conducted, if possible
- uses the procedures proposed for the main study, including such elements as obtaining informed consent
- includes recruitment of the same type of participants.

One major purpose of a pilot study is to assess the feasibility of the main study so that any problems that are identified can be corrected. A pilot study will enable a researcher to evaluate whether:
- the study design is adequate
- the methodology is feasible

- elements are acceptable, such as the recruitment of participants, sampling technique, appropriateness and effectiveness of the procedures, time frame and costs
- the instruments are valid, and if not, which alternatives to choose
- any extra equipment is required that might not have been anticipated
- any unanticipated variables can be identified, what their impact on the study might be and ways in which they can be dealt with.

Preparing for data collection and management

EBP

A data-collection plan should be developed using a flow chart or some other method of laying the research process out and tracking it. This provides a road map of the project that can be used to check the progress of the study.

Acquisition and preparation of equipment and materials

One of the first tasks before commencing with the data collection is to select and acquire any necessary equipment, such as biophysical instruments, computers, modems, telephones, recording equipment and statistical packages, which might involve buying, renting or borrowing pieces of equipment. If equipment is being borrowed it is important to ensure it will be available when required.

It is essential to order any equipment, consumables (consent forms, receipts, information sheets, sticky labels, logbooks) and other materials well before they are expected to be used.

All equipment should be checked to ensure it is complete and in good working order. A final check should be completed immediately before it is taken on site.

Access to the site and participants

Collection of data can be carried out in a range of places, from a **naturalistic setting** to a laboratory. It is mandatory to secure permission to collect data, especially if in a semi-public area, such as a shopping centre, health clinic lobby or hospital waiting room; therefore, it is important to ensure permission is obtained before the study proceeds.

If in a hospital or clinic, ensure that the clinicians in charge will allow access to participants. Before the time of data collection, meeting the clinicians and involving them in the study will improve access, particularly if they are influential. Before entering the research site, it is important to check and make sure that the clinicians or other gatekeepers are still willing to assist.

Preparation of people

When preparing for data collection, it is necessary to prepare the people involved, including the clinicians or gatekeepers, the staff in the clinical area or laboratory and the participants.

Staff

Ensuring the cooperation of staff is crucial to the success of a study. Brief the employees in person by making use of one or more in-service sessions to explain details of the study and how it will affect the staff. Provide a resource folder detailing the study, including any procedures, protocols, patient materials (such as an informed consent document and a plain-language statement) and relevant previous literature that can be left in each participating area.

Recruitment and preparation of participants

Depending on the design of the study, participants may either all be recruited at the beginning of the study, or be recruited in stages. Recruitment carried out by the researcher or by colleagues onsite, is best done by someone involved in the study personally so that all possible potential participants are approached. Depending on the design of the study, clients, members of the public or colleagues can be recruited. It is important to be aware that each of these groups has inbuilt problems.

- Members of the public are often suspicious of strangers.
- Colleagues require special consideration, especially if they are in a junior position, to ensure they do not feel compelled to participate in the study.
- Special consideration is necessary when including participants from other cultures and those who do not understand English. An interpreter is necessary for non-English-speaking participants. Care should also be taken when dealing with special populations, such as the elderly, and any participants who cannot give informed consent on their own behalf, such as children.
- Shorter hospital stays for surgical procedures and childbirth can limit access to participants and decrease the number of potential data-collection days for each participant. The trend for shorter hospital stays has also resulted in fewer nursing staff, which means there is less time for nurses to assist with data collection.
- Participants may refuse to participate because they fear that invasive procedures might be required, be disillusioned with research or have poor health status. Some may have been discouraged by staff who have criticised the project.
  The following actions are useful in addressing such problems.
- Have procedures in place to ensure a biased sample is avoided.
- Approach all the selected potential participants at a suitable time; for example, when they are not heavily medicated.
- Explain the study in plain, simple language (i.e. avoid jargon).
- Provide participants with enough time to consider participating in the study by leaving the information and coming back later. After the participant has consented, the consent form is signed.
- Consider nursing care and other routines when collecting data in the clinical area. It is necessary to be flexible about arranging and rescheduling times.

Researchers and data collectors

The following tips will help when preparing researchers and data collectors.
- Ensure that anyone collecting data is familiar with equipment and research material to ensure a smooth process during data collection.

TIP

It always takes longer than you expect to get the required sample size.

- Brief data collectors about procedures, but prevent biased data by not informing them of the expected outcome.
- Be cooperative with the clinical area at all times. It should be remembered that the researcher is there as a visitor and as a representative of the funding institution, and that client care takes priority over any research project.

The process of data collection

Data collection takes place with the use of a variety of methods, but no matter which method is used, it can be anticipated that the data-collection phase of the study will take longer and be more difficult than anticipated and will require adjustments during the process!

Managing equipment and materials

When managing equipment and materials during the data-collection process, take the following into consideration.

- Whatever hardware is being used, ensure that it is kept in prime condition during the course of the data collection.
- All data should be entered correctly and completely, and procedures should be in place to protect against data loss.
- If the computer is plugged into the mains, it should be protected against power surges with a surge protector. If batteries are being used, the batteries should have sufficient power for the period of data collection. It is also prudent to have at least one set of backup batteries.
- Frequent backup copies of all files should be made with backup copies saved in a safe place that is updated regularly.

Preparing questionnaire materials

The following tips will help when preparing questionnaire materials.

- All of the questionnaire should be carefully read before it goes to the printer. Different coloured paper can be used to identify different sites or to differentiate the original from follow-up questionnaires.
- If a mailing list is being requested it should be done in a timely manner so that other arrangements can be made if the request is not granted. Although, due to privacy and to prevent unwanted requests, organisations may not provide a list of members' names and addresses, some will distribute questionnaire packets to their members on behalf of the researcher (at the researcher's expense).
- A computer should be used to randomise the sample for the study. There is a random-number-generating feature in Excel that can do this relatively easily.
- Self-addressed envelopes will be required for respondents to return the questionnaires. Questionnaires can be distributed by several methods, as shown in Figure 5.4.

In person

- Distribute them yourself to clients or to a contact person to distribute for you.
- If you are using a self-selected convenience sample, leave the questionnaires in a box together with a flyer asking people to take them.

Electronically

- Use a web-based or SMS-based survey design that will deliver questionnaires in electronic form directly to a participant's computer or mobile phone. This is a very effective means of reaching people and enables an easy means of response.
- Another electronic option is to send an email to a list of addresses.

By post

- Identify a contact person at the site who can distribute the questionnaires and then send them to that person by post.
- Alternatively, send them to the individual participants by post.

By telephone

- Use of the telephone saves on the cost of postage but obviously incurs call costs.

By video conferencing

- This enables you to connect virtually with participants when meeting in person is not possible.
- This includes video and audio with the option of recording all interviews.
- Transcribing of interview data is an optional selection (additional cost may involved).

▸ **Figure 5.4** Distribution methods for surveys

Managing the site

To ensure there are no interruptions before commencing an interview, all mobile phones should be turned off and beepers disconnected. The interviewee can be asked to do the same.

Collecting data onsite can give rise to various problems, including:

- unforeseen institutional factors, such as changes of policy that affect the study, industrial action, unplanned closure or reorganisation of a clinical area, transfer of cooperative staff out of the unit and transfer of uncooperative staff into the unit
- with regards to the use of available data, a loss of a patient's charts or incomplete charts which result in a loss of data.

Managing the participants

The way to manage the participants during the data-collection phase is to keep them informed about the study, and to also keep the following in mind.

- Treat participants with respect. Remember, they are not compelled to participate and they can withdraw at any time. It is important to put participants at ease as much as possible during data collection; the researcher should introduce themselves, chat briefly about other things to break the ice, then remind the participant of the purposes and procedures of the research.

- There may be problems with the sample that has been recruited, such as participant mortality or loss of participants from the study. Some people agree to participate and then fail to show up for the interview or do not complete the questionnaire. Phoning a day or two beforehand to remind participants of the interview can improve recruitment into the study.
- Sometimes, clients in the clinical field are transferred to another ward or facility or are discharged before the study is complete. It is a good idea to maintain regular contact with clients and keep note of their home addresses so collection of the data can be arranged for a later date.
- Even if participants complete the study, some produce unusable data, such as obviously flippant or insincere responses to interview questions, blanks on questionnaires or a failure to cooperate with clinical procedures integral to the study. Any of these can render those parts of the data useless.

Managing colleagues

People at the data-collection site must also be managed. Sometimes, staff factors outside their control interfere, such as horrendously busy shifts and roster changes. If an increased workload occurs, naturally the staff will give higher priority to patient care than to the research. Strategies that could be considered include:

- educating the staff about the research
- inducting new people into the project
- securing the support of local managers
- taking over more of the data-collection activity
- modifying your protocols.

Regular feedback to the staff about the project should be provided without influencing the data that is yet to be collected.

Managing the process

It is important to manage the research project so that accurate, complete data can be collected. The importance of accuracy applies to both the measurement and recording of data. Data collectors must be well versed in the necessary procedures to achieve the aims of the study; and even then, unplanned errors can occur. The researcher may forget to turn the recorder on, or an interview recording may be overwritten. Developing procedures to prevent this, such as the routine naming of files, using either version control (version 1, 2 and so on) or the date each time data are saved on a secure server, as per the healthcare facility or university responsible conducting research policies. This is to ensure all data are stored safely during the study, as well as on completion of the project. The accuracy of some methods, such as questionnaires, will depend on the participant carrying out the procedure correctly or giving the correct answers.

Sometimes, researchers come up against a conflict of interest or an ethical problem during data collection. It has been known for a researcher to discover an abuse of clients during this process. This poses a dilemma because if the researcher blows the whistle, the institution and/or staff will probably cease to cooperate with the researcher, and the data collection at that facility will be disrupted. On the other hand, to not report the abuse would be unethical. Client safety must take precedence over research outcomes; therefore, it is important to detail the process that will be followed if a situation does arise during data collection, especially if the research involves exploring a sensitive issue.

EBP

Keep track of events that may affect the data. Sometimes, unforeseen events, such as the death of a colleague or a favourite client, could affect the staff during data collection. Data collection may have to be suspended until things have settled down.

Monitoring the process

In every project, no matter how small, it is important to keep track of the process; that is, to keep a record, such as a logbook, of steps taken during the project. This ensures the researcher is not dependent solely on their memory, which can be unreliable, especially over the long periods of time involved in a large project, such as a thesis. For a small project, record keeping can be done in a simple fashion by writing in an exercise book, ideally with divided sections to keep track of the different parts of the project. For larger projects, it may be worth keeping records on a spreadsheet or by using a computer program designed for project management. Record a diary of visits that includes:

- the date
- length of visit
- impressions
- problems encountered
- data collected
- expenses (for future reference; keep all receipts).

These records will assist the researcher when writing up the procedures for the study.

Entries in the logbook should be checked regularly to make sure that things are going to plan. It is crucial to ensure that the appropriate steps of the data-collection process, such as collecting protocols and making telephone calls, are carried out. It is important to document the arrival of data and to identify any intervening variables that have not been accounted for, and monitor their effect or revise the data-collection plan.

After-care

The data-collection process is incomplete until after the cleaning-up process is finished.

- Any equipment should be cleaned and returned to its owner if it has been borrowed.
- The laboratory or clinical site should be left in an acceptable state, with all equipment packed away and all surfaces cleaned.
- The staff at a clinical site should be thanked. A summary report of the findings and any publications that ensue should be sent on completion of the project.
- Make a final backup or set of backups and store them on the site where all data are held.

SUMMARY

1	Identify the purpose of conducting quantitative research	• Quantitative research is used when researchers want objective conclusive answers to a research question • The goal of quantitative research methods is to collect numerical data from a group of people, so that these results can be generalised to a larger group of people

2	Identify the differences between major types of quantitative research designs	• A research design provides the framework by which a project will answer a particular research question
		• A hierarchy of evidence, which ranks study types based on the rigour of the research method, was developed by the National Health and Medical Research Council (2009)
		 — Level I: evidence from a rigorous systematic review of randomised controlled (Level II) studies
		 — Level II: evidence from properly designed randomised controlled trials
		 — Level III: may include evidence from:
		   o pseudo-randomisation — allocation of subjects may not be blinded (Level III-1)
		   o comparative studies with concurrent controls, including non-randomised experimental trials, cohort studies, case-controlled studies and interrupted time series with a control group (Level III-2)
		   o comparative studies with historical control, two or more single-arm studies or interrupted time series without a parallel control group (Level III-3)
		 — Level IV: evidence from case series, either post-test or pretest and post-test
		• There are various types of research designs, ranging from less-controlled descriptive designs to more-controlled experimental designs
		• Major types of design include:
		 — descriptive designs
		 — observational
		 — surveys
		 — correlational designs
		 — quasi-experimental designs
		 — experimental designs, which include:
		   o cross-sectional designs
		   o longitudinal designs
		   o cohort studies
		   o time series designs

3	Describe the difference between an independent and a dependent variable	• An independent variable is the variable that is changed or controlled in research to test the effects on the dependent variable • A dependent variable is the variable being tested and measured • As the researcher changes the independent variable, the effect on the dependent variable is observed and recorded
4	Explain the importance of validity and reliability when conducting scientific research	• Reliability refers to the reproducibility of the results of a measurement technique; given the same circumstances, the technique will reliably produce the same measurements • Validity in research includes two kinds: external and internal validity • *External validity* refers to the capacity for generalisation, or the extent to which the results apply to situations beyond the original study • *Internal validity* refers to the extent to which the design and data allow accurate conclusions to be made; this depends on the extent to which the measurement tool measures what it is supposed to measure

5	Explain the preparation required, and the process of, data collection	• In preparing for data collection and management, the researcher sets up a data-collection plan, selects and obtains the equipment and materials, prepares the participants, setting and self, and ensures that arrangements for insurance, travel and accommodation are made • Whatever hardware is being used, ensure that it is kept in prime condition during data collection • All data should be entered correctly and completely and procedures should be in place to protect against loss at any time during the process • Frequent backup copies of all files should be made with backups saved in a safe place that is updated regularly

REVIEW QUESTIONS

1   What are the main steps involved in quantitative research?
2   What is the difference between reliability and validity?
3   Why is it important to address both validity and reliability when developing a research project?
4   Define what a variable is and explain the difference between independent and dependent variables in research.

CHALLENGING REVIEW QUESTIONS

1   You have been asked to complete a research project assessing the difference in chest compression pressures generated by one-handed and two-handed chest compression techniques on a paediatric manikin.
   a   Explain how you will identify the best research design for this project.
   b   Explain the steps of the research method selected, including the independent and dependent variables.
   c   Detail the data-collection process that will used to collect data in this study.
   d   Explain how you would prepare for and manage the data during the project.

CASE STUDY 1

Susan is a newly qualified registered nurse who is undertaking a rotation to the child and adolescent mental health unit as part of her graduate year program. Susan is required, as part of the program, to develop a research project. She is interested in evaluating the impact of a mindfulness training program and has decided to adopt a quantitative approach. Susan asks you for help in how to proceed with developing the proposal. Outline what you would advise her in relation to the following issues:
1   the random allocation of participants to groups so that the outcome of the mindfulness program can be measured
2   the use of a validated questionnaire for data collection
3   the information that should be entered into a logbook over the course of the study
4   the advantages of conducting a pilot study prior to undertaking the main study.

CASE STUDY 2

Priya is an Advanced Life Support Paramedic who works in a rural area. Priya is authorised to attain and analyse a 12-lead ECG and to administer thrombolytic therapy in the setting of acute myocardial infarction (AMI). She has administered thrombolytic therapy on 12 occasions, but she does not know the outcome for those patients who received treatment. Priya would like to undertake research to investigate patient outcome following acute myocardial infarction managed with thrombolytic therapy in the rural prehospital environment.

1 Develop a research aim for Priya's study.
2 Develop a research question for the study.
3 Create a short abstract for the study.

REFERENCES

Abutabenjeh, S., & Jaradat, R. (2018). Clarification of research design, research methods, and research methodology: A guide for public administration researchers and practitioners. *Teaching Public Administration, 36*(3), 237–58.

Australian Bureau of Statistics. (2016). Census of Population and Housing. http://www.abs.gov.au/census

Bai, Y.-L., Lai, L.-Y., Lee, B., Chang, Y.-Y., & Chiou, C.-P. (2015). The impact of depression on fatigue in patients with haemodialysis: A correlational study. *Journal of Clinical Nursing, 24*(13/14), 2014–22.

Bhide, A., Shah, P. S., & Acharya, G. A. (2018). A simplified guide to randomized controlled trials. *Acta Obstetricia et Gynecologica Scandinavica, 97*, 380–7.

Bryman, A. (2015). *Social Research Methods* (5th edn). Oxford, UK: Oxford University Press.

Burns, P. B., Rohrich, R. J., & Chung, K. C. (2011). The levels of evidence and their role in evidence-based medicine. *Plastic Reconstructive Surgery, 128*(1), 305–10.

Carter, E. J., Mastro, K., Vose, C., Rivera, R., & Larson, E. L. (2017). Clarifying the conundrum: Evidence-based practice, quality improvement, or research? The clinical scholarship continuum. *JONA, 47*(5), 266–70.

Chaboyer, W., Johnson, J., Harfy, L., Gehrke, T., & Panuwatwanich, K. (2010). Transforming care strategies and nursing-sensitive patient outcomes. *Journal of Advanced Nursing, 66*(5), 1111–19.

Chawla, T., Shahzad, N., Ahmad, K., & Ali, J. F. (2020). Post-operative pain after laparoscopic ventral hernia repair, the impact of mesh soakage with bupivacaine solution versus normal saline solution: A randomised controlled trial (HAPPIEST Trial). *Journal of Minimal Access Surgery, 16*(4), 328–34. https://doi.org/10.4103/jmas.JMAS_50_19

Evans, J., Taylor, J., Browne, J., Ferguson, S., Atchan, M., Maher, P., Homer, C. S., & Davis, D. (2020). The future in their hands: Graduating student midwives' plans, job satisfaction and the desire to work in midwifery continuity of care. *Women and Birth: Journal of the Australian College of Midwives, 33*(1), e59–66. https://doi.org/10.1016/j.wombi.2018.11.011

Grimes, D. A., & Schulz, K. F. (2002). An overview of clinical research: The lay of the land. *The Lancet, 359*, 57–61.

Hogh, A., Baernholdt, M., & Clausen, T. (2018). Impact of workplace bullying on missed nursing care and quality of care in the eldercare sector. *International Archives of Occupational & Environmental Health, 91*(8), 963–70. https://doi.org/10.1007/s00420-018-1337-0

Kim, K., & Lee, I. (2020). Medication error encouragement training: A quasi-experimental study. *Nurse Education Today, 84.* https://doi.org/10.1016/j.nedt.2019.104250

Kuriakose, S., Kaima, R. S., Cherian, V., & Peter, P. (2020). Comparison of incidence of acute respiratory infection in exclusively breastfed infants and not exclusively breastfed infants from 61 to 180 days of age: A prospective cohort study. *Journal of Family Medicine and Primary Care, 9*, 2823-2829.

Marques, A., Pinho, C., De Francesco, S., Martins, P., Neves, J., & Oliveira, A. (2020). A randomized controlled trial of respiratory physiotherapy in lower respiratory tract infections. *Respiratory Medicine, 162.* https://doi.org/10.1016/j.rmed.2019.105861

Melnyk, B. M., & Fineout-Overholt, E. (2011). *Evidence-based practice in nursing & healthcare: A guide to best practice*. Philadelphia, PA: Wolters Kluwer/Lippincott Williams & Wilkins.

Miller, C. J., Smith, S. N., & Pugatcha, M. (2020). Experimental and quasi-experimental designs in implementation research. *Psychiatry Research, 283*.

Mongkuo, M. Y., & Quantrell, S. (2015). The influence of excessive alcohol consumption, gender, age, enrollment status and academic class on risky sexual behavior among predominantly black college students. *Public Health and Preventive Medicine, 1*(4), 144–52.

National Health and Medical Research Council (NHMRC). (2009). NHMRC levels of evidence and grades for recommendations for developers of clinical practice guidelines. https://www.nhmrc.gov.au/_files_nhmrc/file/guidelines/developers/nhmrc_levels_grades_evidence_120423.pdf

National Statement. (2007). *National Statement on Ethical Conduct in Human Research*. National Health and Medical Research Council Act 1992. NHMRC.

Rattray, J. E., Lauder, W., Ludwick, R., Johnstone, C., Zeller, R., Winchell, J., Myers, E., & Smith, A. (2011). Indicators of acute deterioration in adult patients nursed in acute care wards: A factorial survey. *Journal of Clinical Nursing, 20*, 723–32.

Rosen, E., & Tsesis, I. (2016). Classifying scientific evidence as the basis for evidence-based decision making: Is strength of evidence absolute? *Evidence-Based Endodontics, 1*, 5. https://doi.org/10.1186/s41121-016-0005-7

Roulin, M., Jonniaux, S., Guisado, H., & Séchaud, L. (2020). Perceptions of inpatients and nurses towards the importance of nurses' caring behaviours in rehabilitation: A comparative study. *International Journal of Nursing Practice, 26*(4), 1.

Saunders, H., & Vehvilainen-Julkunen, K. (2017). Nurses' evidence-based practice beliefs and the role of evidence-based practice mentors at university hospitals in Finland. *Worldviews on Evidence-Based Nursing, 14*(1), 35. https://doi.org/10.1111/wvn.12189

Savoia, E., Argentini, G., Gori, D., Neri, E., Piltch-Loeb, R., & Fantini, M. P. (2020). Factors associated with access and use of PPE during COVID-19: A cross-sectional study of Italian physicians. *PLoS ONE, 15*(10): e0239024. https://doi.org/10.1371/journal.pone.0239024

Setia, M. S. (2016). Methodology series module 1: Cohort studies. *Indian Journal of Dermatology, 61*(1): 21–5. https://doi.org/10.4103/0019-5154.174011

Sullivan, G. M. (2011). Getting off the 'gold standard': Randomized controlled trials and education research. *Journal of Graduate Medical Education, 3*(3), 285–9. https://doi.org/10.4300/JGME-D-11-00147.1

White, J., Hemingway, S., & Stephenson, J. (2014). Training mental health nurses to assess the physical health needs of mental health service users: A pre- and post-test analysis. *Perspectives in Psychiatric Care, 50*(4), 243–50.

FURTHER READING

Bandyopadhyay, M., Markovic, M., & Manderson, L. (2007). Women's perspectives of pain following day surgery in Australia. *Australian Journal of Advanced Nursing, 24*(4), 19–23.

Casey, D., & Murphy, K. (2009). Issues in using methodological triangulation in research. *Nurse Researcher, 16*(4), 40–55.

Catchpole, K., De Leval, M., McEwan, A., Pigott, N., Elliot, M., McQuillan, A., MacDonald, C., & Goldman, A. (2007). Patient handover from surgery to intensive care: Using Formula 1 pit-stop and aviation models to improve safety and quality. *Pediatric Anesthesia, 17*, 470–8.

Dixon, L., Aimer, P., Fletcher, L., Guilland, K., & Hendry, G. (2009). Smoke free outcomes with midwife lead maternity carers: An analysis of smoking during pregnancy from the New Zealand College of Midwives Midwifery database 2004–2007. *New Zealand College of Midwives, 40*, 13–19.

Erci, B. (2011). The effectiveness of the Omaha System intervention on the women's health promotion lifestyle profile and quality of life. *Journal of Advanced Nursing, 68*(4), 898–907.

Gaffney, K., Douglas, C., Henry, L., & Goldberg, P. (2008). Tobacco use triggers for mothers of infants: Implications for pediatric nursing practice. *Pediatric Nursing, 34*(3), 253–8.

Gray, B., Robinson, C., Seddon, D., & Roberts, A. (2008). Confidentiality smokescreens and carers for people with mental health problems: The perspectives of professionals. *Health and Social Care in the Community, 16*(4), 378–87.

Health Knowledge. (2017). Introduction to study designs – cohort studies. https://www.healthknowledge.org.uk/e-learning/epidemiology/practitioners/introduction-study-design-cs

McGahee, T. W., & Tingen, M. S. (2009). The use of the Solomon four-group design in nursing research. *Southern Online Journal of Nursing Research, 9*(1). Retrieved from http://www.resourcenter.net/images/snrs/files/sojnrarticles2/Vol09Num01Art14.html

Messina, D., Scott, D., Driscoll, A., Ganey, R., & Pinto Zipp, G. (2009). The relationship between patient satisfaction and inpatient admission across teaching and non-teaching hospitals. *Journal of Healthcare Management, 54*(3), 77–190.

Panjari, M., Bell, R., Adams, J., Morrow, C., Papalia, M., Astbury, J., & Davis, S. (2008). Methodology and challenges to recruitment to a randomized, double-blind, placebo-controlled trial of oral DHEA in postmenopausal women. *Journal of Women's Health, 17*(10), 1559–69.

Wong, E., Sung, R., Leung, T. F., Wong, Y., Li, A., Cheung, K. L., Wong, C. K., Fok, T. F., & Leung, P. C. (2009). Randomized, double-blind, placebo-controlled trial of herbal therapy for children with asthma. *Journal of Alternative and Complementary Medicine, 15*(10), 1091–7.

Chapter learning objectives

The material presented in this chapter will assist you to:

1   describe the various types of data and scales of measurement
2   manage the data and products of analysis
3   understand the difference between descriptive and inferential statistics
4   explain probability and hypothesis testing
5   understand how to compare groups for statistical differences and associations.

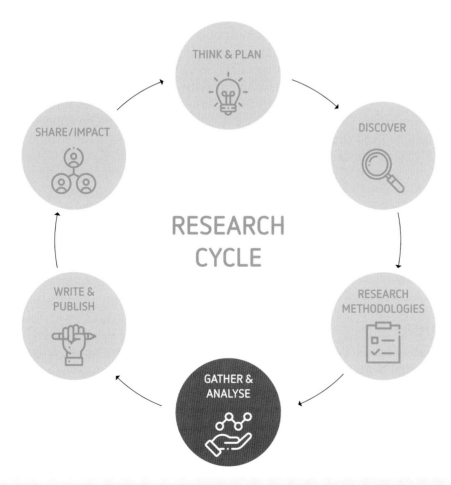

Research cycle

The primary focus of this chapter is analysis of quantitative data. This is a key component of collecting and analysing data, as highlighted in the research cycle above.

Introduction

The purpose of this chapter is to present broad principles of data management and beginning concepts applicable to the analysis of quantitative data. Whether conducting quantitative research or reading about it, knowledge about quantitative data analysis is necessary. Understanding statistics is also essential because researchers use them routinely to present information about quantitative data.

Data come in many forms: numbers, words, even objects. It is important to know what type of data will be managed as a researcher because this will determine how analysis will be carried out and how answers to the research question may or may not be found.

Types of data and scales of measurement

Data occurs in two broad groups – qualitative and quantitative. Within these two groups there are a number of subgroups (Gray, Grove & Sutherland, 2017; Polit & Beck, 2014. Qualitative data can be ordinal or nominal, and numeric data can be discrete or continuous. A scale is a 'measuring stick' or standard reference for comparison of measurements between cases. Measurement is the assignment of numbers or codes to observations of phenomena, and different types of data are measured on different scales. It is important to know exactly what type of data are being collecting and the scale that will be used to measure the variable because this will determine what type of data analysis can be carried out.

Cases

In a research project, every participant is a case. That is, in a study of drug taking among teenage girls, for example, every teenage girl in the research study is a case. But cases do not always consist of data about people. They might consist of data about hospitals, plots of land or streets.

Variables

The information for each case – the person's name and the amount of drugs taken per day – are referred to as 'variables' because their nature varies from case to case. Because not all research is about people, some variables might relate to other types of cases, such as the number of bike accidents, amount of rainfall or number of carjackings in the last year.

Data

The value of a variable for a particular case is referred to as a *datum* (singular); the values for all cases in a sample are referred to as *data* (plural). Data refer to the actual measurements taken, or information collected during the research.

FOR EXAMPLE

TYPES OF QUANTITATIVE AND NUMERICAL DATA

There are four broad types of quantitative or numerical data.

1 **Nominal data** are observable and not measurable; for example, gender, hair colour or state of residency. Objects or people are assigned to categories that may be given a numerical value.

2 **Ranked (ordinal) data** can be ranked in order from first to last in some way. The term usually refers to variables that cannot be measured precisely but can be compared with one another in order to rank them. The scale of measurement used in the collection of these types of data are ordinal. It lends itself to ranking data in some kind of order for a variable. It is the order of the values that is important and significant. For example:
   How do you feel today?
   a   Very unhappy
   b   Unhappy
   c   Okay
   d   Happy
   e   Very happy

3 **Discrete (interval) data** is often obtained in response to questions that relate to quantity (how many). Each datum is a whole number that cannot be broken down into fractions as it is being counted. The scale of measurement used in the collection of this type of data is discrete – it lends itself to the collection of whole number data for a variable. Time is a good example of an interval scale, as it is a measurement of a temperature using a thermometer.

4 **Ratio (continuous) data** can be measured on a scale from zero to infinity, with every possible graduation in between and a potentially unlimited number of decimal places. Each datum can be represented in decimal form or fractions of whole numbers. The scale of measurement used in the collection of this type of data is continuous – it lends itself to the collection of very accurate data for a variable. Height and weight are examples of ratio variables.

Levels of measurement

As we move from categorical measures through interval to ratio scales, there is an increasing amount of definiteness about the relationship between any datum and another. This gives rise to the concept of levels of measurement, with categorical measures as the lowest and ratio scales as the highest.

The mathematical basis of statistical procedures depends on assumptions about the relationship between variable values. More precise or powerful statistical procedures are appropriate for data collected using higher levels of measurement.

The type of data-analysis procedure used depends on the type of measurement procedure used. Data-analysis procedures become more powerful as measurement procedures become more precise.

As data progresses along a continuum of precision, potential analyses progress along a continuum of power (see Table 6.1).

▶ Table 6.1   Data progressing along a continuum of precision

Precision ranking	Level of measurement	Highest level of potential analysis
1	Ratio (continuous)	Parametric statistics
2	Interval (discrete)	Parametric statistics
3	Ordinal (ranked)	Non-parametric statistics
4	Nominal (categorical)	Descriptive statistics
5	Qualitative	Qualitative

As measurement becomes more precise, analysis becomes more sophisticated and more powerful. Parametric tests are based on assumptions about the distribution of the underlying population from which the sample was taken.

Parametric data are data that have come from variables that are based on measurable population characteristics or variables that have a distribution in the given population of interest and that were measured at least on a variable scale. A parameter is a measurement across a population. If the data deviate strongly from the assumptions of a parametric procedure, using the parametric procedure could lead to incorrect conclusions. If it is determined that the assumptions of the parametric procedure are not valid, an analogous non-parametric procedure is used instead. The parametric assumption of normality is particularly worrisome for small sample sizes ($n < 30$). Non-parametric tests are often a good option for these data. Generally, data must be at least at the interval level of measurement and have some sort of distribution before they can be subjected to parametric analysis techniques.

Non-parametric tests do not rely on assumptions about the shape or parameters of the underlying population distribution. Some things are considered to be measurable only in non-parametric forms; that is, they have no distribution. Non-parametric procedures generally have less power for the same sample size than the corresponding parametric procedure if the data truly are normal. Interpretation of non-parametric procedures can also be more difficult than for parametric procedures.

FOR EXAMPLE

LEVELS OF MEASUREMENT

Research conducted on cigarette-smoking behaviour may be possible to collect data across all five levels of measurement, as follows.

Qualitative level of measurement
Why do you continue to smoke cigarettes?

Nominal level of measurement
Please indicate which of the following symptoms you experience by ticking the appropriate boxes:
- ❑ persistent cough
- ❑ poor circulation to feet, legs and/or hands
- ❑ high blood pressure
- ❑ sleep problems.

Ordinal level of measurement
Please rank (from 1 to 7) the importance of the following concerns you have for your own health:
- ❑ diet
- ❑ weight
- ❑ cigarette smoking
- ❑ alcohol
- ❑ exercise and activity
- ❑ sleep
- ❑ stress.

Discrete (interval) level of measurement
Please indicate the number of days per week on average on which you smoke:

Continuous (ratio) level of measurement
Please record your lung vital capacity (in litres) as measured by vitalograph:

ACTIVITY

Write a question that would require data to be provided about someone's weight according to each of the following levels of measurement:
- qualitative
- nominal
- ordinal
- interval
- ratio.

Managing data and products of analysis
Logging the data

It is extremely important to keep good records of data. Coding data in a code book enables the study to be repeated and validated. For more detail on the construction of code books, see Gray, Grove and Sutherland (2017), *Burns and Grove's The Practice of Nursing Research: Appraisal, Synthesis, and Generation of Evidence.*

See Figure 6.1 for the steps in logging data.

It is important to note that the main purpose of storing data is to enable investigation of fraud should that become necessary.

TIP

It is preferable to store data on a secure drive that is consistent with the responsibilities of the researchers outlined in the Australian Code for the Responsible Conduct of Research 2018 (Australian Research Council, 2019).

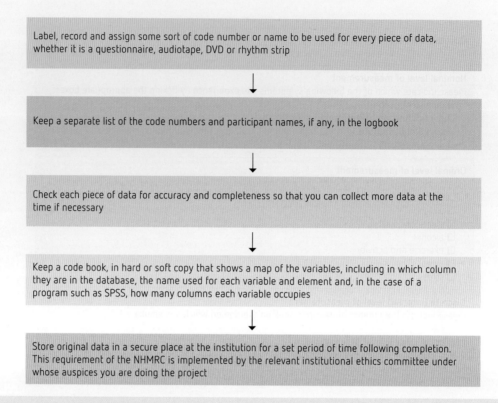

> ▸ **Figure 6.1** Steps in logging data

Source: Lloyd Sealey Library (2017). How to: Write a literature review: Writing a literature review. Retrieved from http://guides.lib. jjay.cuny.edu/c.php?g=322839&p=2162061.

Processing data for analysis

Capturing the data

Some data that have already been put into a computer may not require any further preparation. If, for example, using a database that has been put into a computer already, the researcher only needs to transfer the data into their own program for analysis. Similarly, some researchers can enter their data straight into a portable computer in the field or laboratory directly from an instrument that is hooked up to the computer, or by means of the data collector keying the data into the computer. Questionnaires that have been prepared and responded to in such a way that they can be directly scanned into a computer likewise do not need any further preparation. Gray, Grove and Sutherland (2017) provide a useful discussion of the issues concerning electronic scanning.

If the data involve voice recordings, most researchers prefer to have these transcribed before analysing the data, particularly if they are analysing the meaning of the text. Transcription can be done by the researcher, a research assistant or a keyboard operator who has the requisite skills. If using video recordings, they will need to be edited and the video clips identified using a coding system.

Coding the data

Most questionnaires require some coding. This is the process that usually renders the data into numbers that can be entered into the database in a form in which they can be easily analysed. Data can range from open-ended questionnaires that require a lot of researcher coding to precoded questionnaires that require minimal coding. A precoded questionnaire is easy to produce; however, there is a limited choice of answers.

FOR EXAMPLE

PRECODED QUESTIONNAIRE

On a precoded questionnaire, the respondent must tick one of four boxes (numbered 1 to 4) to answer a question. The researcher enters the number into that person's data entry for that question. An example of a precoded questionnaire is: 'How many hours each week do you spend on study?'

1	1–3 hours	☐
2	4–6 hours	☐
3	7–9 hours	☐
4	more than 10 hours	☐

Actual numbers (e.g. the person's age in years) do not need to be coded. Sometimes data will be from open-ended questions on questionnaires or from text for content analysis. If the researcher wishes to quantify these data, they will have to develop a coding schema to handle it.

The process of coding can be done in either of the following ways.

- Code directly from the data source. With questionnaires, some people like to write the code on each questionnaire, while some prefer to code straight into the computer. The amount of transformation of data required depends on how the questionnaire has been constructed in the first place. If it is precoded by putting the numbers on the questionnaire, then there is little coding to do at this stage.
- Code the data onto a coding sheet and then enter it into the database from the coding sheet.

Each of these methods has advantages and disadvantages. Coding directly from the data source is faster and avoids transcription errors that arise from the double handling of the data, but it is more prone to data-entry errors. The coding sheet method speeds up the data entry process and increases its accuracy, but is more prone to errors of transcription during the coding process.

> **TIP**
> Use participant numbers, not the database row numbers. If you use the latter and sort the data, the database numbers will not change with the data.

Direct data entry

If coding is entered straight into the electronic file, it will need to be set it up first so that it will accept the data. A database file is usually a matrix of rows and columns that intersect to form cells. Each row of the matrix is one person's data, while each column is one variable or answer to one question of the questionnaire. Thus, reading across a row will detail a participant's data, while reading down a column will display every person's data on that one variable. Head each of the columns with the variable name or its abbreviation to make it easier to recognise the variable. In addition, at the beginning of the row, always put a participant number that is also on the raw data.

All programs will need to be instructed on what the variable names are and what the values of the elements that comprise the variables are; for example, '1' equals 'Never married' and so forth. Some data-analysis programs allows keying in the actual element name or part of it, such as 'n' for 'Never married', 'm' for 'Married', 'di' for 'Divorced', 'de' for 'De facto' and so on. However, even though they are typed in as names and they appear as names on the monitor, the computer stores them as numbers. It is useful to have a logical structure for the element labels of the variables; for example, yes = 1, no = 0. This will help later in interpreting the data correctly. It is particularly important where the variable has an underlying numerical structure, such as the Likert Scale. In order to avoid errors in data entry, it is vital to keep to the same code as a precoded questionnaire when entering data. If necessary, the data can be recoded later. An example of a printout from a database is shown in Table 6.2.

▶ Table 6.2   Printout of data in database

Participant	Gender	Age	Marital status	Religion	Education
1	M	30	Married	Prot	Yr 10
2	F	25	Nevmar	RC	Yr 12
3	F	43	Div	Prot	Yr 12
4	F	64	Nevmar	Buddhist	Uni deg
5	M	36	De facto	Prot	TAFE cert/dip
6	M	29	Div	Nil	Yr 10
7	F	21	Nevmar	Muslim	Yr 12
8	M	19	Married	Nil	Uni deg
9	M	53	De facto	RC	Yr 12

Once the data file is set up in the computer, data can be entered. This is part of the drudgery of research, but it is necessary to ensure the data entered onto the spreadsheet is correct.

Using coding sheets

If using a separate coding sheet, it is very important for ease of transfer that it is the same structure as the computer file into which the data will be entered. A blank coding sheet would look like the printout shown in Table 6.2, only without data in it.

It is crucial to check the finished coding sheet against the raw data. If there is only a small amount, then check it all. If there is a large amount, check 10 per cent at random. If it is error-free, assume that the rest will probably be too.

What the researcher needs to ensure

- *Ensure that data coding and data entry are consistent:* changes can occur in the data because the data coder changed the code part way through coding or direct data entry. Resist this, but if it happens, the previous coding will have to be rectified so that it is consistent with the new code.
- *Ensure that data coding and data entry are accurate:* if, for example, there are complicated procedures that require special care during coding and entry, check even more carefully.

In, say, a long questionnaire, the order of items may be reversed in half of the copies to control for respondent fatigue. Extreme caution must be exercised to make sure that all the answers to each item are in the correct column. The accuracy rate should be one that can be worked with, but it must be at least 90 per cent.

- *Missing values are a problem and occur where, for some reason, the data are missing:* let's say that a respondent has not given an answer to a question. If a whole section of data is consistently missing, none of it can be entered. If collecting data on each of the three days following childbirth and most of the mothers have gone home on the second day, delete all data for the third day.
- Some data-analysis programs have a mechanism for handling missing values that gives them a code or does not use that case in the data analysis. If the variable is numerical, it is important not to put zero for a missing value as this will lower the value of the mean. Either leave it missing or put in the median value.

After the data have been entered into the computer, it is extremely important to proofread them. Follow the process shown in Figure 6.2.

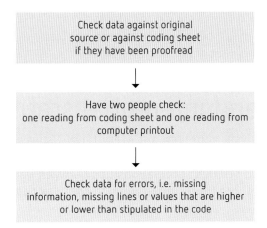

▸ **Figure 6.2** Ensuring the data are correct

ACTIVITY

Design a spreadsheet with columns and rows, in which each column represents a variable and each row represents a participant. Think of four demographic variables (e.g. age, gender, residence and income) and four health variables (e.g. chronic illness, smoking, alcohol use and body mass index) that could be entered into this spreadsheet. What kinds of codes might be necessary to enter these variables?

TIP

Always keep backup master copies of the original computer data as well as the working copy of the transformed data.

Manipulating data

During the process of data analysis, it is almost always the case that there is a need to change the data in some way. This can involve such operations as combining variables, recoding variables to change the values, applying a weighting to a variable and/or applying mathematical formulae. Double-check that the conversion has been done correctly by checking the input with the output. If these operations have been carried out incorrectly, the data will be meaningless. Whenever data is changed, it is vital to note this in the logbook or record it in some other way. Do not rely on memory. When any changes are completed, a fresh backup copy should be made and renamed or renumber the file. Older versions of the data should be kept in an archive, either electronically or as hard copy.

Managing products of data analysis

When generating the data analysis, organise it in some way. A data-analysis program will generate the analysis. Most programs generate output files that can be saved on the computer, or create a word-processed file and copy the data analysis into it. These methods allow organisation of the data analysis. The data analysis should then be saved and a hard copy printed. The word-processed file can also serve as a backup if the hard copy is lost.

Store a hard copy of the data analysis systematically.

Descriptive and inferential statistics

In quantitative data analysis, numbers are everything. Using numbers, it is possible to describe amounts, proportions and patterns in the data. Hypotheses may be tested by investigating the type and strength of relationships between variables. Quantitative data analysis can produce anything from simple sums to complex three-dimensional patterns.

Statistics

A *statistic* is a summary description of information gathered through observation or measurement. Or, to put it another way, it is a numerical summary of a phenomenon. Quantitative analysis is done to generate statistics.

Statistics can be found everywhere. Some statistics, such as those that count the number of people with measles in a population, are simple. Others are quite intricate, such as those that determine the statistical likelihood of high blood pressure causing a heart attack, among all the other known factors to be risk factors.

Data-analysis software is used to carry out statistical operations and enable researchers to analyse data and generate statistics without the drudgery of knowing statistical formulae and how they work. But to carry out the data analysis, it is necessary to be able to understand the language of statistics.

Descriptive statistics

Descriptive statistics are the analysis of data that help describe or summarise data, but that do not allow for conclusions or predictions. In writing up the results of a research project, the researcher will probably want to describe the characteristics of the group or the subgroups that comprise the group.

We will now look at some statistics that describe and summarise data.

Sums

Frequently, the total of something is required; for example, the number of patients that are in a hospital or come to a clinic. To find out, all the elements are counted to calculate the sum of each variable.

Suppose that you want to test a hypothesis that patients in the respiratory clinic where you work are more likely to be heavy smokers than light smokers or non-smokers. By completing a chart audit, the following information for all patients attending the clinic could be captured (see Table 6.3).

▶ Table 6.3   Number of clients who are heavy, light and non-smokers

Heavy	Light	Non	Heavy	Heavy
Non	Non	Light	Heavy	Non
Light	Heavy	Heavy	Light	Light
Heavy	Non	Heavy	Light	Heavy
Heavy	Light	Heavy	Heavy	Light
Light	Heavy	Non	Light	Heavy
Heavy	Heavy	Light	Non	Light
Heavy	Light	Heavy	Light	Heavy
Light	Heavy	Non	Light	Non
Heavy	Non	Light	Light	Non

By counting, it can be established that there were 50 patients who attended the clinic, a statistic that is often given by the computer program in the course of other statistical analysis. It is also possible to find out about the numbers in the different categories of smoking. To get this information, count the numbers of patients in the different categories to calculate the sum or total of heavy smokers to be 21, light smokers 18 and non-smokers 11. This will identify that on the day data was collected, more heavy smokers than light smokers or non-smokers were seen.

Percentages

A percentage is the proportion out of 100 that a group comprises. A percentage is obtained by taking the number, dividing it by the number of elements in the group and multiplying by 100. The beauty of a percentage is that it enables comparisons of groups. It is not possible to meaningfully compare a raw number of one group with a raw number in another group if the totals of the groups are different.

To establish what proportion of clients is in each of the three categories of smokers, as shown in Table 6.3, work out the percentage of the total clients in each category. By dividing each total by 50 and multiplying by 100, it will show that the proportion of heavy smokers is 42 per cent, the proportion of light smokers is 36 per cent and the proportion of non-smokers is 22 per cent. In the same way, it is possible to calculate that the proportion of smokers is 78 per cent.

Frequency distributions

The statistical program can generate the number and percentage of each subgroup by generating a statistic called a 'frequency distribution table'. This is a description of the components in a group that identifies the number and percentage of elements in each subgroup of the main group. A frequency distribution statistic can also be used to generate histograms and pie charts by computer.

The frequency distribution table for the client data will look something like Table 6.4. This table identifies that there are 11 non-smokers, who comprise 22 per cent of the group; 18 light smokers, who comprise 36 per cent of the group; and 21 heavy smokers, who comprise 42 per cent of the group.

▶ Table 6.4   Frequency distribution table for clients who are heavy, light and non-smokers

Bar	Element	Count	Percentage
1	Non	11	22
2	Light	18	36
3	Heavy	21	42

Using graphics to show sums and percentages

In a research report or article, it is possible to show categorical information more dramatically by means of a graphic illustration or figure called a histogram or bar graph. People use graphics to illustrate points in reporting information about data because graphics are easier to interpret than tables, which validates the old saying that a picture is worth a thousand words.

Histograms and bar graphs

Histograms and bar graphs are figures that show the numbers in groups as vertical columns or horizontal rows, which allows for easy comparison of groups. The largest group will have the longest column or bar and the smallest group will have the shortest. A bar graph shows discrete categories, such as types of injuries, while a histogram shows numbers in different categories of a range, such as income groups. In a bar graph there will be space between the bars, while in a histogram there is no space. Figure 6.3 shows a bar graph of the example group of clients broken down into its subgroups of heavy, light and non-smokers.

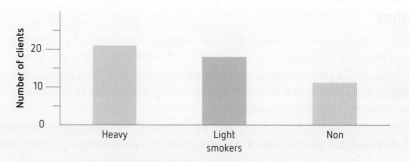

▶ Figure 6.3   Bar graph showing number of clients who are heavy, light and non-smokers

Pie charts

A pie chart is another kind of figure that shows the proportions of subgroups in a group. It divides the total pie into its components, again enabling ease of comparison. Figure 6.4 shows a pie chart of the client data.

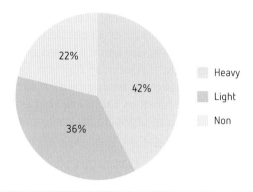

▶ **Figure 6.4** Pie chart showing clients who are heavy, light and non-smokers as percentages of the group

Tables

A table is one of the most common tools that a researcher uses to analyse data. It is a meaningful presentation of numbers in rows and columns. Columns are the vertical arrangement of like numbers, and rows are the horizontal arrangement of like numbers. The intersection of a column and a row is called a cell. Each number will appear in a column and in a row, or a cell.

By analysing the clients in the clinic at the present time, a snapshot has been taken of the data to see whether the hypothesis has any potential for a conclusion. However, conclusion cannot be based on data recorded on only one day, in case that day was atypical. Obtain data for a more extended period. Take a random sample of one day per month and examine all the clients on those specific days, and then organise the data into a table showing the numbers of each group of smokers and non-smokers for each of the days that have been examined. Then construct a table (as shown in Table 6.5) using the numbers that have been obtained.

▶ **Table 6.5** Table showing number, by month, of clients who are heavy, light and non-smokers

Month	Heavy	Light	Non	Total
January	21	18	11	50
February	18	9	8	35
March	14	10	6	30
April	19	14	10	43
May	20	9	15	44
June	7	6	3	16
July	9	6	7	22
August	10	6	9	25
September	11	9	9	29
October	15	9	6	30
November	16	16	12	44
December	15	7	10	32
Total	175	119	106	400
Total as %	44	30	26	100

The raw data shows that there were 400 clients seen on the 12 selected days. Of these, 175, or 44 per cent, were heavy smokers; 119, or 30 per cent, were light smokers; and 106, or 26 per cent, were non-smokers. This is the same pattern that was seen for the one day in January, so it can be concluded that the January day was typical. To see whether each day was typical, calculate the percentage for each group for each of the 12 days. After this is done, construct another table (as shown in Table 6.6) that enables a comparison of the percentages of types of smokers and non-smokers for each month.

▶Table 6.6   Table of percentages, by month, of clients who are smokers and non-smokers

Month	Heavy (%)	Light (%)	Non (%)
January	42	36	22
February	50	27	23
March	48	33	19
April	42	30	24
May	45	20	35
June	48	30	22
July	41	29	30
August	38	25	37
September	40	30	30
October	50	30	20
November	36	36	28
December	48	22	30

Notice that the percentages were not worked out first and then the average calculated from them. For example, 48 per cent for heavy smokers, instead of the 44 per cent calculated from the totals. The reason for this apparent discrepancy is that averaging the percentages gives each month's result the same weight or importance. In our example, the results for January are four times as significant as those for June because we had four times as many observations. It is crucial to look at the raw data before transposing them to percentages, otherwise there is a risk of drawing conclusions that misrepresent what happened. The information in the table of percentages can also be shown in graphic form (see Figure 6.5).

The graph shows that on every day examined, the percentage of clients who were heavy smokers was equal to or greater than each of the other groups, though there is some fluctuation when different months are considered. The first day measured in January may have had a high proportion of heavy smokers compared with the other days. To find out how typical it was, look at what the general picture is. This is explored further in the next section.

Measures of central tendency

Measures of central tendency are the mean, median and mode – statistics that let us see what the most common scores in a group are and how the group did as a whole.

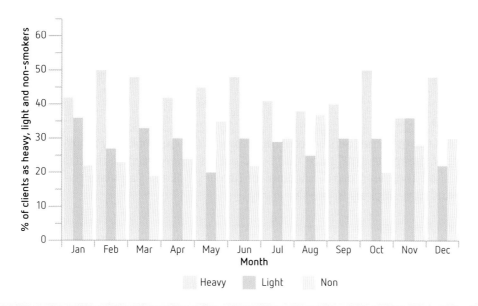

▸ **Figure 6.5** The percentages, by month, of clients who were heavy, light and non-smokers

The mean

The mean score of a group is the average.

To continue our example, it would be helpful to compare the findings for January with the findings for the entire year. This would tell us whether January was a typical month for the percentages of subgroups of clients. To do this, calculate the average, or mean, percentage for the year for each subgroup, which, in this example, means that the total number of clients seen is divided by the number of days, or 400/12 = 33:

- heavy smokers comprised (175/12 = 15)/33 = 44 per cent
- light smokers comprised (118/12)/33 = 30 per cent
- non-smokers comprised (106/12)/33 = 26 per cent.

Now compare each month's percentage with the mean or average percentage and see how typical it was. January's figures were:

- heavy smokers = 42 per cent
- light smokers = 36 per cent
- non-smokers = 22 per cent.

It can be concluded, then, that January's figures were a bit over the average for heavy smokers but under the average for light smokers and non-smokers.

The median

Another useful measure of central tendency is the median. This is the score in the middle. For an odd number of scores, the middle one is the median. For an even number of scores, the median is the average of the two middle ones. In the case of heavy smokers, if the data were rearranged from least to most score, they would look like this:

36, 38, 40, 41, 42, 44, 45, 48, 48, 48, 50, 50.

TIP

Obtain the mean by taking the sum of the elements and dividing it by the number of elements in the group.

Since this set of figures comprises an even number (there are 12 months in a year), the median would be the average of 44 and 45, the two middle scores, or 44.5. In this case, the mean and the median are very close.

Calculate the median of the light smokers and non-smokers in a similar fashion.

The mode

The mode is the most frequently occurring score. In the case of heavy smokers, it can easily be seen that the mode is 48 since that score occurs three times in the dataset. The mode is higher than the mean or the median for heavy smokers. Calculate the mode for light smokers and non-smokers in the same way.

Measures of variability

Sometimes it is required to see how the figures are distributed in a group of scores. Measures of variability help to do this.

The range

The range is a number that reflects the spread of the scores. It is obtained by subtracting the lowest score from the highest score. To follow our example, the highest number of heavy smokers is 50 and the lowest number is 36, so the range is 50 − 36 = 14.

Standard deviation

The standard deviation is a number that is calculated from the data to show the amount of dispersion of the data.

In the temperature dataset in Figure 6.6, the mean is 37°C and the standard deviation is 1. This means that one-third of the temperatures lie between 36°C and 37°C and another third lie between 37°C and 38°C, or two-thirds are between 36°C and 38°C. If the data are normally distributed, then another 14 per cent are between two standard deviations above and below the mean, so that 96 per cent are between 35°C and 39°C.

If the temperatures were more tightly clustered about the mean, the standard deviation would be low. In Figure 6.6, you can see that there are a lot of people with a temperature on or around the mean temperature of 37°C, whereas there are very few people with extreme temperatures.

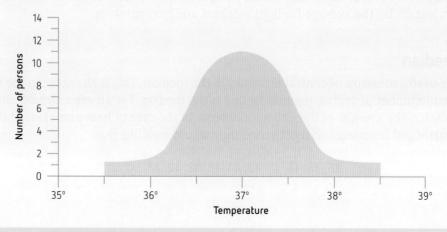

▶ **Figure 6.6** Graph showing temperature, low standard deviation

The standard deviation of these temperatures is 0.6 of a degree. This means that one-third of the observations fall between 36.4°C and 37°C and another third fall between 37°C and 37.6°C and so forth.

If the temperatures were more spread out, the area graph would look like Figure 6.7.

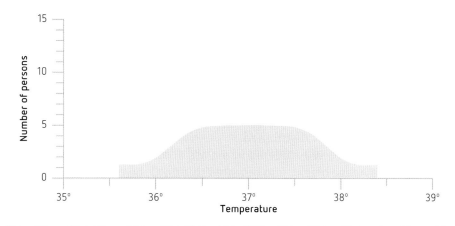

▶ **Figure 6.7** Graph showing temperature, high standard deviation

It can see that there are fewer people with temperatures on or around the mean and more at the extreme temperatures. The standard deviation for this set of data would be higher than the previous example because the temperatures are more dispersed.

Statistical inference

Inferential statistics make it possible for the researcher to arrive at conclusions and predict changes that may occur regarding the area of concern. If a sample is representative of the total population (i.e. it has similar overall characteristics to the total population of interest), inferences can be made about the population from our sample data and the statistics produced from it, such as the average number of cigarettes smoked per day. The process of statistical inference underpins the entire research process in most traditional approaches to health research, and it depends on good sampling and good measurement.

Probability and hypothesis testing

Sampling distributions

The concept of sampling distributions refers to the characteristics of the curve which could be plotted from the means of sets of measurements taken from all possible samples of a population. It is the sampling distribution that underpins most of the techniques used in the statistical analysis of data. Sampling distributions tend to have certain key characteristics and this chapter will deal with a number of these characteristics.

TIP

To use inferential statistics with any validity, base the data on a random sample.

Central limit theorem

All procedures that use **inferential statistics** are based on the assumption that the data being used are based on a random sample taken from the population and is therefore representative of the population data.

Naturally, it is quite possible to draw a number of different random samples from a population and end up with data that are not identical from one sample to the next. In fact, if an infinite number of random samples was drawn and the mean of each was taken, the range of sample means would follow a normal distribution. This phenomenon is known as the **central limit theorem**.

The important thing about the central limit theorem is that it applies to the mean of an infinite number of samples, not to the actual distribution of the parameter in the population. Very few things are normally distributed in nature, but the mean of an infinite number of samples is normally distributed.

If, for example, there are 100 students in a class and one took samples of 10 students and measured their average height, and repeated this until the possible combinations of 10 students were exhausted, there would be millions of average heights. If these were plotted on a curve, it would represent a normal or bell-shaped curve as shown in Figure 6.8.

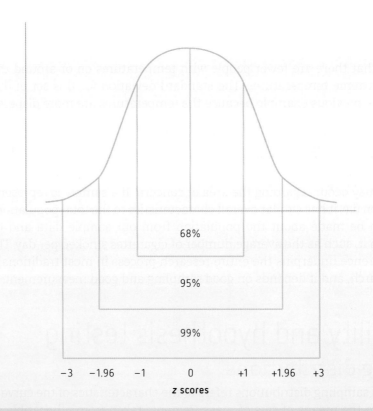

▶ Figure 6.8   A normal curve

A normal sampling distribution has the following characteristics:
- 68 per cent of scores will fall between one standard deviation either side of the mean
- 95 per cent of scores will fall between 1.96 standard deviations either side of the mean
- 99 per cent of scores will fall between three standard deviations either side of the mean.

The total area under the curve represents the total population of possible values for the variable being examined.

It is possible to determine how many standard deviations from the mean a value is by calculating a z *score*. This shows how many standard deviations above or below the mean the value is. The formula for calculating a z score is:

$$z = y - x \div s$$

where y = the value under consideration, x = the mean of the distribution and s = the standard deviation of the distribution.

A z score of 1 means that a score is exactly one standard deviation above the mean.

The probability of a sample mean having a particular value, or z score (z), which falls between two possible values (a and b) is equal to the area under the curve between the two values (where the total area under the curve is taken as 1.0). The value of this probability is automatically calculated by computerised statistics programs. The calculation of z scores is one of the techniques used when inferential statistics are applied to a set of data. Figure 6.9 represents how probability is derived from sampling distributions.

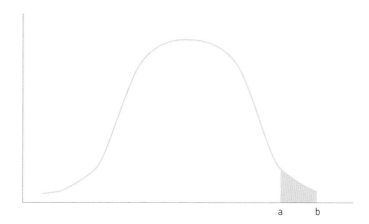

▸**Figure 6.9** Probability and the sampling distribution

Checking sample representativeness

It is possible to calculate the standard error of a sample mean to determine how representative a sample is or to estimate the extent that a sample might vary from the population. The standard error represents the size of a possible sampling error based on the standard deviation and size of the sample. It gives the possible variation in the mean due to sampling error. The formula for calculating the standard error is:

$$Sx = sd \div \sqrt{n}$$

where Sx = standard error of the mean, sd = standard deviation of the sample and n = size of the sample.

It can be seen that the standard error is reduced by increasing the sample size. The larger n is, the smaller Sx is.

Hypothesis testing

When a set of data is used based on a sample of the population to make inferences about the characteristics of the population, there is a certain amount of risk involved. A biased sample might have been accidentally obtained, or the sample tested at a bad time, so data will be obtained that risks making incorrect decisions about the results. Inferential statistics use the formal process of hypothesis testing to reduce this risk.

The errors that might be made have to do with whether the hypothesis was wrongly accepted or rejected. Hypotheses are usually tested by stating them in reverse as null hypotheses and trying to prove them wrong, because it is not possible to actually prove anything using statistics, but it is possible to statistically disprove something. It is not, for example, possible to prove statistically the existence of two-headed wombats if none have ever been found. It is possible to disprove the existence of two-headed wombats by taking a set of observations of a sample of wombats and counting their heads. If 100 wombats are observed to all have only one head, it can be reasonably assumed that two-headed wombats do not exist. In the same way, research hypotheses are tested as null hypotheses because it is statistically easier to disprove something than to prove it.

If the research hypothesis is that there will be a significant difference in attitudes towards drug use between students in private schools and students in state schools, then the null hypothesis would be that there will be no significant difference in attitudes towards drug use between students in private schools and students in state schools. If these attitudes are measured from two samples of children and then compared, the null hypothesis can be either accepted or rejected. The key to hypothesis testing is the fact that the samples are truly representative of the population of interest that they are drawn from.

Type I and type II errors

There are two types of error that might be made when using inferential statistics: *type I error* (alpha error) and *type II error* (beta error).

Type I error (alpha error)

A type I error occurs when it is mistakenly believed that a significant result from a statistical test has been found. In statistical procedures, a null hypothesis can be tested and wrongly rejected, leading to the acceptance of a research hypothesis that is false. It usually occurs because of poor sampling. In other words, the sample is biased in some way and the result was simply due to chance (Pallant, 2016; Saltiker & Whittaker, 2013).

A type I error is controlled by setting significance levels (p values). A p value of 0.05 means a 5 per cent probability of a type I error.

Type II error (beta error)

A type II error occurs when it is mistakenly believed that anything significant has not been found when it really does exist in the population of interest. In statistical procedures, this is usually done by accepting a null hypothesis, which leads to rejecting a research hypothesis that is true. Once again, the result was due to chance and probably based on a biased sample (Pallant, 2016; Saltiker & Whittaker, 2013). It is possible to quantify the likelihood that an error in judgement has been made using probability.

A type II error is controlled by doing power calculations and setting a power level for the study. An 80 per cent power level means an 80 per cent probability that no error has been made.

Both of these types of error are related to sample size.

Power is calculated to ensure that a sample size is large enough to find a significant difference between two or more groups, or an association between two or more variables, if such a difference or association exists in the population. Power is expressed as $1 - \beta$. A 30 per cent probability of making a type II error (β) means a 70 per cent probability of not making the error. A power value of 0.70 or better is normally acceptable in most types of research.

Level of significance

The *level of significance* of the result is the term that describes the likelihood that an error in judgement has been made regarding the result. It is expressed as a probability, such as $p < 0.01$ or $p < 0.05$, which means that the probability of an error being made is less than 1 per cent (1 in 100) or less than 5 per cent (5 in 100). Determine a level of significance whenever a statistical procedure is done to qualify whether the result is statistically significant. The usual minimum accepted level of significance is $p < 0.05$ ($p < 0.01$ or $p < 0.001$ are much more significant). Such levels of significance are based on the size of the sample used; computer statistics programs will automatically determine them for you.

EBP

A randomised controlled trial study prospectively evaluated the effectiveness of a nurse-led intensive educational program on chronic kidney failure patients with hyperphosphataemia. The results found that there were statistically significant differences between the study groups in the decline in serum phosphorus and calcium–phosphorus product levels ($p < 0.001$) and the improvement in the patients' general knowledge three months postintervention. These differences were sustained until the end of the study ($p < 0.001$) (Shi et al., 2012).

This meant that the researchers were confident that their results were statistically significant and that their findings could have occurred by chance less than 5 per cent or 1 per cent of the time in each respective type of deficit.

Degrees of freedom

An indication of sample size is obtained when calculating levels of significance and is referred to as *degrees of freedom* (usually $n = 1$, for the purpose of the calculations). It means the number of measurements that are free to vary and still give the sample the same mean score. Degrees of freedom is an important concept in the process of hypothesis testing because it affects the level of significance of a result and hence the probability that an error in judgement has been made.

The term 'degrees of freedom' is closely related to the sample size; and the sample size is closely tied to the level of significance of a result. You might, for example, correlate amount of cigarette smoking with stress and find a correlation of $r = 0.69$ (a moderately strong correlation). If your sample size was only 10 people, it would be unlikely to be statistically significant. You would have to say, then, that despite the moderate correlation, the result is not significant (because of the high probability of a type I error). If the sample size was 3000, the result would most likely be statistically significant.

One-tailed and two-tailed tests

If your research question requires you to compare for differences between two or more sets of data, you will use a procedure that determines whether there is any statistical difference between two sets of data. The level of significance you choose will enable you to determine the probability of your decision to accept or reject the hypothesis as being correct. Choosing a significance level of $p < 0.05$, for example, means that there is a less than 5 per cent probability that the result was simply due to chance.

It is necessary to identify whether your research hypothesis is directional or non-directional, which means whether you are interested in the direction of the difference or simply whether a difference exists.

FOR EXAMPLE

DIRECTIONAL DIFFERENCE

- Non-directional hypothesis: the mean blood sugar of people with diet-controlled diabetes will be no different to the mean blood sugar of people with insulin-controlled diabetes.
- Directional hypothesis: the mean blood sugar of people with diet-controlled diabetes will be lower than the mean blood sugar of people with insulin-controlled diabetes.

Recall that when the sampling distribution of the means of all the possible random samples drawn from a population is plotted, it has the characteristics of a normal curve. It is then possible to determine what the probability of a value falling between two other values under the curve is. This is done by calculating the area under the curve between the two points as a percentage of the total area under the curve. When you use a non-directional hypothesis, you want to find the probability of your result falling within the level of significance you have set for your test; in other words, whether your result falls in the area under the curve you designate as the 'rejection region', which is the area where a result forces you to reject your hypothesis.

The rejection region is defined by nominating a level of significance that is expressed as a probability. The usual levels are $p < 0.05$ and $p < 0.01$. This means that the probability of the result falling in the rejection region is 5 per cent (5 in 100) or 1 per cent (1 in 100).

When your hypothesis is non-directional, you will have a rejection region at either end of the sampling distribution. Each tail of the curve will have an area under it that is a rejection region, which is why testing a non-directional hypothesis (see **Figure 6.8**) is called a two-tailed test. When your hypothesis is directional, there will be a rejection region only under the end of the curve that relates to the direction of the hypothesis (see **Figure 6.10**), which is why testing a directional hypothesis is called a one-tailed test.

There is a range of statistical tables that automatically tabulate the probabilities of results falling in the rejection regions for a variety of inferential statistics and for one-tailed and two-tailed tests.

There are three things you need to know to test a hypothesis:

1 the size of the sample (degrees of freedom)
2 the level of significance you have set (normally, $p = 0.05$)
3 whether the hypothesis is directional or non-directional (one-tailed or two-tailed test).

A computer statistics program will determine these things for you as part of its calculations.

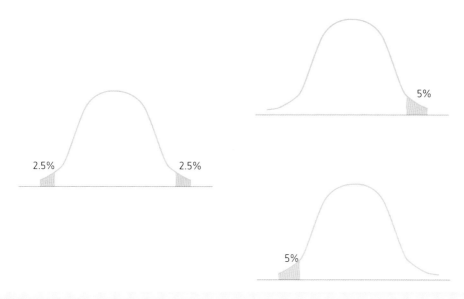

▶ **Figure 6.10** Rejection regions for one-tailed and two-tailed tests

Comparing for differences and associations

When using statistics to compare for differences (e.g. the difference in body fat between men and women) or to compare for associations (e.g. the association between dietary fat and total body fat), inferential statistics are used to determine the differences. Inferential statistics have the following characteristics; they:

- are used to make comparisons to find differences or associations between sets of data
- are used to make inferences about the population from which the sample data were extracted
- can be either parametric or non-parametric techniques.

Associations in one group

Correlation

Some research designs require the researcher to examine relationships between the characteristics of people in a group. You might want to see if postoperative pain levels were higher for clients who had high levels of preoperative anxiety than for those who had low levels. To do this, you would collect data on each person's anxiety and pain. If you had an anxiety scale and a numerical pain scale, you could investigate whether the amount of anxiety was related to, or correlated with, the amount of postoperative pain. You might expect that clients who scored high on the anxiety scale would also score high on the pain scale; however, it is possible that clients who scored low on the anxiety scale could score high on the pain scale. It is also possible that there is no relationship between the two factors.

To test your hypothesis, look at the numerical relationship between the clients' scores on the two scales. To do this, create a plot of each client's anxiety level along one axis of a graph (the X axis) and the pain score along the other axis (the Y axis; see **Figure 6.11**). This concept can be shown pictorially by means of a scattergram, or a graph that shows each person's data as a point on the graph. Note that both variables must be numerical in order to use this test. Each client's datum for where the pain score intersects with the anxiety score will appear as one point on the graph. (You can find what each person's score was on both scales: find a dot and draw a horizontal line from it to the Y or vertical axis and a vertical line to the X or horizontal axis.) The idea now is to fit a straight line that best represents the data. This can be done by eye or by generating the regression line (i.e. the best-fit straight line) via a computer program.

The graph in **Figure 6.11** shows a positive relationship between anxiety and pain. Clients who had high anxiety levels also had high pain levels and clients who had low anxiety levels had low pain levels. This means that anxiety is positively correlated with pain for this group of clients. The regression line is also shown that has been fitted to the data by the computer program.

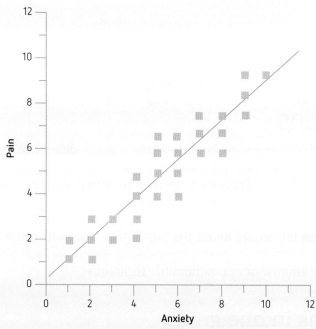

▶ **Figure 6.11**   Scattergram showing positive correlation of pain and anxiety

The extent to which the variables are related to each other is expressed as a correlation coefficient, the symbolic notation for which is an italic r. The r value corresponds to the slope of the line. The most common correlation coefficient used in modern computer analysis is the Pearson correlation coefficient. The Pearson correlation coefficient has a range of scores from −1.0 to +1.0. The more strongly the two variables are correlated with each other, the farther the score will be from zero. A score of 0 in the middle represents no correlation at all.

−1 −0.9 −0.8 −0.7 −0.6 −0.5 −0.4 −0.3 −0.2 −0.1 0 0.1 0.2 0.3 0.4 0.5 0.6 0.7 0.8 0.9 +1

The Pearson correlation coefficient assumes that the data are normally distributed. If they are not, a non-parametric test such as the Spearman rank order correlation (statistical dependence between the ranking of two variables) would be used.

Figure 6.11 shows a strong positive relationship between pain and anxiety, with the participants' scores on one scale similar to their scores on the other scale. This result would give a Pearson correlation coefficient of 0.92, which is a strong positive correlation.

However, if a set of data in which the anxiety scores go up while the pain scores go down, a different result would be seen, as Figure 6.12 shows.

It can be seen in Figure 6.12 that the data points and the regression line run in the opposite direction to those in the previous graph. The high scores on the anxiety scale are matched to the low scores on the pain scale. Participants who were very anxious had a low level of pain after the operation. Conversely, participants who had high anxiety levels before the operation had low levels of postoperative pain. The Pearson correlation coefficient for these data is –0.9.

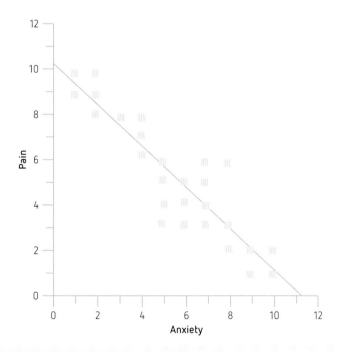

▸ **Figure 6.12**   Scattergram showing negative correlation of pain and anxiety

The third possibility is that there is no relationship between pain and anxiety. Figure 6.13 shows the lack of a relationship when anxiety is regressed upon pain.

Note that the scatter on this graph is random: there seems to be no relationship between anxiety and pain. The Pearson correlation coefficient on these data was near zero, –0.01.

Correlation and significance

In Figure 6.11, a strong positive correlation was seen spread over the whole range of possible responses. What if there were only a few data and they were all grouped at one end but showed the same best-fit line? The r value is the same (i.e. slope) but confidence in the reliability of the data is way down. Or what if the scatter were much wider? Again, the slope of the best-fit line could be the same, but it is not certain.

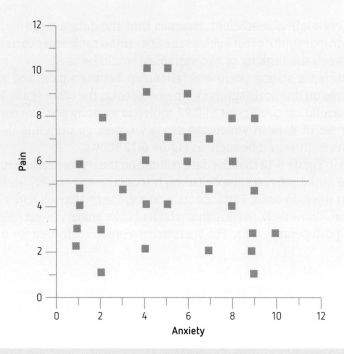

▶ **Figure 6.13** Scattergram showing no correlation of pain and anxiety

At this point, the statisticians provide an almost universally confusing table that relates the number of subjects in the study (the number of data points in this instance) to the value of *r* that must be exceeded for it to pass a certain level of significance. The left-most column is usually headed 'degrees of freedom (df)' and is two less than the number of data points (so, for this example, 'F' or 'f' or 'df' is close enough to the number of data points – say, 30). This determines which row of the table is used. It does not make sense to be too fussy here, provided there is more than a dozen points. Now compare the *r* value (in this case 0.92) with the values in the 'F' or 'f' or 'df' = 30 row. If the value for *r* is bigger (ignoring whether it is positive or negative) than the value in the column for the required level of significance, this result is important. Fortunately, the computer program is able to calculate the *p* value, taking the pain out of the process.

ACTIVITY

List two sets of variables related to health where an association using a correlation coefficient could be established. Have one set demonstrate a positive association and the other a negative association.

Testing for differences in means of two groups of data

Independent groups *t*-test

Some research designs and hypotheses call for testing to see if there is a significant difference between two groups' means on the same variable. Suppose mobile and immobile clients in a long-term care facility were classified as constipated or not constipated. The actual difference in numbers of bowel motions per week for the two groups would be compared. Again, data would be collected on whether each client was mobile or immobile as well as on the number of bowel motions for one week. Then an independent group's unpaired *t*-test would be done to see whether the mean number of bowel actions per week for the immobile clients was greater than that for the mobile clients. The results might look like Table 6.7.

▶ Table 6.7   Unpaired *t*-test

Unpaired *t*-test: X: mobility and Y: bowel actions			
Unpaired *t*-value			Probability
6.8			0.0001
Group	Count	Mean	Std dev.
Mobile	25	6.8	1.1
Bed rest	15	3.9	1.6

Table 6.7 ascertains that there were 25 mobile patients, with 15 bed-rest patients. The mean number of bowel actions per week for the mobile patients was 6.8, while for the bed-rest patients it was 3.9. The results of the *t*-test show that this finding was statistically significant ($p = 0.0001$), which means that there was a probability of less than one in 10 000 that this result could have happened by chance alone.

The independent *t*-test rests on the assumption that the data for bowel motions are normally distributed; that is, they approximate the normal curve outlined earlier. If the data were skewed, a non-parametric test would be used such as the Mann-Whitney U test, which is used to test whether two sample means are equal or not, because it does not require a normal distribution. But how is this found? The best way is to do a histogram to show the distribution of the data. If the data look skewed, it would be better to do the non-parametric test.

Paired *t*-test

Another test that can be done to find relationships in one group is the paired or one-group *t*-test. This test is done when two readings are compared for each participant on the same variable. The paired *t*-test needs at least an ordinal level scale for this test; that is, it is done on data that are numerical. This test is useful where there is a pretest post-test design or more than one post-test measurement. Another example is to see whether preoperative teaching results in less postoperative anxiety. A preoperative pretest of anxiety, an intervention of preoperative teaching and a postoperative post-test of anxiety would be done. A paired *t*-test would be done to see if the postoperative anxiety scores are lower than the preoperative scores. Suppose that the group of participants had a mean preoperative anxiety level of seven and the mean postoperative anxiety level was four, a drop of three. Table 6.8 shows the results for the paired *t*-test.

▶Table 6.8   Results of paired *t*-test

Paired *t*-test	X: preoperative anxiety	Y: postoperative anxiety	
DF	Mean x–y	Paired *t*-value	Prob. (two-tailed)
20	3	14	0.0001

The *p* value shows that these results were highly significant and that the hypothesis that the postoperative anxiety would be less after the intervention of preoperative teaching is probably correct.

ACTIVITY

Assume that there are two groups of people in a study. Describe one type of datum that could be collected for each group related to a single variable that would allow a comparison between the two groups using a *t*-test.

Chi-square test

The chi-square test is a test for determining within-group relationships on nominal variables; that is, variables that are measured by categories rather than numbers. In a chi-square test, there are two variables, each of which is broken down into two levels.

As a simple example, suppose the relationship between bed rest and constipation in long-stay clients is of interest. The hypothesis is that those who are on bed rest are more likely to be constipated than those who are more mobile. Data is collected on 40 clients, classifying each one as either on bed rest or not, and constipated or not. Each person must be classified in both categories. Now there are four possible categories into which the clients can be classified:

- constipated and on bed rest
- constipated and not on bed rest
- not constipated and on bed rest
- not constipated and not on bed rest.

Next, a chi-square test is done. If there was no relationship between bed rest and constipation, it might be expected to have equal numbers of clients in each category and the results might look something like Table 6.9. But if the hypothesis is correct and there is a relationship between mobility and bowel activity, the results might look like Table 6.10.

▸ Table 6.9   Chi-square test: expected values

	Bed rest	Mobile	Totals
Constipated	10	10	20
Normal	10	10	20
Totals	20	20	40

▸ Table 6.10   Chi-square test: relationship between mobility and bowel activity

	Bed rest	Mobile	Totals
Constipated	14	6	20
Normal	5	15	20
Totals	19	21	40

It is clear from looking at Table 6.10 that the clients who are on bed rest are constipated and those who are mobile are not.

The chi-square test will also provide information about percentages of clients in each category. By reading down the columns of Table 6.11, it can be seen that three-quarters of the clients who are on bed rest are constipated and 71 per cent of those who are mobile are not.

Another type of table looks at the percentages from the point of view of the other variable. Table 6.12 shows that 70 per cent of clients who are constipated are on bed rest and three-quarters of non-constipated clients are mobile.

▸ Table 6.11   Chi-square column totals

	Bed rest (%)	Mobile (%)	Totals (%)
Constipated	74	29	50
Normal	26	71	50
Totals	100	100	100

▸ Table 6.12   Chi-square row totals

	Bed rest (%)	Mobile (%)	Totals (%)
Constipated	70	30	100
Normal	25	75	100
Totals	48	52	100

A computer chi-square test will also give a p value, in this case $p = 0.01$. This means that the result probably would have happened by chance alone only 1 per cent of the time, so the findings meet a 99 per cent level of confidence.

Contingency tables

A contingency table is an expanded chi-square used where either variable has more than two categories. In the example above, the variables may be broken down into finer categories. Thus, for example, mobility could be broken down into 'completely mobile', 'partially mobile' and 'bed rest'. Bowel activity could be broken down into 'severely constipated', 'mildly constipated' and 'normal'. In this case, there would be nine categories, with a 3×3 contingency table instead of the 2×2 table shown in Table 6.11. But this would need many more participants to give enough data in each cell.

ACTIVITY

Assume that there are two groups of people in a study. Describe one type of datum that could be collected for each group related to a single variable that would allow comparison between the two groups using a chi-square.

Testing for differences in means of more than two groups

Many research designs call for the determination of whether there is a difference in the mean score for more than two distinct groups. Suppose that the earlier design is expanded, this time to look at the effect of three levels of mobility – bed rest, partly mobile and fully mobile – upon the number of bowel actions. An analysis of variance (ANOVA) would ascertain whether the mean number of bowel motions per week was significantly different in the three groups. This test examines the mean scores and will detect whether there is a significant difference in them. The test actually detects whether there is more difference within each group than between the groups. Note that the independent variable, *mobility*, is nominal, while the dependent variable, *number of bowel actions*, is numerical.

To do this test, more participants would be needed since three levels of mobility are being studied. Suppose the study was redone with more clients, classifying them as 'bed rest', 'partially mobile' and 'fully mobile patients', and again collected data on the number of bowel motions for the week. The results, using ANOVA, would look something like Table 6.13.

▶ Table 6.13   Analysis of variance

One factor ANOVA: X: mobility and Y: bowel actions ($p = 0.0001$)			
Group	Count	Mean	Std dev.
Bed rest	15	2.9	1.2
Partially mobile	22	5.3	0.8
Fully mobile	23	7.8	1.0

Table 6.13 shows that there are 15 bed-rest patients, 22 partially mobile patients and 23 fully mobile patients. It also shows that there was a statistically significant difference in the mean number of bowel motions per week for the two groups. The bed-rest patients had a mean of approximately three bowel motions per week, the partially mobile had a mean of five and the fully mobile had a mean of eight. This finding is statistically significant ($p = 0.0001$) with only a 1 in 10000 possibility that this finding would have occurred by chance. From these results, it could be concluded that, all other things being equal, mobility makes a difference to the bowel activity of patients.

If the data are skewed, use a non-parametric test. A Kruskal–Wallis test could be used for three groups; however, as these data have a reasonably normal distribution, a parametric test is indicated.

Methods involving more than one variable

The advent of computers and statistics-analysis programs has meant that increasingly sophisticated techniques of data analysis have been demanded by researchers and devised by statisticians. This chapter is not intended to teach complex statistical analysis, but it is important to understand some advanced quantitative techniques so that it is possible to recognise the terms included in research reports or articles.

Condensing data into scales: factor analysis

Some research projects use questionnaires that have a considerable number of items. Using the methods so far outlined, only the independent variables are able to be tested on each item individually, which would leave a large mass of data that it would be hard to make sense of. One way of handling the data is to group the items into scales.

In the context of a questionnaire, a scale is a group of items that are conceptually related. There are various ways of developing scales, one common way being factor analysis. All the items can be entered into a factor-analysis program that tests each item to determine with which group of items it conceptually belongs and clusters the related items into factors, or groups of items with a similar focus. The researcher can then treat each factor as one dependent variable.

Tests involving more than one independent variable

More complex tests must be done if a researcher wants to test the effects of two or more independent variables upon the dependent variable. The researcher can test each independent variable individually using the techniques outlined earlier in this chapter; indeed, this is one way to eliminate from the analysis variables that have little or no effect. Individual analysis will not tell the researcher how the variables interact with one another though, or which variable has the most powerful effect. To do this, use a test that will allow the entry of a group of independent variables into the analysis. Some of these statistical tests are described briefly below.

Multiple regression

If the independent variables are numerical and the dependent variable is also numerical, a more complex regression called a 'multiple regression' can be used. A researcher might want to analyse the relative effects of intelligence and socioeconomic status (SES) upon the ability of clients to learn information about diabetes mellitus, or the researcher could administer an intelligence quotient (IQ) test and a test of diabetes knowledge to the participants in the study and also determine their score on an index of SES. The researcher could then use a multiple regression with the test of knowledge score as the outcome variable and the SES and IQ scores as the research variables. This would tell the researcher what effects SES and IQ have and whether they are linked.

Two-way and three-way ANOVAs

If there is more than one nominal-level independent variable and one interval-level dependent variable, the researcher would need to use a more sophisticated ANOVA. A two-way ANOVA will handle two independent variables, a three-way ANOVA will handle three independent variables and so forth. Continuing our earlier example, suppose that a researcher wanted to examine the effects of mobility and gender on the mean number of bowel motions per week in nursing home clients. The researcher would use a two-way ANOVA with three levels of mobility and two levels of gender. If the researcher wanted to examine the effect of type of diet along with mobility and gender, a three-way ANOVA would be indicated.

Logistic regression

Log-linear analysis is a type of logistic regression analysis in which all the variables are measured on a nominal scale (Saltiker & Whittaker, 2013). Logistic regression examines the relative effect of more than one nominal-level independent variable upon a nominal-dependent variable, a kind of expanded chi-square test. A researcher might, for example, want to examine the effect of gender and mobility upon whether clients are selected for placement in a particular nursing home. An example of this type of statistical analysis can be found in a study that examined medication refill adherence among pregnancy women living with HIV in Nigeria (Omonaiye et al., 2020). The study found that the availability of a treatment supporter was significantly associated with antiretroviral therapy refill adherence ($p = 0.001$).

Discriminant analysis

Discriminant analysis is a technique that allows the researcher to use numerical independent variables to predict whether participants will belong to different groups. The independent variables must be interval-level and the dependent variable is nominal level. If a researcher wanted to see whether SES and IQ would predict if a person was a smoker or a non-smoker, they would do a discriminant analysis.

Tests involving more than one dependent variable

Some research designs have more than one dependent variable. If the dependent variables are unrelated, they can be examined using separate ANOVAs (allowing only one dependent variable to be analysed at one time). If, though, the dependent variables are related in some way, they can be examined together by using more advanced statistical techniques. One such technique is the multivariate analysis of variance (MANOVA).

Confidence intervals

Confidence intervals are often used in health research to demonstrate the level of 'confidence' that a finding is true and not the result of a sampling error. While p values tell us the probability that the result we have is a true estimate of the given statistic in the real population, they can vary according to the sample size and the actual effect size being measured (the size/strength of difference or association between two sets of measurements). In health research, we are more concerned with the real strength of an effect, and not so much with the sample size needed to make it statistically significant. This refers to the *clinical significance* of an effect.

Confidence intervals provide the range of likely estimates for an effect. p values are *point estimates*; that is, the significance of a single point of measurement is calculated. The difficulty of relying on p values in clinical research is that they may obscure the clinical significance of a finding by relying totally on the statistical significance of a single point. A real health benefit or health problem may be ignored because the sample size was small, while a clinically insignificant result may be considered important simply because an extremely large sample produced a statistically significant result, based on a small effect level.

Confidence intervals are a way of discriminating between statistical significance based purely on p values and actual clinical significance of a result. A 95 per cent confidence interval will tell us where 95 per cent (19 out of 20) of the likely results would fall from all possible samples used. Confidence intervals are calculated as follows.

1 Upper and lower limits are calculated to demonstrate 95 per cent confidence in the result.
2 These are then added and deducted from the mean to give the 95 per cent confidence interval.

Formulae for confidence intervals:

$$\text{lower} = (\text{mean} + [1.96 \times \text{std dev.}]) \div \sqrt{n}$$

$$\text{upper} = (\text{mean} + [1.96 \times \text{std dev.}]) \div \sqrt{n}$$

(The number 1.96 in these formulae corresponds to a z score of 1.96 either side of the mean, which covers 95 per cent of the area under the normal curve; n is the size of the sample.)

Summary of tests for comparing for differences

Table 6.14 provides a summary of those statistical tests that can be used to compare groups of data to see if there is a statistically significant difference between the groups. These tests will tell you if the mean of one group is higher than the mean of one or more other groups of data, other than by chance alone.

▶ **Table 6.14** Tests for comparing for differences

	Nominal data (non-parametric)	Ordinal data (non-parametric)	Interval or ratio data (parametric)
Two independent groups of data	Chi-square test	Mann-Whitney U test	*t*-test (independent groups)
Two dependent groups of data	McNemar test	Sign test	*t*-test (dependent groups)
Three or more groups of independent data	Chi-square test	Kruskal–Wallis test	ANOVA (independent groups)
Three or more groups of dependent data	Cochran's Q test	Friedman two-way analysis of variance	ANOVA (dependent groups)

Summary of tests for comparing for associations

Table 6.15 is a summary of those statistical tests that can be used to compare groups of data to see if there is a statistically significant association between the groups. These tests will tell you if one variable is associated with one or more other variables, other than by chance alone.

▶ **Table 6.15** Tests for comparing for associations

	Nominal data (non-parametric)	Ordinal data (non-parametric)	Interval or ratio data (parametric)
Two groups of data	Logistic regression or log-linear analysis	Spearman rank order correlation	Pearson correlation coefficient
Three or more groups of data	Logistic regression or log-linear analysis	Logistic regression or log-linear analysis	Multiple 95% or factor analysis

SUMMARY

This chapter has presented the management of quantitative data.

1	Describe the various types of data and scales of measurement	• Sound procedures should be implemented for handling, entering and analysing data and dealing with the products of data analysis

2	Manage the data and products of analysis	• Quantitative data analysis:
		  – usually involves the use of statistics to describe the data
		  – enables inferences to be made about the relationships expressed in hypotheses
		  – shows the results of hypothesis testing

3	Understand the difference between descriptive and inferential statistics	• Descriptive statistics are those that describe a phenomenon • Inferential statistics are those that enable us, through a process of hypothesis testing, to make inferences about the population from which the data were collected
4	Explain probability and hypothesis testing	• These estimate the probability that a relationship observed in the data occurred only by chance; that is, the probability that the variables are really unrelated in the population • Tests for statistical significance are used
5	Understand how to compare groups for statistical differences and associations	• Inferential statistics are used to determine the differences • A number of tests are used for determining associations in one group

REVIEW QUESTIONS

1 Describe the different scales and levels of measurement.
2 What are the commonly used descriptive statistics?
3 What is the purpose of hypothesis testing in statistical analysis?
4 What is meant by statistical significance?

CHALLENGING REVIEW QUESTIONS

1 Discuss the difference between parametric and non-parametric tests.
2 What conditions are necessary to enable the use of parametric data analysis techniques?
3 In what situations would multiple regression analysis be utilised?
4 What is a correlation coefficient and when is it used?

CASE STUDY 1

At the monthly meeting of the nursing practice committee of the residential aged-care facility where you work, the issue of physical health status among the residents is raised by a member of staff. As the chair of the committee, you suggest a research project to examine the effects of an exercise program on health-related quality of life in older residents.

1   If you want to establish a cause and effect relationship between physical activity and quality of life, what research design approach should be used?
2   What would be the independent variable?
3   What would be the dependent variable?
4   What other factors might modify, confound or bias your findings?
5   What would you need to do if you wanted to be able to generalise the results of your findings to all nursing homes in Australia?

CASE STUDY 2

You want to investigate the use of soap bubbles as a distraction technique in the management of pain, anxiety and fear in children who are admitted to the emergency department. You have determined that there are many independent variables, such as age, gender, blood pressure, respiratory rate, heart rate, oxygen saturation, pain fear and anxiety scores. You have decided to use the first and last recordings at each stage of the child's progress through the continuum of care – from pre-treatment, to post treatment, to discharge from hospital.

1   How will the data be coded for each of the variables?
2   Which statistical test would be the most appropriate for analysis of the data?

REFERENCES

Australian Research Council. (2019). Research data management. Australian Government. https://www.arc.gov.au/policies-strategies/strategy/research-data-management

Gray, J. R., Grove, S. K., & Sutherland, S. (2017). *Burns and Grove's The Practice of Nursing Research: Appraisal, Synthesis, and Generation of Evidence* (8th edn). St Louis, MO: Elsevier.

Omonaiye, O., Nicholson, P., Kusljic, S., Mohebbi, M., & Manias, E. (2020). Medication-based refill adherence among pregnant women living with HIV in Nigeria. *Clinical Therapeutics, 42*(11), e209–19. https://doi.org/10.1016/j.clinthera.2020.08.014

Pallant, J. F. (2016). *SPSS Survival Manual: A Step by Step Guide to Data Analysis using IBM SPSS* (7th edition.). Allen & Unwin.

Polit, D. F., & Beck, C. T. (2014). *Essentials of Nursing Research: Appraising Evidence for Nursing Practice* (8th edn). Wolters Kluwer Health / Lippincott Williams & Wilkins.

Saltiker, J. B., & Whittaker, V. J. (2013). Selecting the most appropriate inferential statistical test for your quantitative research study. *Journal of Clinical Nursing, 23*, 1520–31.

Shi, Y. X., Fan, X. Y., Han, H. J., Wu, Q. X., Di, H. J., Hou, Y. H., & Zhao, Y. (2012). Effectiveness of a nurse-led intensive educational programme on chronic kidney failure patients with hyperphosphataemia: Randomised controlled trial. *Journal of Clinical Nursing, 22*, 1189–97.

FURTHER READING

Bryman, A., & Cramer, D. (2011). *Quantitative Data Analysis with SPSS 17, 18 and 19*. Routledge.

Fan, L., Hou, X., Zhoa, J., Sun, J., Dingle, K., Purtill, R., Tapp, S., & Lukin, B. (2016). Hospital in the Nursing Home program reduces emergency department presentations and hospital admissions from residential aged care facilities in Queensland, Australia: A quasi-experimental study. *BMC Health Services Research*, *16*, 46. http://doi.org/10.1186/s12913-016-1275-z

Mannix, J., Wilkes, L., & Daly, J. (2015). Good ethics and moral standing: A qualitative study of aesthetic leadership in clinical nursing practice. *Journal of Clinical Nursing*, *24*, 1603–10.

McKenna, B., Furness, T., Oakes, J., & Brown, S. (2015). Police and mental health clinician partnership in response to mental health crisis: A qualitative study. *International Journal of Mental Health*, *24*, 386–93.

Salkind, N. J. (2011). *Statistics for People Who (Think They) Hate Statistics* (4th edn). SAGE Publications.

Salcedo, J., & McCormick, K. (2020). *SPSS Statistics for Dummies* (4th edn). John Wiley & Sons, Inc.

Taplin, J., & McConigley, R. (2015). Advanced life support (ALS) instructors experience of ALS education in Western Australia: A qualitative exploratory research study. *Nurse Education Today*, *35*, 556–61.

Chapter learning objectives

The material presented in this chapter will assist you to:

1 differentiate between interpretive and critical forms of qualitative methodologies
2 describe the four common forms of qualitative interpretive methodologies
3 describe the three common forms of qualitative critical methodologies
4 understand how to use multiple qualitative methodologies
5 discuss the rationale for choosing congruent methods in qualitative research
6 know the importance of research contexts and participants
7 discuss some data collection methods that may be used in qualitative research.

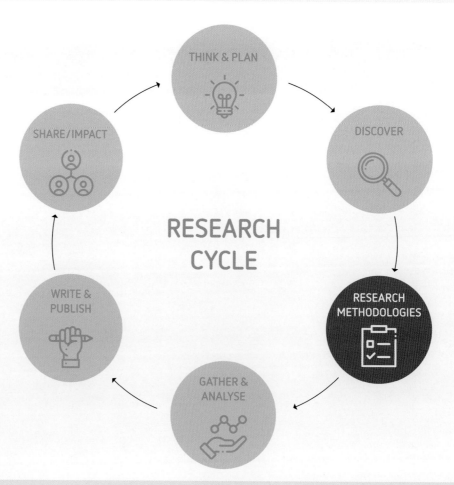

Research cycle

The primary focus of this chapter is qualitative methodologies. This is a key component of research methodologies.

Introduction

This chapter presents the key ideas and methods of qualitative interpretive methodologies and critical methodologies. Following this, a list of methods that can be used in qualitative research can be found. All the methods are briefly discussed by way of introduction and a direction to further reading. Qualitative research is used in a number of health disciplines with examples of this research presented throughout this chapter.

Interpretive and critical forms of qualitative methodologies

The major difference between interpretive and critical qualitative research is the primary intention of what the researcher hopes to achieve through the research process. **Interpretive research** mainly aims to generate meaning (i.e. tries to explain and describe) in order to make sense out of things of interest. **Critical research** aims to bring about change in the status quo by systematically working through research problems to find answers and to cause change activity considering those answers. In doing what they intend to do as their priority, interpretive and critical researchers also manage to do other things, such as generate meaning and bring about change, but they differ in the intensity of their intentions.

The methodologies of **grounded theory**, phenomenology, **ethnography** and **historical research** will be discussed further on in the chapter as examples of qualitative interpretive research approaches.

Common forms of qualitative interpretive methodologies

Grounded theory

Grounded theory is an inductive methodology that attempts to make sense of issues of importance in people's lives and seeks to convert these statements to construct theory. Researchers start with a topic of interest then collect data and allow the relevant ideas to develop. Initially, the approach taken is **inductive**; consequently, hypotheses and tentative theories emerge from the dataset. Existing theory is not imposed on the data, but is utilised to support the emergent theory, creating possibilities for multiple theoretical frameworks to be applied to the research interest (Rieger, 2018).

The approach identifies and relates factors that might be used to define and explain relatively unknown situations. Thus, the methodology assumes that problem identification and solution generation are within the realms of interpretive research. This means that practical solutions can be found to problems generated by nurses and other healthcare workers. Constructivist theory fosters reflexivity on behalf of the researcher, culminating in the co-construction of a theory that is a combination of the researcher's and the participant's stories and views. Constructivist theory acknowledges that reality is a social construction and facilitates a researcher's understanding of how people negotiate and manipulate social structures, how a shared reality is created and how meaning is developed through the social interactions with others within defined contexts. Constructivist grounded theory researchers acknowledge the subjectivity of data and data analysis (Rieger, 2018).

EVIDENCE FOR BEST PRACTICE

CONSTRUCTIVIST GROUNDED THEORY RESEARCH AND ITS IMPLICATIONS FOR PRACTICE

Butler, Copnell and Hall (2018) employed constructivist grounded theory to explore bereaved parents' judgements of healthcare providers when their child died in the paediatric intensive care unit.

The results of this study have clear implications for clinical practice. Bereaved parents' judgements of healthcare staff provide landmarks for staff behaviours, attitudes and interactions when a child is dying in the paediatric intensive care unit. Healthcare staff should endeavour to include the family in the care of the child; they should care for the parents emotionally and practically and demonstrate respect for the child as a living person.

In an occupational therapy study by Walder and Molineux (2019), stroke survivors' perception of their relationship with their healthcare team as they adjust to life following stroke was explored.

The results of this study have clear implications for occupational therapists. The relationship with healthcare providers is important for the person who has survived a stroke experience and will impact on their needs, motivation, confidence and goal setting. Clients need to be understood in relation to their hopes, goals and priorities.

The method

Various modes of data collection may be used, such as unstructured interviews, media items, personal observations and informal conversations. The researcher transcribes the interviews as soon as possible after the interview; data analysis commences within the first interview to facilitate the simultaneous collection, coding and analysis of the data and to provide a focus for subsequent data collection. Data collection and analysis are done jointly, guided by the constant comparative method and theoretical sampling (Chun Tie, Birks & Francis, 2019; Polit & Beck, 2020).

Theoretical sensitivity refers to the insight of the researcher. It is the ability of the researcher to identify a data segment that is important to their theory (Chun Tie, Birks & Francis, 2019). By being theoretically sensitive and using insight, the researcher is able to develop a theory that is grounded, theoretically dense and cohesive. The researcher interacts with the data; that is, they ask questions of the data, which are in turn modified by the emerging answers. Each emerging category, idea, concept or linkage informs a new look at the data to elaborate or modify the original construct. It is theoretical sensitivity that enables one to develop a theory that is grounded, conceptually dense and well-integrated, and to do so quicker than if this sensitivity were lacking (Achora & Matua, 2016; Chun Tie, Birks & Francis, 2019). A literature review may be done as a preliminary look into the area being researched, but the insights complement rather than direct the grounded theory project. Undertaking an early literature review does not refute the point that a researcher should try to approach the research with a mind that is sufficiently open to allow new, perhaps even contradictory, findings to emerge from the raw data (Timonen, Foley & Conlon, 2018). Grounded research requires researchers to eradicate or minimise their own preconceptions because personal biases can affect the data (Achora & Matua, 2016; Chun Tie, Birks & Francis, 2019). Researchers' presuppositions about the area of interest are acknowledged at the outset and set aside to allow the data to speak for themself.

Theoretical sampling occurs as the project progresses. Initially, there will be purposive sampling in which particular people who fulfil certain criteria, such as gender, age, professional experience or experience of the phenomenon to be studied, will be intentionally recruited to the research. Theoretical sampling allows the researcher to follow leads in the data by sampling new participants or material, thus aiding the evolving theory and ensuring the final theory is grounded in the data (Chun Tie, Birks & Francis, 2019). As the codes and categories start to emerge, the researcher may need to return to the data, the participants and possibly the literature to extend categories and increase their depth of understanding (Achora & Matua, 2016).

Constant comparative analysis is an analytical process used for coding and category development (Chun Tie, Birks & Francis, 2019) and is a flexible and open-ended feature of grounded theory (Achora & Matua, 2016). The researcher works with the data from the beginning of the project in a process of analysis to constantly compare all new data that emerge from participants' accounts of their experiences, to identify similarities in codes and categories and to facilitate the conceptualisation of higher-order categories by comparison of codes, categories and their properties. Interpretations and codes arising from the data analysis are clarified during the interview or later and are substantiated during subsequent interviews. Analysis and data collection continually inform one another.

The coding and categorisation of data occur during constant comparative analysis to identify patterns and events in the data, akin to subthemes in a **qualitative analysis** process. This iterative process involves inductive and deductive processes and sets grounded theory apart from a purely descriptive analysis. The codes create categories (akin to themes) when they are assembled into similar groupings. Charmaz (2014) uses the terms 'initial coding' and 'focused coding' to analyse data. Initial coding occurs line by line and is the step between collecting data and theory speculation. The coding occurs at three levels: open, axial and selective; these are explained in more depth in Figure 7.1.

Category saturation is reached when there are no new codes or categories identified during the analysis of subsequent data. That is, no new ideas are raised in the data. This process results in the emergence of a core category that appears frequently in the data, explains most of the variation in the data, links easily with all categories and has implications for the theory, enabling it to become known and progress with maximum variation in the analysis (Strauss & Corbin, 2008).

Theoretical memos and diagrams are aids to the analysis process. Memos are notes and diagrams are drawings recorded by the researcher as memory aids and conceptual imagery tools that assist in generating categories at each stage of the analysis. Memos are the theorising write-up of ideas about codes and their relationships.

Literature as a data source is useful in grounded theory but, as with qualitative projects involving participants, it is not imposed on the data because the participants' accounts of their experiences are what the research reveals. The existing literature is not used as a theoretical background, but instead as data to be used in analytic strategies of the research (Timonen, Foley & Conlon, 2018). This differs from other research as a literature review precedes data collection and analysis. The development and integration of theory occurs throughout the analysis with deep immersion in the data and through the processes of category reduction and selective sampling of the literature and of the data. Category reduction means clustering large numbers of categories and subsuming them until they are reduced to their smallest number without losing their uniqueness (Chun Tie, Birks & Francis, 2019). Selective sampling of the literature refers to the integration of existing literature with the emerging codes and categories. Selective sampling of the data occurs when more data are collected from participants to test hypotheses and reveal the properties of the categories.

OPEN CODING (LEVEL I CODING)

Generating initial concepts from the data
Occurs when raw data are first given conceptual labels using words spoken by participants

Labelling occurs line by line to thoroughly reduce and analyse the data

As the process becomes more familiar, it can occur in sentences and sometimes paragraphs

↓

AXIAL CODING (LEVEL II OR THEORETICAL CODING)

The linking of concepts into conceptual categories

Occurs when data are put back together to form links to emerging categories

↓

SELECTIVE CODING (LEVEL III CODING)

The formalising of these relationships into theoretical frameworks

Identifies categories and attempts to make links with other categories through a cyclical process that moves between the levels of coding to sort the data into meaningful connections from which a theory can be generated

▶ **Figure 7.1** The three levels of coding

Source: Strauss, A., & Corbin, J. (2008). *Basics of Qualitative Research: Techniques and Procedures for Developing Grounded Theory* (3rd edn). Thousand Oaks, CA: SAGE.

EVIDENCE FOR BEST PRACTICE

GROUNDED THEORY AND CULTURAL SAFETY

McGough, Wynaden and Wright (2017) employed grounded theory method to develop a substantive theory to describe the experiences of mental health professionals caring for Aboriginal people in Western Australia.

RELEVANCE TO CLINICAL CARE IN MENTAL HEALTH NURSING

Practicing cultural safety is vital in ensuring meaningful care and in moving towards improving the mental health outcomes for Aboriginal people. Insights into the provision of cultural safety in the mental health setting may be facilitated by greater collaboration with Aboriginal families and communities, which may provide an opportunity to review care and practices.

FOR EXAMPLE

EXAMPLES OF GROUNDED THEORY

Bloxsome, Bayes and Ireson (2019) used Glaserian grounded theory to underpin a new middle-range theory of retention of midwives in Australia that will be of interest to healthcare leaders.

Another example is the study undertaken by McDonald (2018) who developed a substantive theory of 'integration of the examination of the newborn into holistic midwifery practice' that contributes to a greater understanding of midwives' roles and responsibilities in the newborn infant physical examination.

Phenomenology

Phenomenology is defined by Neubauer, Witkop and Varpio as a 'an approach to research that seeks to describe the essence of a phenomenon by exploring it from the perspective of those who have experienced it' (2019, p. 91). Its prime intent is to discover, explore and describe 'uncensored phenomena' (Spiegelberg, 1970, p. 21) of the things themselves, as they are immediately experienced. Phenomenology enables nurses and other health professionals to explore the **lived experience** of any person in their care and the people with whom they work in order to explain the nature of that existence (being).

Phenomenologists believe that knowledge and understanding are embedded in our everyday world. Although this belief is shared among phenomenologists, they have developed more than one approach to gain an understanding of human knowledge. While there are several schools of phenomenological thought, descriptive phenomenology and interpretive or hermeneutic phenomenology are presented.

Descriptive or Husserl's phenomenology

The concepts of **phenomenological reduction** and **bracketing** are central to descriptive phenomenology. Using the technique of phenomenological reduction allows for reflection in research while at the same time ensuring that the findings are not overly influenced or directed by the researcher's agenda (Carpenter, 2014). Bracketing is the process in which the researcher recognises and sets aside preconceived notions of the phenomena of interest, thereby enabling objective description of the phenomena under study. Another assumption is that there are many features of any lived experience that are common to all persons who have lived the experience.

Interpretive or hermeneutic phenomenology

Interpretive phenomenology focuses on describing the meanings given by individuals of their 'being' in the world and how these meanings influence the choices they make. Interpretive phenomenology can also be described as Heideggerian phenomenology. There is an overall emphasis on the interpretation of experience rather than description alone, and this is a major point of difference between interpretive phenomenology and descriptive phenomenology. In interpretive phenomenology bracketing of prior knowledge is not required, as the researcher's prior knowledge is considered a useful feature.

LeBlanc and colleagues (2018) drew on van Manen's hermeneutic phenomenology, which combines both descriptive and interpretive phenomenology. Their research asked the question: 'What is the lived experience of intensive care nurses caring for patients with dementia?'

Ethics

EVIDENCE FOR BEST PRACTICE

PHENOMENOLOGICAL RESEARCH AND THE IMPLICATIONS FOR PRACTICE

Delany, Edwards and Fryer (2018) used hermeneutic phenomenology to explore how physiotherapists perceive, interpret and respond to ethical challenges in their work context and how professional codes of conduct are used in their practice.

IMPLICATIONS FOR PRACTICE

The codes of conduct need to be dynamic documents that assist physiotherapists to interpret and integrate ethical ideals into their diverse workplace contexts, and for ethics education to focus on cultivating and nurturing ethics capability in physiotherapy practitioners.

The methods

There are no absolutes when it comes to phenomenological methods; the very nature of phenomenology makes it a nebulous task that defies sure and certain methods of grasping and representing the phenomena. Phenomenological methods differ according to the kinds of theoretical assumptions on which they are based. Phenomenologists ask questions about the lived experience. Purposive sampling for recruitment is used as large numbers are not necessary to generate rich data (Gullick, Monaro & Stewart, 2016). Researchers have selected various methods for collecting, analysing and verifying phenomenologically informed research.

Phenomenological researcher Max van Manen (1990) developed a method that is useful in understanding how to go about phenomenological research. It involves six steps, as shown in Table 7.1.

▶ **Table 7.1** The process of phenomenological research

Turning to the nature of the lived experience	• What experience do you want to research? • Access the people who can tell you about it from their experience, including yourself if it is also your experience
Investigating experience as we live it rather than as we conceptualise it	• The experience is told, as it is lived, straight from a spontaneous source of telling through thoughts on direct observations, stories and impressions, usually in creative writing, interviews and any other ways of exposing fresh and immediate insights
Reflecting on the essential themes that characterise the phenomenon	• What is the nature of the phenomenon I am gaining from these accounts? • Search visual data sources such as transcripts, creative writing, photographs and so on for illumination of the essence of the directly expressed phenomenon (the thing about which you wanted to know)
Describing the phenomenon through the art of writing and rewriting	• Work with participants' transcripts to create themes or exemplars, or, if you are the person giving an account, perhaps work with your own writing to create clear, direct synopses of your lived experience

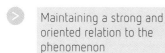

| Maintaining a strong and oriented relation to the phenomenon | • Keep your thoughts and attention on the phenomenon for richer and deeper insights, which will come when the eloquent clarity of simplicity and directness illuminate the research interest |
| Balancing the research context by considering the parts and the whole | • All things (phenomena) exist in relationship with other phenomena; keep this in mind when considering all the features of the research setting to which this phenomenon relates |

Source: van Manen, M. (1990). Beyond assumptions: Shifting the limits of action research. *Theory into Practice, 29*(3), 152–7. Taylor & Francis Online.

FOR EXAMPLE

PHENOMENOLOGICAL RESEARCH

Kelly and Henschke (2019) used Heideggerian phenomenology to explore the experiences of Australian Indigenous nursing students. Indigenous students included in this study responded to the same teaching and learning strategies and methods as non-Indigenous students.

Thompson, Cook and Duschinsky (2017) drew on the work of van Manen's hermeneutic phenomenology to explore nursing home nurses' experiences and views of work identity.

ACTIVITY

Imagine an area in your work or student experience that could be researched using a phenomenological approach. Develop a concise statement of purpose or question, and list some possible methods for data collection you could use.

Ethnography

Ethnography is a research methodology that focuses on the scientific study of the lived culture of groups of people (Polit & Beck, 2020). There are several approaches to ethnography including focused ethnography, institutional ethnography, ethnonursing, autoethnography (Polit & Beck, 2020) and critical ethnography (Gray, Grove & Sutherland, 2017).

A comprehensive approach to ethnography in all its forms and focusing on field work can be found in Paul Atkinson's 2015 book, *For Ethnography*.

The method

Ethnographical research uses observation or participant observation as the method of data collection, with semi-structured focus and group interviews to confirm the researchers' interpretation of the behaviour observed (Laging et al., 2018; Sharp, McAllister & Broadbent, 2018). Visual techniques including photography and film may also be used for data collection. Also, purposive sampling is used, whereby the researcher chooses a specific group or setting to be studied (Moser & Korstjens, 2018).

FOR EXAMPLE

ETHNOGRAPHIC STUDIES

Laging and colleagues (2018) explored the recognition and assessment of resident deterioration in the nursing home setting using critical ethnography. In another study, Harmon, Summons and Higgins (2019) used focused ethnography to explore the older hospitalised person (those aged over 65 years) in relation to the perceptions and experiences of pain care provision by nurses in acute care.

ACTIVITY

Imagine an area that could be researched using an ethnographic approach. Write an aim and some objectives, and list some possible methods you could use for data collection.

Historical research

This is a form of research because its methods seek to discover new knowledge about what has happened in times past in relation to specific portions of time and foci of interest. Certain theoretical assumptions are forwarded as to the value of historical knowledge, including the need for the representation of historical accounts through interpretation. The retrospective nature of the documentation of history has been open to the interpretations of the historian.

The compilation of a valid history relies on the legitimacy of its sources. The two kinds of historical sources are primary and secondary (Schafer, 1980). Primary sources are provided by the original sources of the information, such as participants and observers. Secondary sources are all other accounts, once removed from participation.

The methods

For conducting traditional historical research, a systematic set of steps, fashioned on the rules and procedures of empirical science (Schafer, 1980), is advocated, including:

- defining a topic by using a hypothesis or a set of questions
- locating texts and compiling a bibliography
- researching other sources
- analysing and compiling information
- writing a research article.

The researcher decides on the appropriate means of presenting the data. The completed historical research document may appear deceptively simple to the reader, who is unaware of the painstaking work that was needed to create the final product. The intention is to reconstruct from primary and secondary sources, with due attention to a rigorous research process, a faithful historical account of the area of interest that can be judged to be an accurate and truthful record of events over time.

Oral history

One form of historical research is oral history. Oral evidence is gathered from a primary source whose accounts act as raw historical data that can stand alone as their own account or be synthesised with other sources for further analysis and interpretation. The benefits of oral history include the validity of the primary oral source as the person who has lived the experiences and the potential for the historian to crosscheck interpretations with the person providing the oral history.

Reflective topical autobiography

Reflective topical autobiography is an autobiographical method that can be used by nurses to retrace the events of their lives and the sense they have made of them through reflection. Johnstone (1999) suggests that this form of historical research 'is an important research method, one which promises to make a substantive contribution to the overall project of advancing nursing inquiry and knowledge' (p. 24). She explains that the 're-visioning' of an original topical self-life story 'demonstrates the enormous creativity of the reflective topical autobiographical method' and 'leaves open to the self-researcher the opportunity to return at will to his or her life story again to re-read, re-vision and re-tell the story in the light of the new insights, understandings and interpretations of meaning acquired through ongoing lived experience' (p. 25). Such a suggestion situates reflective topical autobiography in the interpretive paradigm in a place that integrates storytelling with history.

FOR EXAMPLE

HISTORICAL RESEARCH

An example of historical research is presented by Jeffries, Duff & Nichols (2017). Their historical analysis identified the experience of women admitted to a psychiatric hospital in Sydney with psychosis or mania following childbirth after World War II (1945–1955)

Another example is Tierney and colleagues (2018) who presented the history of the governance and accreditation of Australian midwifery programs, with a particular focus on the evolution of the continuity of care experience as a now mandated clinical practice-based experience.

ACTIVITY

Imagine an area that could be researched using a historical approach. Write an aim and some objectives and list some possible methods you could use for data collection.

Common forms of qualitative critical methodologies

Critical social science is of the view that collective social action can be successful in recognising and dealing with oppressive relationships, systems and conditions. Therefore, the critical research methodologies derived from critical social science apply to research that adopts this assumption about the nature and effects of power in human relationships. Critical research activity can be geared directly and strategically towards freeing people from forces and agents that cause human oppression and domination. Freedom from oppression comes from being aware that it is happening and in finding the motivation and means to do something about it.

In healthcare arenas, this means that critical approaches can address the power imbalances in disciplinary conditions, relationships and organisations, and turn upside down some taken-for-granted assumptions about the way things are and the way they need to be. Many of the circumstances in which healthcare workers find themselves can be attributed to events and influences over time. Due to the often-subtle historical changes in the events inside and outside practice, clinicians may develop the impression that they cannot change their work conditions and relationships, and that little can be done about the social and political injustices they face as part of their chosen work.

ACTIVITY

Think about the work constraints – economic, cultural, historical, political and so on – that operate in your professional group and describe the ways in which you think that research based in critical social theory has a chance of changing your work conditions.

Invariably, critical methodologies involve research methods that encourage people to come together to share collaboratively, to bring forward their personal and collective concerns and to make group efforts for changes through their research. The intention is to decrease possible power differences between researcher and participants so that the people in the group take on co-researcher identities, thus attempting to own more equally their research problems, processes and outcomes.

In the section that follows, examples of qualitative critical methodologies, including action research, feminisms and critical ethnography, will be described in terms of specific methodological assumptions and methods.

Action research

Action research is a methodology designed to engage people meaningfully in change processes that affect them and to empower them to shape the changes that are made. Action research goes to the site of the concern or practice and works with the people there as co-researchers to generate solutions to the problems, which they are keen to deal with. This form of research involves action that is directed towards showing the problems in the present situation and then facilitating improvements and sustaining changes.

Action research is categorised into three types, summarised in Table 7.2.

▶ **Table 7.2**   The three types of action research

Technical action research with empirico-analytical underpinning	This research aims to improve techniques and procedures by having practitioners work collaboratively to test the applicability of results generated elsewhere
Practical action research with interpretive underpinning	This research aims to improve existing practices and develop new ones; the emphasis here is on reflecting and interpreting to take deliberate strategic action
Critical action research with critical theory underpinning	This involves a group of practitioners taking responsibility for freeing themselves from the constraints of their practice through understanding and transforming the political, social and economic conditions that keep them from doing their work as they would ideally choose

The method

The method of action research involves four stages of collectively planning, acting, observing and reflecting. This phase leads to another cycle of action, in which the plan is revised, and further acting, observing and reflecting is undertaken systematically to work towards solutions to problems of a technical, practical or emancipatory nature (Taylor et al., 2014). Focus group discussions are used in the initial phase when establishing the action research group (Xiao, Kelton & Paterson, 2012).

Even though there are some underlying principles based on researchers working together through action research cycles, there is more than one way of doing action research. Researchers are free to interpret the methods of action research differently, according to the needs of the collaborating research group. Madden and colleagues (2017) identified the cyclic process for action research as shown in Figure 7.2. There is a full description of the approach elsewhere (see Taylor, 2006), but there are 13 basic steps as shown in the following Activity box 'Steps for action research'.

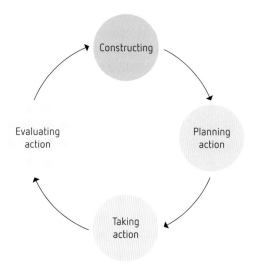

▶ **Figure 7.2**   Activities of the action research cycle (ARC)

Source: Adapted from Madden, D., Sliney, A., O'Friel, A., McMackin, B., O'Callaghan, B., Casey, K., Courtney, L., Fleming, V., & Brady, V. (2017). Using action research to develop midwives' skills to support women with perinatal mental health needs. *Journal of Clinical Nursing, 27,* 561–71.

ACTIVITY

STEPS FOR ACTION RESEARCH

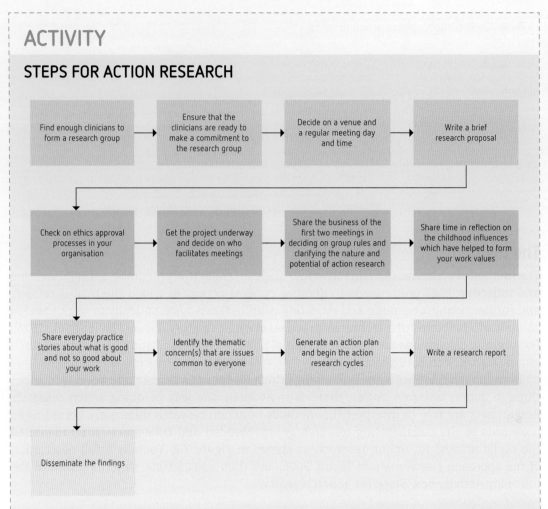

Source: Taylor, B. J. (2006). *Reflective Practice: A Guide for Nurses and Midwives* (2nd edn). Maidenhead, UK: Open University Press.

Using Taylor's 13 steps, set up and undertake an action research project. If you do not intend to undertake the research, you could plan a theoretical project up until the point of ethics clearance, which will at least show you how much interest there is in forming an action research group with your colleagues.

- Describe the ways in which the people and situations of your work setting are problematic to you and your practice.
- Do other clinicians have similar concerns?
- Do you think others would be prepared to work with you to use an action research approach to work collaboratively through these problems?
- Ask them. You may find that you have made the first step towards setting up an action research project.

FOR EXAMPLE

ACTION RESEARCH

Hickey, Kildea, Couchman and colleagues (2019) used participatory action research to improve maternity care for Aboriginal and Torres Strait Islander women and families. The project was to improve clinical and cultural safety of the maternity service throughout the pregnancy, labour and birth and postnatal journey.

Madden and colleagues (2017) employed action research using cooperative inquiry to identify and develop midwives' skills to support women with mental health needs during pregnancy.

Feminist research

Feminist researchers agree that 'women are the major focus of feminist research from the beginning to the end of *whole* research projects', and that therefore feminist methodology 'concerns research *by* and *for* women … putting feminist theory into practice … by applying feminist principles directly from feminist premises' (Glass, 2000, p. 368). Pervading much of feminist literature are the key ideas of embodiment, **empowerment** and emancipation. Empowerment and emancipation in feminist research are of relevance in using participatory research processes to work towards the attainment of women's power and freedom.

A feminist poststructuralist approach offers ways of identifying how language and **discourse** exercise power, showing how oppression operates by creating and affecting the possibilities for resistance (Weedon, 1991), and of identifying women's participation in multiple discourses of everyday life (Davies, 1994). Feminist poststructuralism allows women to recognise and change the cultural patterns of oppression inherent in dominant patriarchal society through constantly renewed ways of seeing and repositioning themselves.

The methods

Feminist research not only emphasises *what* is done in terms of methods, but also *how* projects are done, in faithful reflection of feminist processes. Methods are not prescriptive, but they may include group work, storytelling, interviews, participant observation and so on, depending on the focus of the research interest. The main consideration is keeping to the important principles of feminist research, listed by Glass (2000, pp. 368–9), including the importance of a transforming and empowering focus, and research *with*, never *on*, women, based on mutual respect and sharing. Interpersonal interactions are 'based on equality, reciprocity, and promote mutuality among all women involved' (p. 369). Feminist research values women's unique experiences and stories and recognises and respects 'the inherent sensitivity in collecting data from women' (p. 369). Feminist research methods and designs 'benefit the women involved either whilst actively participating in the research or in the longer term' (p. 369).

FOR EXAMPLE

A POSTMODERN FEMINIST STUDY

Olivier, Ashton and Price (2019) employed feminist poststructuralism to critique, understand and improve sexual health care and policy in healthcare settings.

Another study by Olivier, Ashton and Price (2018) employed feminist poststructuralism to critique and analyse current health research and practice surrounding postpartum sexual health. Agency, subjectivity, gender and sex considerations, relations of power, and discourse are essential to understanding postpartum sexual health in a more holistic, woman-centred way.

ACTIVITY

Explain what sort of work concerns might be best managed by a feminist research process in your healthcare setting. Keep in mind the extent to which the possible research concerns reflect some fundamental principles of feminism, such as those covered in this section.

Critical ethnography

Critical ethnography not only has the exploratory and descriptive mission of ethnography, but it also has the emancipatory aims of critical research approaches. This means that it can go further than descriptive or interpretive ethnography, which seeks only to describe the cultural features of a particular group of people in order to understand their symbols, rituals and practices (Bidabadi, Yazdannik & Zargham-Boroujeni, 2019).

Critical ethnography can create a dialogue with research participants so that they can examine the personal, political, social, cultural, historical and economic aspects of their contexts to develop local knowledge of use in their own situations, and also the power relations and influences affecting and determining the nature and consequences of human behaviour.

The methods

Although there are no prescriptive rules to follow in planning and undertaking a critical ethnography, the methods used will be congruent with certain interests of critical inquiry, such as power and power relations. The methods used to ensure that issues of power are addressed may include group processes such as discussion and debate, participant observation, and reflective-practice strategies such as keeping diaries, writing **narratives** and engaging in individual and group critiques.

The clinical setting and some of the rituals and practices are possibilities for a critical ethnographic study.

FOR EXAMPLE

CRITICAL ETHNOGRAPHY

Examples of critical ethnography research include Bidabadi, Yazdannik and Zargham-Boroujeni (2019), whose study aimed to uncover the cultural factors that impeded maintaining patients' dignity in the cardiac surgery intensive care unit.

Digby, Lee and Williams (2017) used critical ethnography to explore the perspectives of nurses caring for people with dementia to evaluate the reasons behind the widely reported poor care received by such patients.

ACTIVITY

Explain in what ways work rituals and practices are taken for granted in your workplace and to what extent clinicians are aware of those aspects of their work. Discuss whether there are political struggles, either out in the open or behind the scenes, and if there is any interest among colleagues in working together to set up systematic, politically active research processes and methods to raise awareness, questions and critique about selected practices in the culture.

Using multiple methodologies

Creating flexible approaches to methodologies

Multiple methodologies offer wider frames of reference with a greater likelihood of generating many more options for public debate. Previously, a purist approach dictated that certain methodologies fitted into particular paradigms, and that they could not be combined because they contain inherent theoretical contradictions that clash with one another. The rationale for a purist approach was, and to some extent still is, that a carefully selected single methodology (e.g. grounded theory) can adequately act as a vehicle to carry the data collection and analysis methods and will be sufficient to fulfil the research objectives. In today's research climate, it is possible to open up methodologies to creative combinations and move them along paradigmatic continuums. Table 7.3 shows how the methodologies can move across paradigmatic positions. As shown in this table most of the research methodologies extend across paradigmatic positions, which means that they can take on the theoretical assumptions of any of the positions.

Combining qualitative methodologies

Just as it is possible to mobilise methodologies across paradigmatic positions, it is also possible to imagine many combinations of methodologies, depending on the aims and objectives of the research.

▸Table 7.3   Mobilising qualitative methodologies

Examples	Potential mobility in paradigmatic positions		
	Interpretive	Critical	Postmodern
Grounded theory	→→→→→		
Phenomenology	→→→→→→→→→→→→→→→→→→→→→→→→→→→→→→→→		
Ethnography	→→→→→→→→→→→→→→→→→→→→→→→→→→→→→→→→→→		
Historical research	→→→→→→→→→→→→→		
Action research	→→→→→→→→→→→→→→→→→→→→→→→→→→→→→→→→→→→→		
Feminist research	→→→→→→→→→→→→→→→→→→→→→→→→→→→→→→→→→→→→		
Critical ethnography	→→→→→→→→→→→→→→→→→→→→→→→→→→→→→→→→→→→→		
Narrative/storytelling	→→→→→→→→→→→→→→→→→→→→→→→→→→→→→→→→→→		

Newnham, McKellar and Pincombe (2017) investigated the personal, social, cultural and institutional influences on women making decisions about using epidural analgesia in labour. They employed ethnographic methodology underpinned by Foucauldian and feminist theory. Lea and colleagues (2015) used a quasi-experimental mixed methods design within an action research framework to identify the potential for aged care placements to deliver benefits for second-year nursing students when conducted within a supportive framework with debriefing and critical reflection opportunities.

Although methodologies can be combined, this is not necessary if one methodology is sufficient to carry the needs of the project, in terms of the research methods and processes.

Methods for data collection and analysis are based on the assumptions a particular methodology makes about the nature of knowledge generation and validation. Table 7.4 presents the differences between methods, processes and methodologies.

▸Table 7.4   Differentiating between methods, processes and methodologies

Methods	• Strategies by which data are sought and analysed, such as interviews, participant observation, reflective journal writing, focus groups and so on • Data analysis methods could include manual or computer program thematic analysis

Processes	• How data are collected shows the embodied values of researchers, such as respect, patience and thoughtfulness, honouring, acknowledgement and a host of other ways of being mindful of the human nature of the research
	• When thinking about the research process, the main questions are:
	  – How will I undertake these methods?
	  – How will I conduct myself as a researcher in this project?

Methodologies	• Research approaches that can be chosen to act as overarching theoretical concepts for the selection of the methods; that is, methodologies have within them certain theoretical assumptions about the nature of knowledge

Choosing congruent methods is a creative part of the research proposal process and it is the focus of the next section.

Choosing congruent methods

Methods may be chosen that collect information that is language-based and specific to people's particular experiences. The attention paid to choosing congruent methods is based on the assumption that if a methodology is a set of theoretical assumptions, and a method is a means for generating a certain type of knowledge, then it seems reasonable to assume that there needs to be a degree of fit between the type of knowledge that is to be generated and the means that are available to achieve it.

A research project that seeks to explore the lived experiences of nurses and patients, for example, would need to select some methods through which those people would have the best chance to express their experiences. In such a case, participant observation and participant interviews would be consistent with the epistemological (knowledge-producing and proving) assumptions.

ACTIVITY

Explain what is meant by congruent methods. For each of the following methodologies, suggest congruent data collection methods and the reasons why these are most probably suitable. Remember, though, that the methods are not strictly connected to any one methodology, so you may notice repetition in your choices.

Methodology	Possible methods	Reasons for suitability
Grounded theory		
Phenomenology		
Ethnography		
Historical research		
Action research		
Feminist research		
Critical ethnography		

Research contexts and participants

People are central in qualitative research because it is through the expression of their life stories that we come to understand their experiences. People's experiences may not seem significant to them because they may be regarded as simply part of living their lives, but qualitative research has an interest in commonplace experiences. It encourages people to delve into their experiences and to show that it is through their accounts that personal and practical knowledge may be generated for themselves and for others.

A general principle of qualitative research is that people are placed in time and space, and where they are placed has a bearing on how they will interpret their situations. It is important to bear this in mind when asking people to speak of their experiences.

Applying this principle to nursing practice, nurses and patients will make sense of their experiences in relation to the situations they find themselves in, such as the ward or unit they are in, the time of day and their unique set of circumstances, including the social, political, economic, physical, emotional and spiritual aspects of their lives.

Qualitative researchers value people and the accounts these people give of their experiences because it fits with the relativistic view that knowledge changes and that an understanding of human existence resides in people's lives.

Rigour in qualitative research

Qualitative research is no less rigorous than quantitative research, but it uses different words to demonstrate the ways of making explicit the overall processes and worthiness of a project because it is based on different epistemological assumptions. There is not one accepted test of rigour in qualitative research, just as there is not one way of doing qualitative research, which means that researchers must use the most appropriate means of assessing rigour that reflect the methodological assumptions of the project.

Researcher such as Sundler and colleagues (2019) argue that reflexivity, credibility and transferability must be considered to engender rigour. Further, rigour can be judged based on how the research is presented to the reader.

ACTIVITY

Discuss why it follows that the criteria for judging the rigour of quantitative and qualitative research projects must, of necessity, differ. Use the line of argument that it does differ to explain why reliability is, in the strictest quantitative sense, not possible in qualitative projects.

Data collection methods in qualitative research

This section introduces a variety of methods that may be used alone or in combination in qualitative research projects according to the requirements of the research question or area. For ease of access, the methods are listed alphabetically. Bear in mind that methods are used to gather information considered most likely to be of assistance in fulfilling the aims and objectives of a research project. This means that they have been considered carefully and put into place and used with thoughtfulness in relation to what they may offer.

Archival searches

Archival information consists of original hard copies of aged documents such as logs, diaries, government agency agendas and minutes, reports, photographs, newspapers, books, private papers donated by families to the archives and so on. This method involves going to archival repositories, such as purpose-built archival buildings and libraries, to seek specific research information of a historical nature. For more information on how to do archival searches, refer to Streubert and Carpenter, *Qualitative Nursing Research: Advancing the Humanistic Imperative* (2011, 5th edition).

Artistic expression

Data collected through artistic expression can be particularly useful in research aimed at determining certain conditions, states or perspectives from the unique viewpoint of individuals. Participants may be invited to use a variety of artistic expressions to represent themselves and issues in their lives through creative images. Alternatively, the researcher may decide to express some of their observations through an artistic medium, such as poetry, to add further richness to the other sources of data.

In the area of artistic expression, the researcher is limited only by their own imagination, but the unlocking of creative potential needs to be related to the aims and objectives of the project, otherwise it may be fun but without practical application.

Case studies

The case study method fully describes selected foci of research interest, such as individuals, in groups or institutions. The researcher uses a case study method to try to understand as much as possible over time about the area in focus, so the method is characterised by intensive analysis of all the determinants involved.

In planning a case study, consider the research question and how it might be best answered. This may mean that a variety of strategies in sequence will be needed that will ensure a comprehensive approach to the area of inquiry.

Read widely to see how other researchers have organised their case studies, and be prepared to critique those methods and designs that could have been more creative and/or comprehensive in their approaches. An example is Adams, Gardner and Yates (2016), who used a multiple exploratory case study design to examine private sector nurse practitioner service. Another example is Lea and Cruickshank (2017), who investigated the nature and timing of support available to new graduate nurses within a rural transition to practice program.

Field work

Field-work methods may vary according to the intentions of the research, but they usually consist of combinations of observation, participation, documentation and analysis. A common form of data collection in field work is the documentation of field notes, which are selective notes made by the researchers to themselves that will form part of the data when the entire project is drawn together. They need to be made as soon as possible so that the events are still fresh in the researcher's mind.

An alternative for researchers who prefer oral rather than written accounts is to use a portable recording system; in this way, observations can be recorded rapidly and with the relative spontaneity of spoken words. All recordings should be identified with details of the date, time and general content, so that they can be easily organised for later analysis.

Field work and observation or participation observation are related methods, in that field work can be taken to mean broader activities such as those undertaken in ethnographic studies. Here, the emphasis is on the methods observation researchers use when they are undertaking qualitative projects.

Focus groups

A focus group is a collection of research participants who have given their consent to be involved in the project, having been deliberately invited due to their knowledge and/or skills in the area to which the research relates. The group is facilitated by the researcher or by a research assistant with the necessary skills to keep the group focused on its aims and objectives. Focus groups help research by getting several people together to solicit their contributions.

The process usually involves a brainstorming session in which the focus group members respond to questions and comments made by the facilitator and/or in response to group discussion. Responses are recorded on an object visible to the group, such as a blackboard, whiteboard, or butcher's paper. The facilitator calls for all spontaneous responses with no holds barred, then the group works together to collate and prioritise ideas and to remove duplications, off-the-wall remarks, or responses that are judged by the group to be of minimal help or relevance to the research question, aim or context.

The disadvantages of focus groups include the following:

- less-vocal members can be overlooked if they are not drawn out carefully by the facilitator
- responses may not be as rich and full as they might be in the privacy of an interview
- it is difficult to track an individual's perceptions among the group's responses, leaving the interpretations broad and relevant only to the collective responses of the group.

Researchers can use focus groups as their sole method of data collection, or they can use focus groups in combination with other methods.

FOR EXAMPLE

USING FOCUS GROUPS FOR DATA COLLECTION

Simpson and colleagues (2017) used focus groups to explore the decision-making processes used by paramedics when caring for older people who fall. Their study was informed by constructivist grounded theory.

ACTIVITY

Read the article by Pilkington and colleagues (2017), 'Perspectives of Aboriginal women on participation in mammographic screening: A step towards improving services', and then make notes on how the researchers used focus groups in their research.

Describe what other methods were used in this project and how these methods were integrated to generate the project results.

TIP Sim and Waterfield present some ethical challenges in the use of focus groups for data collection:
- Sim, J., & Waterfield, J. (2019). Focus group methodology: some ethical challenges. *Quality and Quantity, 53,* 3003–22. https://doi.org/10.1007/s11135-019-00914-5
  The following is an excellent text for a comprehensive account of focus groups:
- Morgan, D. (2019). *Basic and Advanced Focus Groups.* Sage Publications.

Group work

Group work is particularly suited to collaborative research, such as action research and feminist research, because it involves groups of people working together to create shared meaning. In these cases, the underlying assumptions of the research are that:

- people need to be empowered to find and use their voices
- multiple perspectives are valued
- group members have agreed on the research problems
- those members are the best people to solve the problems through their own collective processes.

Some methods for collecting information may include note taking, audio recording, video recording or by collective review processes at the end of the session. Encourage the group to generate ideas and write them up clearly on a whiteboard as the meeting progresses so that members can decide collectively on the main ideas, areas to be prioritised and areas for further action. Sometimes it is useful to create smaller groups that present their main ideas to the whole group at the conclusion of the session. Another method is for group members to take responsibility for contributing to a brainstorming or ideas-collating exercise at the end of the session.

Whatever occurs, ensure the most important ideas are gathered so that the perspectives of the group can be adequately represented. It is also vital that the group members validate their ideas by confirming that the interpretations that have been made faithfully reflect the meaning that was intended.

Group members comprise a purposive sample because they have the experiences needed to offer insights into the research topic. At the outset of the project, it is important for all members to speak openly within the group to express their preferences for how group members will work together.

Skills in group processes are many and varied; read beyond this text for more suggestions on how to effectively conduct this process.

Interviews

Interviews can be conducted with a structured list of set questions or they can be relatively unstructured with little more than an invitation being issued by the researcher for the participant to talk about an area of interest. In between these is a semi-structured interview, a conversation in which the researcher invites the participant to talk and encourages a free flow of words and ideas while at the same time keeping the interviewee relatively on track in the conversation if that person tends to wander off the point.

TIP

The best way to collect interview data is via an audio recording, although video may be advisable in cases in which non-verbal cues are important.

Audio recordings of the interview can be transcribed to form written text for analysis or may be replayed to allow for the recognition of themes. If participants are shy of the audio equipment, it might be necessary to spend some time in general conversation with the recording device turned on in order for people to become more comfortable with it.

Interviews may be focused or non-directive, depending on how the participant is invited to respond. Some guiding questions may be necessary to maintain a clear direction in a focused interview, but it is particularly important that the questioning does not extend to a long list, as the depth of responses may be sacrificed for breadth of coverage. Some lead-up conversation may be necessary to emotionally settle the interviewee and to ascertain that they are clear about the focus of the research and how the information they provide can contribute. Participants may also be given a list of guiding questions that will be asked to engage the interviewee in a storytelling and/or conversational process.

When a research participant is invited by an interviewer to tell a story, the researcher's directive may be as simple as:

- 'Tell me about your experience of …'
- 'I understand that you have experienced … Would you tell me about that please?'
  When an interviewee requires prompts, simple encouraging words may help, such as:
- 'What happened then?'
- 'Where or when did that happen?'
- 'How were you involved?'
- 'How did that make you feel?'

As with all good communication, listening attentively and responding appropriately are important skills for unfolding effective conversations and stories. Do not underestimate the power of silence. Remaining silent gives the participant a chance to think and to speak without haste and pressure.

For many helpful and practical details on the 'how, why, when, where and with whom' of interviewing, refer to *Interviews in Qualitative Research* (2nd edition) by King, Horrocks and Brooks (2018).

Journal keeping

The journal form of data collection is useful for research in which the researcher and participants are conversant with, and willing to indulge in, reflective writing for the purposes of the research. There are several good reasons for keeping a journal.

- *As a research student*: a journal of this nature might record impressions of meetings with the research supervisor, the joys and pains of being a researcher, and any thoughts, insights and inspirations along the way.
- *The role in the research*: this can describe how to manage being a nurse researching some aspect of nursing or health.
- *Research participants for information gathering*: ensure that participants are willing, able and eager to write reflectively. Build some time into the project to coach participants in the methods and processes of reflection. These skills can be acquired, especially if the participant need to go beyond descriptive accounts of their personal stories to make sense of their experiences.
- *Reflective journal of your experiences*: this can describe how a co-researcher can share equally in group processes.

In using a journal, all participants need to be clear about the objectives of the activity, otherwise many words may be written that do little to inform the research. Journals may be private or semi-private, and therefore participants may decide on what they choose to divulge for the research data. Group processes or discussions with individuals can clarify expectations about the use of journal entries as data. Participants need to agree to disclose material, with the amount and level of privacy they choose. Indeed, there may be excerpts that are so deeply personal that they are known only to the writer, who may use them as aids for working through personal and professional issues. Areas that can be shared publicly can be spoken about in meetings and/or photocopied for incorporation into research articles and papers using pseudonyms.

The amount of material that can be generated will depend on the objectives of the exercise and the amount of disclosure that is required, but journal keeping is likely to amass a substantial amount of information that needs to be sorted in some way in order for it be useful. Interpretations will be most useful if they are made by the person doing the writing, in collaboration with another person, possibly the researcher, who acts as a critical friend, asking constructive questions to bring out the richness of the content.

TIP   Research projects that have used reflective journal keeping as a method of data collection and reflexivity include:
- Irving, M., Short, S., Gwynne, K., Tennant, M., & Blinkhorn, A. (2016). 'I miss my family, it's been a while...': A qualitative study of clinicians who live and work in rural/remote Australian Aboriginal communities. *Australian Journal of Rural Health, 25*(5), 260–7. https://doi.org/10.1111/ajr.12343

ACTIVITY

Locate and read one of the references cited in the tip above and take note of what kind of reflective writing the researcher used and their impressions of the relative merits of journal keeping as a method of data collection.

Literature searches and reviews

Part or all of a research project will involve searching for literature. In applied research, literature features as background data when it is used to show how the findings relate to published accounts of the same area of interest. In pure research, the project may consist of literature entirely, such as in the scholarly critiques expected in philosophical or evidence-based projects that critically appraise the extant literature. Literature in the form of books and refereed journal articles is collected from all the likely sources and repositories, such as electronic and library databases. (See Chapter 2 for a detailed account of literature search and review skills.)

Observation and participant observation

Observation and participant observation usually involve systematically watching and attending to a setting, then retreating for some time to write up the impressions. If there are no technological aids, such as computers, impressions can be audio recorded or written into a logbook or some other permanent record system.

Types of observation can be structured or relatively unstructured; they can also be solely by observation or by varying degrees of participant observation.

Structured observation

Structured observation or non-participant observation requires strict attention to objectivity via checklists of events and behaviours. A structured observation may be part of a larger, issue-based, participatory action research project in which the observation component of an action cycle has an intention to identify predetermined categories of events and behaviours. Duxbury and colleagues (2010) employed structured observations to describe current practice in the administration of medication in an acute psychiatric unit and explore factors that influence nurses' decisions regarding the administration of medication during 'rounds'. Walshe (2020) employed non-participant observations in investigating the role of the district nurse in the provision of palliative care. The study aimed to gain an understanding of how district nurses enact their role with palliative care patients.

Unstructured observation

In an unstructured observation, the researcher observes a context systematically, carefully and with an open mind as to what may occur, with no predetermined categories in mind. The researcher's attention is drawn to what is happening, where, when, how, why and with whom, without actual involvement in the setting as a participant. This means that the observation periods are flexible in relation to the place in which the observation of the participants and events occurs, as well as the time of day, length of observation and expectations about the aspects to be observed. Observations are documented as field notes that describe the broad features of the setting. de Lange, van Eeden and Heyns (2018) used unstructured participant observation of patient handover practices between emergency care practitioners and healthcare practitioners in an emergency department.

Ethics

As with all human research, the researcher must be aware of ethical considerations, such as who has given their consent to be observed during interactions; exclude anyone who has not consented. Attending to ethical issues means not only having informed consent to observe people, but also changing the names and identities of people and places to pseudonyms to maintain privacy and anonymity.

Having gained consent, it is important that the researcher blends in as much as possible so that people are unaware or become less aware of their presence, except in specific cases where they need to make their presence known for ethical or methodological reasons. Done well, participant observation is not conspicuous and as such has less chance of disrupting the usual features of the setting. As the work of observation begins, the researcher may take a little time to settle into the situation, to enable people to get used to having you around in a researcher capacity. Develop a watchful approach to what is happening around you. Learn to observe sensitively to enable as many details in the situation to be seen as possible. Use a systematic approach to observing and documenting what is seen, and think carefully before writing field notes (see **Figure 7.3**).

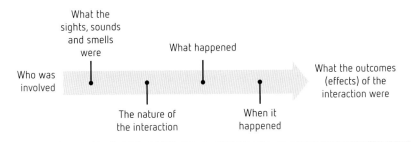

Who was involved — **What the sights, sounds and smells were** — **The nature of the interaction** — **What happened** — **When it happened** — **What the outcomes (effects) of the interaction were**

▸ **Figure 7.3** Unstructured observation: Field notes

Write up the field notes as soon as possible after the interaction. The data are best written in a richly descriptive form and read easier if they are written in the present continuous tense; for example, 'I take a wash bowl to the bed and the other nurse draws the curtains around the bed. Suddenly, Mr Green holds his chest and winces with pain'.

Ensure that there is a selection of interactions occurring over time with the people involved. Thus, various people will be involved over many shifts or times of day. Participants need to be assured that their names will not be used in the accounts and that other identifiable information will be hidden. Be careful in this respect: refer only to 'the nurse', 'the patient', 'the relative', 'the doctor' and so on.

Photography

Photographs can be taken that represent the features of the research setting and/or participants and be highly significant sources of data. If, say, a project involved exploring the routines of a nursing home, other sources of data such as participant observation and interviews could be augmented well by selected pictorial images. Sort photographs into categories, label them accordingly and then select the best images – ideally the most descriptive photos – for inclusion in the research article. Details of the photographs could also be analysed to contribute to informing the research questions. Make sure participants have given consent before their photograph is taken.

Organisations may have strict rules about the use of cameras and videos with respect to the anonymity of their clients and the workplace. Certain groups, such as Aboriginal and Torres Strait Islander people, may have strong cultural taboos about having their images caught on camera; taking and using photographs has the potential to violate sacred beliefs. As a general principle, it is wise to seek permission from people whose photograph is needed and have them sign a release form.

Ethics

Moving pictures captured on video or DVD technologies can offer more scope and dimension than still photographs for data, so their value as sources of data is self-evident. The same precautions apply to video recording as have been outlined for photography. It is imperative that ethical clearance is gained before video recording begins, and that participants give consent for their involvement. Exceptions to this may be in the use of such recordings when the researcher is the focus of the project and wants to make a compilation of personal data of an archival nature that may be used in an autobiography or oral history.

Storytelling

Whether as a single story or as in the organising scheme of a narrative, data for qualitative research can be gathered easily and effectively through having people relate accounts of their experiences relevant to the research. It is an effective way of involving people in research, as they may respond well to the invitation to tell a story.

The story can be audio recorded for later analysis, but some participants who are shy of this method may feel happier writing their stories and adding illustrations. In some cases, stories may be enacted in traditional ways, such as dance or rituals, and other creative means, such as poetry, music, singing and film. If creative means are used, it is important that the artist is the interpreter of their own story, the accounts of which are stored by a recordable means that the artist agrees to.

As with all effective communication, if a storyteller has the optimal conditions for speaking, the likelihood of a rich and deeply thoughtful story is enhanced through listener silence and attention. Once the storyteller has clear parameters for the story, resist the impulse to interject unless the narrator is wandering right off the track and looks like becoming lost in irrelevancies.

> **TIP** For further reading on storytelling and narrative inquiry, refer to:
> - Klages, D., East, L., Jackson, D., & Usher, K. (2019). A four-stage framework for conducting feminist storytelling research. *Nurse Researcher*. https://doi.org/10.7748/nr.2019.e1624

SUMMARY

This chapter has discussed various qualitative research methodologies.

1 Differentiate between interpretive and critical forms of qualitative methodologies	• Interpretive research aims mainly to generate meaning by explaining and describing • Critical research aims to bring about change in the status quo by working systematically through locally generated research problems to find answers and create change in light of identified constraints
2 Describe the four common forms of qualitative interpretive methodologies	• Grounded theory • Phenomenology • Ethnography • Historical research
3 Describe the three common forms of qualitative critical methodologies	• Action research • Feminist research • Critical ethnography
4 Understand how to use multiple qualitative methodologies	• Combining methodologies is dependent upon the aims and objectives of the course
5 Discuss the rationale for choosing congruent methods in qualitative research	• There needs to be a degree of fit between the type of knowledge that is to be generated and the means available to achieve it
6 Know the importance of research contexts and participants	• People are central in qualitative research • The context of the participant relates to the interpretation of the situation
7 Discuss some data collection methods that may be used in qualitative research	• Data collection methods include: – storytelling – focus groups – field-work methods (observation, participation, documentation and analysis) – case study – unstructured interviews – semi-structured interviews – in-depth interviewing

REVIEW QUESTIONS

1 What are the main philosophical features of critical methodologies?
2 In what ways has critical social theory been criticised, especially its weaknesses as applied to research approaches?
3 Describe the types of interviews most conducive to generating rich accounts of human experience.

CHALLENGING REVIEW QUESTIONS

1 Discuss the value of action research to evidence-based practice.
2 Discuss the development of the debates relating to rigour in qualitative research.
3 Why is it considered important to choose congruent data collection methods in qualitative research?

CASE STUDY 1

You met Angela, a physiotherapist in a multidisciplinary team in a large city hospital, in Chapter 4. She has enrolled in a Master of Physiotherapy Studies. The study itself was not a daunting prospect for Angela; however, deciding on how to research her chosen area gave her some concern. In Chapter 4, Angela noticed in her work that elderly women are often not listened to when they approach members of the health team and that they are seldom given adequate emotional support when they receive negative news about their health status. Therefore, in her research, Angela wants to 'give a voice' to elderly women and to sensitise staff to their unique needs. This study involves other members of the interdisciplinary team.

1 Generate some alternatives for a methodology or combination of methodologies that could carry Angela's project. Explain the rationale for your choice.
2 What can the methodologies offer Angela in terms of their theoretical assumptions about the kind(s) of knowledge she is seeking to generate?

CASE STUDY 2

Karen is undertaking a Master of Clinical Education to further her knowledge and expertise as a clinical facilitator at a busy metropolitan public hospital. Karen provides clinical education support to midwifery students from each year level, but is particularly interested in understanding the experience of the first-year students. As part of her studies, Karen decides to undertake a qualitative research project to describe the lived experiences of first-year midwifery students undertaking their first clinical placement in a postnatal ward. Karen aims to explore the following questions.

- How well do first-year students feel prepared before their first placement?
- What anxieties do students experience before, during and after their placement?
- What stressors do they experience on placement and how well do they feel supported by the registered midwives with whom they work?

1 Why would a qualitative approach be appropriate for Karen's research?
2 Which type of qualitative research design would you suggest Karen use?
3 What methods of data collection would be appropriate for Karen to use in her research project?

REFERENCES

Achora, S., & Matua, G. A. (2016). Essential methodological considerations when using grounded theory. *Nurse Researcher*, *23*(6), 31–6. https://doi.org/10.7748/nr.2016.e1409

Adams, M., Gardner, G., & Yates, P. (2016). Investigating nurse practitioners in the private sector: A theoretically informed research protocol. *Journal of Clinical Nursing*, *26*(11–12), 1608–20. https://doi.org/10.1111/jocn.13492

Atkinson, P. (2015). *For Ethnography*. London: SAGE.

Bidabadi, F. S., Yazdannik, A., & Zargham-Boroujeni, A. (2019). Patient's dignity in intensive care unit: A critical ethnography. *Nursing Ethics*, *26*(3), 738–52. https://doi.org/10.1177/0969733017720826

Bloxsome, D., Bayes, S., & Ireson, D. (2019). 'I love being a midwife; it's who I am': A Glaserian Grounded Theory Study of why midwives stay in midwifery. *Journal of Clinical Nursing*, *29*(1–2), 208–20. https://doi.org/10.1111/jocn.15078

Butler, A. E., Copnell, B., & Hall, H. (2018). The development of theoretical sampling in practice. *Collegian*, *25*(5), 561–6. https://doi.org/10.1016/j.colegn.2018.01.002

Carpenter, C. (2014). Phenomenology and rehabilitation research. In *Research Methods in Health*. Oxford University Press.

Charmaz, K. (2014). *Constructing Grounded Theory*. Sage.

Chun Tie, Y., Birks, M., & Francis, K. (2019). Grounded theory research: A design framework for novice researchers. *SAGE Open Medicine*, *7*, 205031211882292. https://doi.org/10.1177/2050312118822927

Davies, B. (1994). *Poststructural Theory and Classroom Practice*. Geelong, Victoria: Deakin University Press.

de Lange, S., van Eeden, I., & Heyns, T. (2018). Patient handover in the emergency department: 'How' is as important as 'what'. *International Emergency Nursing*, *36*, 46–50. https://doi.org/10.1016/j.ienj.2017.09.009

Delany, C., Edwards, I., & Fryer, C. (2018). How physiotherapists perceive, interpret, and respond to the ethical dimensions of practice: A qualitative study. *Physiotherapy Theory and Practice*, 1–14. https://doi.org/10.1080/09593985.2018.1456583

Digby, R., Lee, S., & Williams, A. (2017). The 'unworthy' patient with dementia in geriatric rehabilitation hospitals. *Collegian*, *25*(4), 377–83. https://doi.org/10.1016/j.colegn.2017.10.002

Duxbury, J., Wright, K. M., Hart, A., Bradley, D., Roach, P., Harris, N., & Carter, B. A. (2010). Structured observation of the interaction between nurses and patients during the administration of medication in an acute mental health unit. *Journal of Clinical Nursing*, *19*(17–18), 2481–92.

Glass, N. (2000). Speaking feminisms and nursing. In *Nursing Theory in Australia: Development and Application*. Pearson.

Gray, J. R., Grove, S. K., & Sutherland, S. (2017). *Burns and Grove's The Practice of Nursing Research: Appraisal, Synthesis, and Generation of Evidence* (8th edn). St Louis, MO: Elsevier.

Gullick, J., Monaro, S., & Stewart, G. (2016). Compartmentalising time and space: A phenomenological interpretation of the temporal experience of commencing haemodialysis. *Journal of Clinical Nursing*, *26*(21–22), 3382–95. https://doi.org/10.1111/jocn.13697

Harmon, J., Summons, P., & Higgins, I. (2019). Experiences of the older hospitalised person on nursing pain care: An ethnographic insight. *Journal of Clinical Nursing*, *28*(23–4), 4447–59. https://doi.org/10.1111/jocn.15029

Hickey, S., Kildea, S., Couchman, K., Watego-Ivory, K., West, R., Kruske, S., Blackman, R., Watego, S., & Roes, T. (2019). Establishing teams aiming to provide culturally safe maternity care for Indigenous families. *Women and Birth*, *32*, 449–59.

Jefferies, D., Duff, M., & Nicholls, D. (2017). Understanding the experience of women admitted to a psychiatric hospital in Sydney with psychosis or mania following childbirth after World War II (1945–1955). *International Journal of Mental Health Nursing*, *27*(2), 702–11. https://doi.org/10.1111/inm.12357

Johnstone, M.-J. (1999). Reflective topical autobiography: An under utilised interpretive research method in nursing. *Collegian*, *6*(1), 24–9. https://doi.org/10.1016/s1322-7696(08)60312-1

Kelly, J., & Henschke, K. (2019). The experiences of Australian Indigenous nursing students: A phenomenological study. *Nurse Education in Practice*, *41*, 102642. https://doi.org/10.1016/j.nepr.2019.102642

King, N., Horrocks, C., & Brooks, J. (2018). *Interviews in Qualitative Research*. (2nd edn). Sage.

Laging, B., Kenny, A., Bauer, M., & Nay, R. (2018). Recognition and assessment of resident deterioration in the nursing home setting: A critical ethnography. *Journal of Clinical Nursing*, *27*(7–8), 1452–63. https://doi.org/10.1111/jocn.14292

Lea, J., & Cruickshank, M. (2017). The role of rural nurse managers in supporting new graduate nurses in rural practice. *Journal of Nursing Management*, *25*(3), 176–83. https://doi.org/10.1111/jonm.12453

Lea, E., Marlow, A., Bramble, M., Andrews, S., Eccleston, C., McInerney, F., & Robinson, A. (2015). Improving student nurses' aged care understandings through a supported placement. *International Nursing Review*, *62*, 28–35.

LeBlanc, A., Bourbonnais, F. F., Harrison, D., & Tousignant, K. (2018). The experience of intensive care nurses caring for patients with delirium: A phenomenological study. *Intensive and Critical Care Nursing*, *44*, 92–8. https://doi.org/10.1016/j.iccn.2017.09.002

Madden, D., Sliney, A., O'Friel, A., McMackin, B., O'Callaghan, B., Casey, K., Courtney, L., Fleming, V., & Brady, V. (2017). Using action research to develop midwives' skills to support women with perinatal mental health needs. *Journal of Clinical Nursing*, *27*, 561–71.

McDonald, S. (2018). Integration of examination of the newborn into holistic midwifery practice: A grounded theory study. *Evidenced Based Midwifery*, *16*(4):128–35.

McGough, S., Wynaden, D., & Wright, M. (2017). Experience of providing cultural safety in mental health to Aboriginal patients: A grounded theory study. *International Journal of Mental Health Nursing*, *27*(1), 204–13. https://doi.org/10.1111/inm.12310

Moser, A., & Korstjens, I. (2018). Series: Practical guidance to qualitative research. Part 3: Sampling, data collection and analysis. *The European Journal of General Practice*, *24*(1), 9–18. https://doi.org/10.1080/13814788.2017.1375091

Neubauer, B. E., Witkop, C. T., & Varpio, L. (2019). How phenomenology can help us learn from the experiences of others. *Perspectives on Medical Education*, *8*(2), 90–7. https://doi.org/10.1007/s40037-019-0509-2

Newnham, E., McKellar, B., & Pincombe, J. (2017). 'It's your body but…': Mixed messages in childbirth education. Findings form a hospital ethnography. *Midwifery*, *55*, 53–9.

Ollivier, R. A., Aston, M. L., & Price, S. L. (2019). Exploring postpartum sexual health: A feminist poststructural analysis. *Health Care for Women International*, 1–20. https://doi.org/10.1080/07399332.2019.1638923

Ollivier, R., Aston, M., & Price, S. (2018). Let's talk about sex: A feminist poststructural approach to addressing sexual health in the healthcare setting. *Journal of Clinical Nursing*, *28*(3–4), 695–702. https://doi.org/10.1111/jocn.14685

Pilkington, L., Haigh, M. M., Durey, A., Katzenellenbogen, J. M., & Thompson, S. C. (2017). Perspectives of Aboriginal women on participation in mammographic screening: A step towards improving services. *BMC Public Health*, *17*(1). https://doi.org/10.1186/s12889-017-4701-1

Polit, D. F., & Beck, C. T. (2020). *Nursing Research: Generating and Assessing Evidence for Nursing Practice.* (11th edn). Wolters Kluwer.

Rieger, K. L. (2018). Discriminating among grounded theory approaches. *Nursing Inquiry*, *26*(1), e12261. https://doi.org/10.1111/nin.12261

Schafer, R. J. (1980). *A Guide to Historical Method*. Dorsey Press.

Sharp, S., McAllister, M., & Broadbent, M. (2018). The tension between person centred and task focused care in an acute surgical setting: A critical ethnography. *Collegian*, *25*(1), 11–17. https://doi.org/10.1016/j.colegn.2017.02.002

Simpson, P., Thomas, R., Bendall, J., Lord, B., Lord, S., & Close, J. (2017). 'Popping nana back into bed' – a qualitative exploration of paramedic decision making when caring for older people who have fallen. *BMC Health Services Research*, *17*(1). https://doi.org/10.1186/s12913-017-2243-y

Spiegelberg, H. (1970). On some human uses of phenomenology. In *Phenomenology in Perspective*. Martinus Nijhoff.

Strauss, A., & Corbin, J. (2008). *Basics of Qualitative Research: Techniques and Procedures for Developing Grounded Theory* (3rd edn). Sage.

Streubert, H., & Carpenter, D. R. (2011). *Qualitative Nursing Research: Advancing the Humanistic Imperative* (5th edn). Philadelphia, PA: JB Lippincott Co.

Sundler, A. J., Lindberg, E., Nilsson, C., & Palmér, L. (2019). Qualitative thematic analysis based on descriptive phenomenology. *Nursing Open*. https://doi.org/10.1002/nop2.275

Taylor, B., Roberts, S., Smyth, T., & Tulloch, M. (2014). Nurse managers' strategies for feeling less drained by their work: An action research and reflection project for developing emotional intelligence. *Journal of Nursing Management*, *23*(7), 879–87. https://doi.org/10.1111/jonm.12229

Thompson, J., Cook, G., & Duschinsky, R. (2017). 'I'm not sure I'm a nurse': A hermeneutic phenomenological study of nursing home nurses' work identity. *Journal of Clinical Nursing*, *27*(5–6), 1049–62. https://doi.org/10.1111/jocn.14111

Tierney, O., Sweet, L., Houston, D., & Ebert, L. (2018). A historical account of the governance of midwifery education in Australia and the evolution of the Continuity of Care Experience. *Women and Birth*, *31*(3), e210–15. https://doi.org/10.1016/j.wombi.2017.09.009

Timonen, V., Foley, G., & Conlon, C. (2018). Challenges when using grounded theory. *International Journal of Qualitative Methods*, *17*(1), 160940691875808. https://doi.org/10.1177/1609406918758086

van Manen, M. (1990). Beyond assumptions: Shifting the limits of action research. *Theory into Practice*, *29*(3), 152–7. https://doi.org/10.1080/00405849009543448

Walder, K., & Molineux, M. (2019). Listening to the client voice – a constructivist grounded theory study of the experiences of client-centred practice after stroke. *Australian Occupational Therapy Journal*, *67*(2), 100–9. https://doi.org/10.1111/1440-1630.12627

Walshe, C. (2020). Aims, actions and advanced care planning by district nurses providing palliative care: An ethnographic observational study. *British Journal of Community Nursing.* 25(6), 276–86.

Weedon, C. (1991). *Feminist Practice and Poststructuralist Theory*. Basil Blackwell.

FURTHER READING

Bunkenborg, G., Samuelson, K., Akeson, J., & Poulsen, I. (2013). Impact of professionalism in nursing on in-hospital bedside monitoring practice. *Journal of Advanced Nursing, 69*(7), 1466–77.

Cooper, L., Ells, L., Ryan, C., & Martin, D. (2018). Perceptions of adults with overweight/obesity and chronic musculoskeletal pain: An interpretative phenomenological analysis. *Journal of Clinical Nursing, 27*(5–6), e776–86. https://doi.org/10.1111/jocn.14178

Flanagan, B., Lord, B., Reed, R., & Crimmins, G. (2019). Listening to women's voices: The experience of giving birth with paramedic care in Queensland, Australia. *BMC Pregnancy and Childbirth, 19*(1). https://doi.org/10.1186/s12884-019-2613-z

Hegney, D. G., & Francis, K. (2015). Action research: Changing nursing practice. *Nursing Standard, 29*(40), 36–41. https://doi.org/10.7748/ns.29.40.36.e8710

Hitchcock, M., Gillespie, B., Crilly, J., & Chaboyer, W. (2014). Triage: An investigation of the process and potential vulnerabilities. *Journal of Advanced Nursing, 70*(7), 1532–41.

Irving, M., Short, S., Gwynne, K., Tennant, M., & Blinkhorn, A. (2016). 'I miss my family, it's been a while…': A qualitative study of clinicians who live and work in rural/remote Australian Aboriginal communities. *Australian Journal of Rural Health, 25*(5), 260–7. https://doi.org/10.1111/ajr.12343

Klages, D., East, L., Jackson, D., & Usher, K. (2019). A four-stage framework for conducting feminist storytelling research. *Nurse Researcher.* https://doi.org/10.7748/nr.2019.e1624

McKittrick, J. T., Kinney, S., Lima, S., & Allen, M. (2018). The first 3 minutes: Optimising a short realistic paediatric team resuscitation training session. *Nurse Education in Practice, 28*, 115–20. https://doi.org/10.1016/j.nepr.2017.10.020

Miller, J., Vivona, B., & Roth, G. (2017). Work role transitions – expert nurses to novice preceptors. *European Journal of Training and Development, 41*(6), 559 74. https://doi.org/10.1108/ejtd-10-2016-0081

Morgan, D. (2019). *Basic and Advanced Focus Groups.* Sage.

Sim, J., & Waterfield, J. (2019). Focus group methodology: Some ethical challenges. *Quality and Quantity, 53*, 3003–22. https://doi.org/10.1007/s11135-019-00914-5

Urban, A. M. (2014). Taken for granted: Normalizing nurses' work in hospitals. *Nursing Inquiry,*

8 COLLECTION, MANAGEMENT AND ANALYSIS OF QUALITATIVE DATA

Chapter learning objectives

The material presented in this chapter will assist you to:

1 identify forms of qualitative data and align data collection methods with different qualitative methodologies
2 prepare for data collection and use strategies for collecting the data, including the storage of data
3 identify approaches to analysing qualitative data
4 code the data
5 discuss methods of thematic analysis, including content analysis
6 describe other methods of text analysis such as narrative and discourse analysis
7 identify computer software that can manage qualitative data
8 discuss analysis of images as qualitative data.

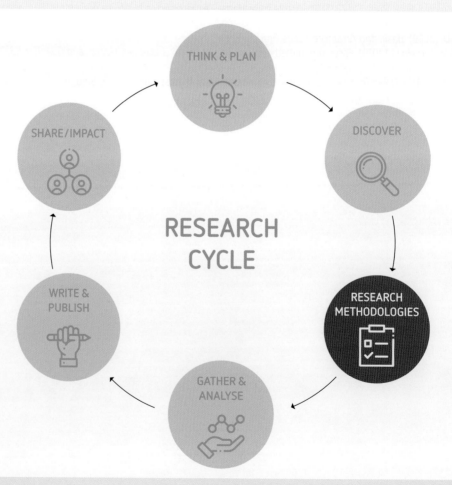

Research cycle

The primary focus of this chapter is analysis of qualitative data. This is a key component of collecting and analysing data, as highlighted in the research cycle above.

Introduction

This chapter introduces you to the various methods and processes of data collection used in qualitative research and discusses the different forms of qualitative data. It discusses the usefulness of qualitative data in relation to context, lived experience, subjectivity and potential for change. This discussion is followed by some strategies that can be used when preparing for data collection and deciding which data forms and combinations to use, consistent with the chosen methodology. Some practical hints for qualitative analysis are then provided. There are hints on pitfalls to avoid in the process and ideas for storing and coding the data. The chapter concludes with an introductory discussion on the use of computers in collecting and managing qualitative data.

Forms of qualitative data

The tools or data for building new knowledge in qualitative research are usually words, because they are the main medium through which people express themselves and their relationships to other people and things, in and beyond their lives. Other data forms in qualitative research include the demonstration and interpretation of artistic expression such as painting, drawing, montage, poetry, dance, music, symbols and singing. Still photographs and videos are also counted as data. Predominantly, though, qualitative research data are collected and stored in the form of words, whether they be from archival searches, case studies, field notes, group process outcomes, interview transcriptions, journal entries, literature searches, observation notes or written accounts of stories. Know ahead of time the data forms you are collecting so you can make appropriate preparations for collecting them.

Data collection

Deciding on data forms and combinations

For the sake of continuity, the distinctions between *interpretive* and *critical* forms of qualitative research will be used. For each methodology, some methods and forms of data will be suggested (see Table 8.1). This does not mean that these combinations are the best or only ways of looking at choosing forms of data; rather, they are meant to be guidelines when decisions are made concerning the nature of the research.

ACTIVITY

Imagine a clinical question you would like to explore using a qualitative research approach. Describe what data forms and combinations would best serve this question.

From undertaking the above activity in setting out some of the possibilities for using qualitative data forms, you may see that data forms are basically combinations of words, images and numbers that act as pieces of information that need to be analysed and interpreted with the research questions, aims and objectives in mind. The choice of data forms will depend on the nature and intentions of the research and the willingness to use combinations of methods, which will in turn produce certain combinations of data. Think about what you want to know and why, before a decision is made on what data will be collected and how. Sources of qualitative data include interviews, observations, and documents in the form of narrative (text) scripts, commonly gathered from interviews, survey questions, journals, recorded observations or existing documents, among other sources.

▶ Table 8.1   Methodologies, methods and possible data forms

Methodology	Possible methods	Possible data forms
Interpretive research methodologies		
Grounded theory	• Participant observation • Interviews	• Words, photographs • Words
Phenomenology	• Participant observation • Interviews • Creative writing	• Words, photographs, video • Words • Words
Historical research	• Archival searches • Interviews • Document analysis	• Words, photographs • Words • Words
Ethnography	• Participant observation • Field notes	• Words, photographs, video • Words
Critical research methodologies		
Action research	• Surveys • Questionnaires • Interviews • Participant observation • Group processes • Reflective journal	• Words, numbers • Words, numbers • Words • Words, photographs, video • Words • Words, drawings
Feminist research	• Group processes • Interviews • Reflective journal • Surveys • Questionnaires • Creative expression	• Words • Words • Words, drawings • Words, numbers • Words, numbers • Words, painting, poetry, dance
Critical ethnography	• Participant observation • Interviews • Group processes • Reflective journal	• Words, photographs, video • Words • Words • Words, drawings

Some qualitative approaches allow for a mixture of people and paper sources. In an oral history, for instance, the person's story of their life might be augmented with some personal and public domain documents and photographs. These data not only add strength to the oral account but may also give validation to what has been said and add visual interest to the story.

Having decided on the data forms that would best serve the research questions, aims and objectives, consider how each of the data forms will be analysed and how the various forms of analysis will be integrated into producing interpretations that best express the findings of the research. Thinking about possible ways of analysing data should begin at around the same time that the decision is made on what forms of data to collect. There is little point in collecting data that may have little or no relevance in fulfilling the aims and objectives of the research.

Strategies for collecting the data

The method of data collection will vary according to what you want to achieve in the research, and can include single or multiple data collection methods. A selection of data collection methods was described in Chapter 7.

Choose the appropriate method

Be confident that the chosen methods will gather the data required. Audio record interviews of one hour or more to ensure that all the ideas expressed by the participant are captured. Similarly, if non-verbal cues are important in understanding the participants' experiences, use video facilities that record all the visual and auditory cues.

Check the usefulness of the method

It is important at this stage to check the validity of the chosen method. Asking yourself the questions shown in Figure 8.1 will help you to ascertain this.

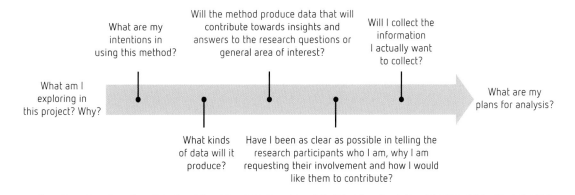

▸ **Figure 8.1** Checking the reliability of the data analysis method

Pitfalls to avoid

People, place and equipment problems

Essentially, qualitative research is people-oriented, so have respect for and include all the people involved. This means that prior to collecting the data, basic steps must be taken, such as obtaining full ethical clearance from the institutions involved, prepared consent forms and plain-language statements for participants to read and sign.

The key people at the research site need to be informed as to who is collecting the data, when the data are being collected and the expectations of the researcher regarding the involvement of staff at the research site. Sometimes, several phone calls need to be made or several letters written to confirm the details of the research and all the arrangements. Even then, people may not show up or, if they do, have little or no idea of who the researcher is and why they are there to talk with them. The researcher is responsible for being clear and concise and to be prepared for any contingencies that may arise. Make sure that people in the setting who are not involved in the project know who the researcher is and why they are there. First impressions are very important in face-to-face interviews so if an appointment time has been made for the interview, be punctual.

Find a place to collect data that is conducive to the methods being used. If staff or patients are being interviewed, a quiet and private place must be organised that provides privacy and ensures there are no interruptions to ensure they can speak freely and be heard clearly on the recording equipment. Generally, avoid busy places that have high traffic flows, lots of background voices, banging doors and ringing phones. If admission to restricted areas cannot be gained, another place to meet participants needs to be negotiated.

It is critical to check that all equipment (e.g. audio recorders, video recorders) works before being taken to the research setting and then again once set up at the location. If one power point does not work, try another. Take extra batteries. Have a backup pen and paper in case there is no power or the power goes out. Ensure the recording device is close enough to record the conversation.

Other practical hints

Some other practical hints to consider during the information-gathering sessions are presented in Table 8.2.

▸**Table 8.2** Practical hints

Introduce yourself	Reiterate your gratitude for the participant's involvement
Spend some time in conversation	Put the participant at ease by creating a relaxed and open setting for the data collection; explain the purpose and the format of the interview and advise how long this will usually take; ensure the consent form is signed and discuss confidentiality and anonymity
Label the data	Record the participant's name, time, date of interview and the setting
Communicate effectively	Communicate clearly and openly during the data collection; ask one question at a time and listen actively; provide transition between major topics
Check that the equipment works properly	Ensure the equipment will work during the data collection; check this occasionally throughout the interview
Keep on track	Keep focused on what it is you are doing so that the data you collect are what you want; don't lose control of the interview
Keep to time	Negotiate if more time is needed
Inform the participant when the collection is over	Explain what happens next in the project and how the participant will be involved
Express your thanks	Participants' contributions to your research are an act of generosity on their part and are worthy of sincere acknowledgement
Immediately after the interview	Add to written notes if these were taken during the interview; write down any observations if written notes were not taken

Approaches to analysing qualitative data

The orientation of the qualitative researcher

Qualitative research analysis requires a personal approach, with an attitude of respect for people, their experiences and words, and with confidence that meaning will be found in them. If the methods have been chosen wisely and the research participants know what knowledge is wanted and why, the data you collect are likely to provide some insights and answers to your research questions.

Being physically and emotionally prepared

Qualitative analysis requires that the researcher read, look at and listen to language with alertness. This means the researcher needs to feel physically and emotionally fresh before attempting the analysis. For example, choose a time of day when you know you will feel your best. It might also help to use some sort of centring technique to get you into a mood that allows you to be fully present.

Getting started

Maintaining data security and integrity

The data collected are tantamount to a rich, raw resource; it is imperative to maintain their security and integrity.

Security relates to ensuring that data are stored according to agreed guidelines. The National Health and Medical Research Council (NHMRC) regulations regarding the storage of data dictate that they be stored in a locked area under the supervision of the researcher for five years after collection. Any copies of the data should be likewise stored.

Integrity refers to keeping data stored in such a way that they are maintained in their best state for use and possible review. The main copies are the heart of the research and should be treated carefully. Store transcripts, documents, photographs, computer files, hard copies of items of artistic expression and other forms of data in a safe place. The integrity of the data should be checked from time to time; if the hard copies that contain the data begin to deteriorate, then steps must be taken to amend the storage plan. This same principle applies to any data stored digitally, such as on a computer hard drive.

Copies of all the data should be made, in whatever form they are stored. Ensure that the original copy is kept to one side, with identifying details and the date written clearly on it, then store carefully. Duplicated copies can be labelled 'Working copy 1' and so on to differentiate them as the copies on which the analysis will be done. Update and label copies as the work progresses so that there is no confusion among differing versions of the same electronic document.

Decide on an organising system

Paper files should be stored in their appropriate bundles, or code and name computer files according to their data content. The principal thing to keep in mind is the need to be practical and careful in preparing the data for analysis. An appropriate organising system should be chosen that suits best but be prepared to make adaptations to that system if it is not serving you well.

Have confidence in words as data

If you are careful about the choice and implementation of the research methods, you can be confident that within the words collected as data there will be answers to the questions posed. If the research participants have responded well to the invitation to speak of their experiences and you have been careful to ask the sorts of questions that will give them a chance to supply the answers needed to fulfil the research objectives, then the magnitude and richness of the textual information that people will offer will be found.

ACTIVITY

Using audio equipment, interview a friend for 5 to 10 minutes on a topic of your choice. Ensure that the topic explores your friend's experience of something that can be analysed – it could be about the experience of being healthy, unwell, fulfilled, hopeful, grieving, being a research student and so on.

The essential research question then becomes: 'What is your experience of ...?' When you are both ready and the audio equipment is recording, ask your friend to 'Think of a time when you felt/were ... Tell me about it please'. If your friend needs help to keep talking, give conversational prompts, such as 'You were saying before that ... Tell me more about that please'.

Coding the data

Ethical requirements demand that data maintain the anonymity and privacy of the research participants and places. There are several ways this can be complied with.

Pseudonyms

Participants may suggest a pseudonym by which they would like to be known and code names for organisations mentioned in the data. If they are hesitant, the researcher makes up names. When the data are ready to be analysed, they can be organised according to the order that they were collected or according to the alphabetical ordering of the pseudonyms.

Ethics

Numbering

A more impersonal way of coding the data for anonymity and privacy is to use a numbering system and to eradicate proper nouns in relation to places. For example, the text could read: 'Participant 1 referred to her experience at the local hospital'. Manual and computer codes can be used to hide the identities of participants and places. The researcher decides on the construction of the code and then stores the main key to the code with the data in the locked area. Manual and computer codes can use letters, words or numbers, alone or in combination. It does not really matter what system is used if it is logical and consistent throughout and has the potential to represent the data in their entirety.

Coding for analysis

Coding is one way of analysing qualitative data, but it is not the only way. Coding involves making sense of the texts from interviews, observations and documents and enables artful and creative interpretation and analysis of the data (Skjott Linneberg & Korsgaard, 2019, p. 260). Coding attributes interpreted meaning to each individual datum for later purposes of pattern detection, categorisation, assertion or proposition development, theory building and other analytic processes. Rarely will anyone get coding right the first time. Qualitative inquiry demands meticulous attention to language and images, and deep reflection on the emergent patterns and meanings of human experience (Saldana, 2021). Since the number of codes can accumulate quite quickly and change as analysis progresses, keep a record of your emergent codes in a separate file as a codebook – a compilation of the codes, their content descriptions and a brief data example for reference. The utilisation of a codebook allows a more refined, focused and efficient analysis of the raw data in subsequent reads (Skjott Linneberg & Korsgaard, 2019).

Methods of thematic analysis

Nursing researchers frequently use qualitative **content analysis** and **thematic analysis** as two analysis approaches (Nowell et al., 2017). The two methods have similarities but they also have important differences. (Brough, 2019) Content analysis is a general term for several different strategies used to analyse text. It is a systematic coding and categorising approach used for exploring large amounts of textual information unobtrusively to determine trends and patterns of words used, their frequency, their relationships and the structures and discourses of communication. The purpose of content analysis is to describe the characteristics of the document's content by examining who says what, to whom and with what effect.

Thematic analysis is a qualitative research method that can be widely used. It is a method for 'identifying, analysing, organising, describing and reporting themes and essences, found within a data set' (Nowell et al., 2017, p. 2). Thematic analysis is simple to use, and therefore lends itself to use for novice researchers who are unfamiliar with more complex types of qualitative analysis. It allows for flexibility in the researchers' choice of theoretical framework. Some other methods of analysis are closely tied to specific theories, but thematic analysis can be used with any theory the researcher chooses. Through this flexibility, thematic analysis allows for rich, detailed and complex description of the data.

Methods appropriate to intentions

The qualitative analysis of words may be by manual or computer-assisted means. The intentions of the analysis will determine what is done with the words. Researchers with exploratory and descriptive intentions, for example, may use analysis methods that produce groups of themes and subthemes. Although there is no strict prescription, these methods are helpful because they enable a descriptive interpretation of human experiences to be made. Practical guides for manual and computer-assisted methods of data analysis are described later in this chapter.

Researchers who intend to bring about changes may prefer critical analyses of discourses and the other economic, political, cultural, social and historical determinants. These analyses may involve thematic approaches, but with extra scrutiny to bring about awareness of the silences and gaps in the discourse as well as issues of power and domination. Methods that provide analysis for qualitative critical research approaches based on critical social science, as well as research influenced by post-structural thinking, are described later in this chapter.

ACTIVITY

Transcribe the audio recording of the 5- to 10-minute interview you undertook with your friend for the previous activity. This process will work best if you type sections of text straight into a word-processing document on your computer. If you are not a touch-typist, you will soon see why the instruction was to keep the interview to 5 to 10 minutes – transcribing takes quite some time and effort.

A visual representation of the coding process is presented in **Figure 8.2**.

Finding explicit and implicit themes

Themes can be known by other names, but they are essentially the same thing. In grounded theory, for example, a subtheme is similar to a code and a theme is similar to a category.

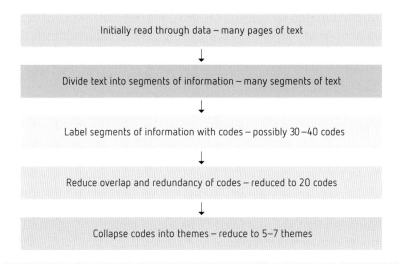

Initially read through data – many pages of text

↓

Divide text into segments of information – many segments of text

↓

Label segments of information with codes – possibly 30–40 codes

↓

Reduce overlap and redundancy of codes – reduced to 20 codes

↓

Collapse codes into themes – reduce to 5–7 themes

▸ **Figure 8.2** The coding process in qualitative analysis

In approaches such as phenomenology, themes can also be called 'essences' or 'aspects'. The following advice on how to find themes, whatever they are named, may be of assistance, regardless of whether a manual or a computer-assisted method of thematic analysis is used.

Know what is being looked for

Before the researcher begins looking for themes, they review the research proposal. What is the research project's aims and objectives? The researcher keeps those ideas firmly in mind as they go about finding themes. This is so that they will recognise a theme when it is seen. It is easy for the researcher to become sidetracked once they get in among the thick undergrowth of data. Keeping the aims and objectives in mind will assist in finding what is being looked for.

Locate specific words for explicit themes

If specific words or combinations of words are searched for, it is a relatively simple task to look for their appearance within sections of the text. The word 'health', for instance, will feature frequently in a discussion about health promotion. This is an **explicit theme** in that it will float with relative ease to the top of a well of words when doing an analysis. Explicit themes are apparent because they provide direct answers to direct research questions, so they speak out loudly when reading, so much so that it is difficult to miss them.

Look closely for implicit themes

It is important to recognise that a theme will not always be stated as a direct word or words, or even as an easily recognisable concept. Take the example of health. People might talk about feeling 'good', 'well', 'happy', 'energised' and so on, but there may be little or no mention at all of health words; rather there might be a story, an innuendo, a hint or a fine wisp of language that portrays a health-related situation.

TIP

Data should be organised in a way that makes it easy to look at and allows the researcher to go through each topic to pick out concepts or themes.

So how is an **implicit theme** recognised? It will be recognised because of the way it fits into the total context of what has been said. By being very familiar with the transcript, the researcher will be ever watchful for what it can tell them. Once located, the fine threads that are its components will be connected to other parts of the text, and where they began and where they finished will be seen.

Be sure it is a theme

The researcher will know a theme has been located because it bears a resemblance to what was thought might be found. It might not look exactly like the whole thing they are looking for, but they will know that it is related because it comes into their awareness in answer to the questions that have been posed as the text has been analysed for signs of it. It is part of the pattern of answers that are intending to be found within the text and it is relevant because its identity is connected directly, or sometimes indirectly, to the stated research aims and objectives.

ACTIVITY

Review everything from the heading 'Getting started' (see page 203) up until this point. Prepare yourself and the transcribed document from previous activities as suggested in this text.

Manual approaches

If not using a computer, then the great many words that qualitative research tends to produce will need to be stored on a lot of paper. Therefore, if a manual method of analysis is chosen there needs to be a systematic approach to handling the data. To chart a course through these data, analytical progress must be documented by using a tagging system called 'thematic identification' that will show the pathway by which sense of the words is made and will put them into some order for interpretation.

Review the aims and objectives

It is important that the aims and objectives of the research are reviewed. What was the purpose of the research? What, why and how was being undertaken in the research? Revisit the words written in the proposal and focus on the key ideas to ensure there is clarity about what it is that needs to emerge from the information amassed from the research participants. The statements made about the aims and objectives of the research should be looked at again and kept in in mind while the analysis is carried out.

Read and reread

Once the view of the research objectives and strategies has been refreshed and refocused, begin by reading and rereading the text. There is likely to be a lot of information in the transcripts, some of which is directly useful, some of which may need to be stored away for another time and some of which will never be used again. There are many ways to proceed at this point. There is no one correct way to do this; as long as the researcher is quite clear about the research aims and objectives, the analysis methods may be adjusted to fit the unique requirements of the project and its participants.

The manual method

As you prepare text-based qualitative data for manual (i.e. paper-and-pencil) coding and analysing, lay out printed interview transcripts, field notes and other researcher-generated materials in double-spaced format on the left half or left two-thirds of the page, keeping a wide right-hand margin for writing codes and notes. Number the pages of the transcript either sequentially from 1 or use a number–number (1-1, 1-2 etc.) or alpha–number (A-1, A-2 etc.) combination to number each transcript or each group of transcripts.

Make multiple copies of the transcripts and ensure that one copy is kept untouched as a guide. It may be useful to have the audio recording of the interview playing as the transcripts are read so the intonations and emphases of the speakers' words can be captured.

Colour-coding is another method, whereby a wide range of coloured pens are used to mark the text in colour codes according to specific words, ideas, sections and/or nuances that appear to be connected. A word or words are written in the margin beside each colour or font to capture the main idea represented. The words are listed then reviewed and the list reduced so that similar ideas merge into groups.

The limits of the reduction are reached when ideas can no longer be moved without losing some of their specialness in relation to the research. What remain (because they defy further movement into groupings) are the distinct themes.

Know the text thoroughly

Read the transcripts one by one and be alert to picking up the nuances in the text. They allow the reader to come to know the text thoroughly. The transcripts may have to be read many times over to get to this stage of familiarity. Keep the research question and/or objectives in mind so that the attention falls on the relevant words, phrases, sections of dialogue and strong and subtle connections between parts of the document.

Allow time for it to come together

It is important not to try to catch the whole of the meaning in an instant or even in the first protracted sitting. Allow the information to percolate and incubate in the mind for a while. This allows for connections to start to emerge, sometimes at the most unexpected moments. Researchers have spoken of waking during the night and writing down an insight or making a hurried note on a paper serviette in a restaurant.

ACTIVITY

To undertake an analysis of your friend's experience, use the suggestions in the section 'Manual approaches' (page 208). Try any or all the methods suggested to analyse what the experience was like for your friend. When you have completed the manual analysis, show it to your friend to see if the themes resonate.

Computer-assisted approaches

Computer-assisted strategies for finding themes may be used instead of paper. An electronic copy of the main text to be analysed is first made.

Tidy the transcript

When working with a transcript of an interview it is important to eliminate any extraneous matter from the copy, such as side conversations or comments not central to the research and any 'ums', 'ahs' and 'ohs'. Some researchers are loath to drop these linguistic hesitations, but they serve no purpose except to make the participant sound awkward, to impinge on the flow of language and to impede the text with irrelevancies. Keep in mind that participants often read their own transcript for validation purposes.

Read and section

The researcher starts from the beginning of the sequence to be analysed and read as they scroll through the text. As parts of the text relating to the research interests appear, they are sectioned off under a descriptive subheading. In a practical sense, sectioning is as simple as pressing the computer's enter key several times to push a block of text several lines down to isolate it for separate consideration.

As progress is made through the document, it may be found that sectioning it through the use of headings and subheadings can better help to organise the text and create connections between themes that are raised in one part of the text and reiterated in another.

Subheadings and general labels may contain some of the words that appear in the text or a short phrase that reflects most closely the explicit content and implicit meaning of the sectioned text.

Look for themes

As the text is being read the researcher asks themselves:
- What is the text saying?
- Is there anything here that relates to my research aims and objectives?
- Is anything here implicitly connected to what I have read before?

    It may be possible to locate themes straight away as the analysis proceeds, or subthemes may be found. Subthemes are related to the main themes; they are subsections or further elaborations of a theme.

Being aware of personal feelings

As the analysis is scrutinised you need to be aware of any emotions you may be feeling. Analysis can be a taxing and tiring experience, so it is important to be sensitive to your feelings and why you might be having them. Do not become too disheartened if you feel you are not finding enough. As mentioned above, one or two themes could be hidden under a mountain of other data and remain out of reach for a while. Just remember that it is quality you are after, not quantity.

    If the analysis process seems to be overwhelming, take a break, go for a walk or create some other relaxing space away from the task. Also, remember not to let personal feelings get in the way of the task at hand; be diligent to ensure that the analysis is what the participants' accounts reflect.

TIP

During the first run-through, do not be overly concerned about trying to find all there is to find; some of the subthemes and implicit themes will remain hidden until later.

Collating the themes

The working document still looks a bit messy with headings, subheadings, themes and subthemes, alone or in combinations, but it is the essence and basis of the final analysis. Now it is time to tidy the working document and collate the actual themes. It is at this point that a computer is useful because you can copy the entire working document easily, ready for its transformation.

Copy the entire analysis of what has just been done and create a new file. Thus, there is a duplicated working document for the next round of refinements.

The next stage is to go through and delete everything in the duplicated copy of the analysis to date except for the headings, subheadings, themes and subthemes that were previously generated.

Review the list and concentrate on the research area again by asking what this says about the research interest. The answers to this question, or others phrased in a similar vein, will provide the themes for the research.

As the list is reviewed the following questions can be posed to look for connections between the words and phrases listed there.

- Do some of these words and phrases look similar?
- If so, are they similar enough to be merged without losing their essential identity?

If the answer to the second question is yes, the words or phrases are put together; if it is no, they are left separate.

This process of thinking, shifting and collating continues until everything settles into the place it fits best in relation to the original questions posed in the project and the aims and objectives in relation to them.

Once this work is complete, what is left are the themes.

Name the themes

The researcher may name the themes whatever they choose. However, they should spare a thought for the readers of their research by not making the theme names too obscure or exotic. Humour and/or simplicity are permissible in naming themes; however, the heading needs to reflect the nature of the text that follows.

ACTIVITY

Use the suggestions in the section 'Computer-assisted approaches' (see page 210) to undertake an analysis of your friend's experience. When you have completed the computer-assisted analysis, show it to your friend to see if the themes resonate. Which analysis method do you prefer – the manual or the computer-assisted method? Why?

Combining to form common themes

The method of analysis thus far is useful for a single-text analysis. But if many people have been interviewed, it may be more appropriate to analyse each transcript separately and then combine the group accounts to find common themes. This involves the simple matter of attending to each transcript as described above and making a document for

TIP

The aim of the collective analysis is to find the ideas that are different enough to remain in their own categories.

each participant. Each document is gone through and the analysis undertaken is described. When all the documents have been separately analysed, they are combined to find common themes by duplicating the final versions of the separate analyses on a computer and putting them together in one file.

Next, similar themes are merged; for example, if participants all say that they are happy, sad, confused and so on, the researcher knows that these are all emotions. Hence, these ideas are placed under one heading, 'Emotions', with the description of the theme, what the term means and what elements are included.

When naming common themes, it is a good idea to write a short phrase consisting of a verb and noun that reflects the participant's experience and is consistent with the project's focus.

Tobler-Ammann and colleagues (2020) undertook a qualitative study that focused specifically on the patients' experience of unilateral spatial neglect between stroke onset and discharge from inpatient rehabilitation, in which thematic analysis following the method described by Braun and Clarke (2006) was employed. **Table 8.3** presents the process Tobler-Ammann and colleagues used.

▶**Table 8.3**   The five phases of analysis and a description of the process involved

Phase	Description of process
1. Each of the seven authors followed Braun and Clarke's (2006) recommendations	• Each author read and reread the transcripts and made notes on their initial interpretations
2. Authors met together for an analysis session to consider the codes and themes generated by each author	• A meeting was set up and the authors described their interpretations of the data individually • Only after consensus was reached between the authors, data analysis moved forward to its next phase • The final themes were agreed on
3. Final reviews of the data to further validate the findings	• Each author then read through the transcripts again to ensure the final themes were truly reflective of the data
4. The report was produced	• Each theme was written up into a report and data extracts were selected to be used as examples when describing each theme
5. Validation from a mental health nurse educator	• A mental health nursing educator read over the themes and considered the credibility of the findings

Source: Based on Tobler-Ammann, B. C., Weise, A., Knols, R. H., Watson, M. J., Sieben, J. M., de Bie, R. A., & de Bruin, E. D. (2020). Patients' experiences of unilateral spatial neglect between stroke onset and discharge from inpatient rehabilitation: A thematic analysis of qualitative interviews. *Disability and Rehabilitation*, 22 November, 1–10, http://doi.org/10.1080/09638288.2018.1531150

Other methods of text analysis

In qualitative research, words make up the texts, language and discourses that carry the meaning of human experience. Qualitative data analysis seeks to scrutinise and organise words in light of the research objectives and the particular methodological assumptions about the approach taken. Methods of data collection and analysis are not bound by methodologies; that is, a qualitative approach such as ethnography does not own participant observation any more than action research does not own participatory group processes. Even though these two examples are known to often use selected methods, they do not always use them; nor do they exclude other possible methods. With this in mind, there are other analytical methods, such as **narrative analysis** and **discourse analysis**, that can be used in a variety of approaches that stretch across and beyond methodologies and research paradigms.

Narrative analysis

Storytelling is a popular method of qualitative data collection. Sense can be made of the stories via a variety of methods (Flanagan et al., 2019; Gould et al., 2017), including thematic analysis, as described in this chapter. If a storytelling or narrative approach is chosen for the project, time should be spent searching the literature for the particular approach that best suits the research questions, aims and objectives.

EVIDENCE FOR BEST PRACTICE

STORYTELLING

Research undertaken by Pilkington and colleagues (2017) examined perspectives on breast screening among Aboriginal women in Western Australia. Factors which impacted on participation in breast screening were explored and potential initiatives to address lower participation in screening were sought. The results argued that making breast screening programs more accessible to Aboriginal women can reduce the current disparity between the screening participation rates of Aboriginal and non-Aboriginal women.

NARRATIVE ANALYSIS

Marsh and colleagues (2019) studied childbearing women's and professionals' experiences of Assumption of Care at birth to increase understanding of individual participants' stories, how they made sense of meanings and how these experiences framed their lives. The researchers used interviews guided by a narrative inquiry framework with four groups: childbearing women, midwives, social workers and Family and Community Services case managers. Holistic form was used for reading, interpreting and analysing the narratives. The findings of the research found unwanted emotional (isolation, shame, guilt, loss, disenfranchised grief) and physical consequences (depression, substance abuse complications) for women experiencing an Assumption of Care at the time of birth. There were also conflicting ethical and moral positions for the professionals involved. The use/abuse of power, concealment of facts and disenfranchised grief were identified as intertwined plots that caused or increased tensions.

The results of this study have implications for practice with a need for a twofold change to maternity care for women at risk of an Assumption of Care: a therapeutic justice model of maternity care and continuity of midwifery care with a dedicated midwife. Introducing these changes could increase women's and children's safety and wellbeing.

Another way of looking at narrative analysis is to consider the ways that stories told in interviews can be analysed. An interview can be converted into a story by amending the text to make the participant's words paramount. If creating stories from interview transcripts, a useful method of 'core story creation' as described by Petty, Jarvis and Thomas (2018), can be used (see Figure 8.3).

1	• Interview transcripts read several times to absorb and understand the content
2	• All interviewer contributions deleted from the transcript
3	• All unnecessary words or sentences that detract from the key ideas of the participant sentence are deleted
4	• Remaining text reread for sense
5	• Steps 3 and 4 repeated so only key ideas are retained
6	• Text reconfigured – divided into events that are reordered chronologically. The end result is now a series of events (emplotment)
7	• Cross-checking between the reconfigured text and the original transcripts to ensure meanings are revalidated
8	• Events / plots combined to create a single coherent story for each participant in chronological order
9	• Verification by returning the transcripts and stories to the participants. If necessary, make final chapter changes or corrections
10	• Core story creation complete

TIP

Having created a core story, the next analysis task is to provide an underlying plot structure or meaning to the story. Petty, Jarvis and Thomas (2018) provide a discussion on employment.

▶ **Figure 8.3**   Summary of procedures used in core story creation

Source: Adapted from Petty, J., Jarvis, J., & Thomas, R. (2018). Core story creation: Analysing narratives to construct stories for learning. *Nurse Researcher, 25*(4), 16 March, 47 – 51. http://doi.org/10.7748/nr.2018.e1533

There are many ways of doing narrative analysis – one of which is presented in Figure 8.4 – just as there are many reasons for, and modes of, telling stories. If you intend to use a narrative approach in your research, explore the literature to locate descriptions of specific forms of narrative analysis; then you will be able to apply the most appropriate one to your research data.

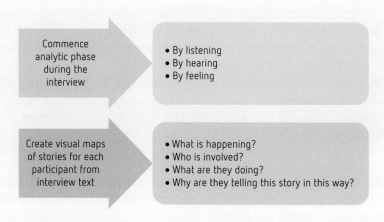

Commence analytic phase during the interview
• By listening
• By hearing
• By feeling

Create visual maps of stories for each participant from interview text
• What is happening?
• Who is involved?
• What are they doing?
• Why are they telling this story in this way?

▶ **Figure 8.4**   Narrative analysis method

Source: Lapum, J., Angus, J. E., Peter, E., & Watt-Watson, J. (2010). Patients' narrative accounts of open-heart surgery and recovery: The authorial voice of technology. *Social Science & Medicine, 70,* 756.

ACTIVITY

Audio record yourself telling a story or a series of stories about an experience that was of great significance to you. Use the Emden (1998) approach to develop a core story. Remember that interview transcription takes time and effort, so decide how long you will take to tell the story (or stories) and keep to the allocated time.

Discourse analysis

Discourse and discourse analysis have different meanings according to the contexts in which they are applied. In a general sense, *discourse* means a series of written or spoken utterances with a formal and organised connotation, such as in a dissertation, lecture, sermon, conversation or text on a certain subject. In effect, discourses, as systems of statements, can be on any topic. In nursing and healthcare, there are multiple discourses on the knowledge and skills clinicians need to practise effectively, such as evidence-based practice (EBP) guidelines and various diagnostic approaches.

Although opinions vary on the constitution of discourse analysis, one name that appears almost routinely in discourse analyses is that of French philosopher Michel Foucault, whose work has had a profound influence on researchers in many disciplines since the 1980s. Also, the terms 'discourse' and 'discourse analysis' are used in many ways in research articles.

FOR EXAMPLE

DISCOURSE ANALYSIS

Cook and colleagues (2017) explored the ethical positions that inform conceptualisations of and responses towards intimacy and sexuality in residential aged care (RAC) through the following question: 'How can analysis of discourses shaping accounts of staff, family and residents of aged care facilities advance theoretical and ethical insights into intimacy and sexuality, in the context of residential care?' The researchers used a discursive methodology, drawing on social constructionist and postmodernist discourses shaping the diverse meanings of intimacy, sexuality and ageing. The results indicated that intimacy and sexuality were everyday RAC matters, involving often tacit moral judgements. The data highlighted the potential value of RAC staff developing the reflective and communicative skills inherent in a narrative ethics approach. The authors suggest that flexible responses that focus on person-centred wellbeing rather than a risk management approach are desirable.

Interpretations of some Foucauldian thought

Foucault's focus was on questions of how some discourses have shaped and created meaning systems that have gained the status and currency of 'truth' and dominate how we define and organise both ourselves and our social world, while other alternative discourses are marginalised and subjugated yet potentially 'offer' sites where hegemonic practices can be contested, challenged and 'resisted'. In Foucault's view, this involves looking at the social context in which certain knowledges and practices have emerged as either permissible and

Ethics

desirable or changed. The rules of discursive practices form and maintain discourses that in turn constitute power and knowledge relationships. Ethical requirements in research projects, for example, maintain the power bases of people on committees who may favour particular design approaches and methodologies and thus obstruct the passage of those projects that do not fit the discourse judged by them to be important and appropriate.

Knowledge that counts as truth is that which has won recognition in a **culture** as being successful and thus has gained and exercised power. Biomedical technology, for example, has been so highly successful in treating diseases that the powerful discourse of medicos has influenced other members of the health team to the extent that biomedical discourse is the benchmark by which effective patient management is judged. The power knowledge of biomedical discourse is immersed in the culture of healthcare settings, especially those organised around hierarchies and bureaucracies that exercise the power of ownership of human healthcare by experts.

Power can operate in many directions at the micro-levels of a culture, but people, through their knowledge, can change their subject positions to disrupt and challenge power relations. Therefore, power knowledge not only maintains the existing 'truth', but it can also shift, circulate, spread and change it. Nurses, for instance, are not necessarily bound by biomedical discourses, as they too can exercise their power knowledge by changing their subject positions in the healthcare team as individuals capable of resistance against injustice.

ACTIVITY

Describe some of the rules of discursive practices (the way people talk and relate together) in your work setting. In what ways are these discursive practices maintained and how do they form and direct power and knowledge relationships?

Post-structural process

There is no one particular way of doing a discourse analysis. But if you are attempting to undertake a thorough process that reflects Foucauldian thought, you will need a comprehensive understanding of his discourse on knowledge and power.

TIP If you are intending to use a **Foucauldian-style discourse analysis**, you would be well advised to read Foucault widely (Foucault, 1965, 1972, 1975, 1978, 1979, 1980, 1981, 1991) as well as authors who have interpreted his writing (Evans, Pereira & Parker, 2008; Richardson-Tench, 2007, 2008, 2012; Springer & Clinton, 2015).

Essentially, a discourse analysis asks questions about the knowledge and power inherent in all kinds of spoken and written life texts. Bear in mind that 'texts' may be interview transcripts, all kinds of academic and general publications, professional and public documents, and other media sources such as films and videos.

FOR EXAMPLE

DISCOURSE ANALYSIS

- *Description of the text:* examination of the organisation, structure and vocabulary of written or spoken text.
- *Interpretation of the interaction process:* includes a moment-by-moment account of how people produce and interpret a text to make visible the discursive practices in play, including the order [in which] they occur. This requires an analysis of where the text originates, the text itself and the reception of the text. It is the interplay between these elements that is of primary analytic concern.
- *Explicatory social action:* the aim of the explanatory dimension is to understand the social processes generated by the text, including the social conditions and context in which these processes occur.

Note: In the third phase, other questions could be raised to facilitate further discourse analysis of the textual comparisons, as shown in the following diagram.

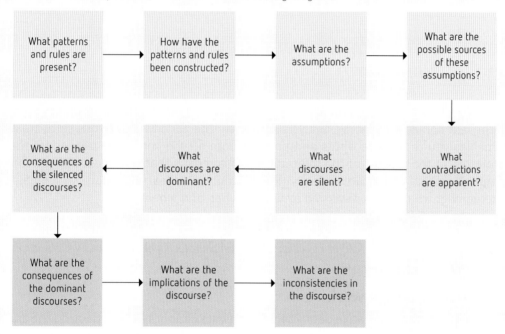

Source: McClosky, R. (2008). A guide to discourse analysis. *Nurse Researcher, 16*(1), 34–5.

In summary, research articles use the terms 'discourse' and 'discourse analysis' in many ways. There are many interpretations of discourse analysis. One textbook that provides a number of interpretations is Meyer and Wodak's *Methods of Critical Discourse Studies* (2016). One of the most accepted interpretations of discourse analysis is to undertake a thorough analysis of texts using Foucault's ideas about knowledge and power.

Computer software that manages qualitative data

Another avenue is the almost exclusive use of a computer to locate the themes through the use of qualitative data analysis software. NUD*IST (Qualitative Solutions and Research) and Ethnograph (Siedel) are two software packages that can group and order the conceptual categories that have been decided progressively by the researcher. These types of software manage the qualitative data with greater and lesser degrees of success, depending on the aim of the researcher who is using them.

ACTIVITY

Locate other examples of computer software that manage qualitative data.

Benefits of computer-assisted qualitative data analysis software

Computer-assisted qualitative data analysis software enables whole transcripts and groups of transcripts to be merged and matched, which gives the researcher the potential to merge all the text and do a collective analysis with ease. The added value of this software is that it enables you to retrieve words and phrases from all the combined transcripts that are connected to the context of the information. This means that sentences and phrases can be moved around and located later, with their contextual features intact, which helps you to remember what words were said by whom, when and where.

Constraints of computer-assisted qualitative data analysis software

It will not do all the work

Computer-assisted qualitative data analysis software cannot read the data, do the analysis or tell the researcher what these things mean because qualitative research data are words and the understanding of language relies on the researcher immersing themself in the text. Even with computer assistance, the researcher is active in feeding in the transcripts as text, locating the meaningful sections, naming and coding them according to their interpretive possibilities, and looking for finer nuances in meaning that a computer cannot detect.

It cannot locate finer nuances

When using any data analysis software for qualitative analysis, the resultant analysis and interpretation of the data are only as rich as the meaning that is tagged to the words through a thorough analysis of the text. If the researcher relies entirely on the word search ability of the system (sophisticated as it may be) and does not look between the words to find the implicit meanings within words, phrases and sections of text, the finer nuances of the text might be missed. In qualitative research, the richest and finest meanings may be hiding within the total context of the words, so it is only through protracted and clear-minded attention to the text that these connections can be made.

Analysing images as qualitative data

Researchers may create images, such as photographs, videos or computer graphics, or research participants may create them as forms of expression to describe their experiences, such as drawings, paintings and collages, photographs, videos and sculpture. This being so, it follows that the images will be analysed most accurately by the people who created them, which means that participants analyse and describe the images they created according to their intentions for creating them in relation to the research. Researchers discuss with participants their analysis of the content of images and create a dialogue with them to make connections to the research aims and objectives. The analyses of images as data are, therefore, made in relation to the aims and objectives of the research and the intentions of the researcher and/ or participant. The interpretations that result from the analysis of the images are what the person creating them says they are. These analyses and interpretations are admissible as they are relevant to the person involved and, as such, add to the richness of the research findings. The research project report will need to show clearly that these analyses and interpretations are acknowledged as being those of the respective participants.

Examples of completed qualitative analyses

The main publication sources for qualitative analysis methods are books, journal articles, theses and published conference presentations.

Books

Books about qualitative research can be in the form of teaching texts, such as this book; accounts of research that have been undertaken (Benner, 1984; Lawler, 1991; Tucakovic, 2005); or a combination of both (Creswell & Creswell, 2018; Flick, 2018).

Reading research books that describe projects in detail provides the chance to see the finished project as literature; that is, as a literary work unrestricted by the constraints of a reduced word count. The other advantage of reading research books of this nature is that they are not bound by the requirements of a research thesis or report and so are more likely to be reader-friendly and engaging.

ACTIVITY

Locate and read a qualitative research book and then discuss how the researcher or author presents the analysis of the data.

Research and thesis documents

Libraries keep holdings of research theses for honours and masters degrees and PhD awards. Some of these theses have been copied electronically and others are available as full-text hard-back copies for reading in the library. Some universities compile digital holdings of theses. Locate theses whose titles and abstracts suggest adherence to a particular approach, such as an interpretive or critical methodology, or postmodern influences. The methods of analysis contained within these theses have been judged by examiners to be of a quality sufficient to warrant the academic award, so a certain amount of trust can be placed in them as guiding documents.

There is no one best method of qualitative analysis and it is permissible to amend and recreate some methods as long as there is consistency with the methodological assumptions of the research approach and the analysis method is described fully and clearly.

Research project presentations

Oral accounts of qualitative analyses may be given by researchers presenting their projects at professional conferences. Conference presentations may be published in a book of proceedings, which may be a good source of worked examples of research analysis. Many successful researchers are willing to share their techniques and strategies for data analysis, and a great deal may be learnt from them.

SUMMARY

This chapter explained the qualitative research process and discussed the collection, management and analysis of qualitative data.

1 Identify forms of qualitative data and align data collection methods with different qualitative methodologies	• Qualitative data forms consist of combinations of words, images and sometimes numbers that act as pieces of information that need to be analysed and interpreted with the research questions, aims and objectives in mind • Be clear about what is to be explored and why the methods chosen will give relevant and appropriate data
2 Prepare for data collection and use strategies for collecting the data, including the storage of data	• Pitfalls to avoid in data collection include being aware of potential people, places and equipment problems • These can be minimised with adequate foresight and planning
3 Identify approaches to analysing qualitative data	• Data are a rich, raw resource • Maintain data security and integrity • Develop an organising system
4 Code the data	• Code data with useful and uncomplicated pseudonyms and numbering systems

5 Discuss methods of thematic analysis, including content analysis	• To find explicit and implicit themes within the text:
	  − know what you are looking for
	  − locate specific words for explicit themes
	  − look closely for the nuances of implicit themes

6 Describe other methods of text analysis such as narrative and discourse analysis	• A discourse analysis systematically and thoroughly asks questions about the knowledge and power inherent in all kinds of spoken and written life texts in relation to:
	  − the nature and construction patterns and rules present
	  − the kinds of assumptions and their possible sources
	  − the contradictions, silences, dominance and inconsistencies in the discourse

7 Identify computer systems that manage qualitative data	• Specific computer systems for qualitative data analysis can manage large amounts of data tagged to participants' identities and dialogue

8 Discuss analysis of images as qualitative data	The analyses of images as data are made in relation to the:
	  − aims and objectives of the research
	  − intentions of the researcher and/or participant
	  − what the person creating them says they are

REVIEW QUESTIONS

1 Given that words are the main form of qualitative data, how are they best collected and stored?
2 Discuss how language conveys lived experience.
3 How can you ensure that your main data sources are safely stored?
4 Describe the aspects of getting started when embarking on qualitative analysis.

CHALLENGING REVIEW QUESTIONS

1 Discuss how you will avoid the main people, place and equipment pitfalls when collecting qualitative data.
2 Discuss why effective communication is essential in collecting qualitative research data.
3 Discuss the difference between thematic analysis and discourse analysis.
4 Discuss the value of coding data.

CASE STUDY 1

Prisha is an undergraduate nursing student beginning her third year. Prisha is considering her options for a graduate position after she completes her course. As a student nurse, Prisha is aware that stress and burnout are important considerations for hospital nurses and would like to ensure she is fully prepared.

Prisha has determined there is a large volume of quantitative research related to the nursing work environment. Prisha feels that qualitative research will contribute a valuable perspective related to the types of strategies she will require to cope with working as a registered nurse after graduation. Prisha critically appraised a research article by Cope, Jones and Hendricks (2016); however, the critical appraisal raised many questions that Prisha would like to explore to increase her understanding and knowledge of qualitative research.

1   What are the different types of data collection methods appropriate for qualitative research?
2   Describe the different methods that could be used to analyse qualitative data.
3   Describe how narrative analysis may be used for qualitative research.

CASE STUDY 2

We revisit Karen, the clinical facilitator from 'Case study 2' in Chapter 7. Karen is using phenomenology as her research methodology to explore the lived experiences of first-year midwifery students undertaking their first professional experience placement in the postnatal ward. After gaining ethics approval from her university, Karen prepares to undertake focus group discussions with small groups of first-year students.

1   Karen is quite nervous about facilitating her first-ever focus group discussions. What practical advice would you provide to Karen in facilitating an effective focus group discussion?
2   What are the disadvantages of focus group discussions?
3   Karen has completed her focus group discussions. Each discussion was digitally recorded and the data transcribed verbatim into Microsoft Word documents. Karen has completed a workshop to learn how to use the university's software program to manage and analyse qualitative data. She is very keen to use this software to code her research data. What are the benefits and constraints in using computer systems for qualitative data analysis?

REFERENCES

Benner, P. (1984). *From Novice to Expert: Uncovering the Knowledge Embedded in Clinical Practice.* San Francisco, CA: Addison-Wesley.

Braun, V., & Clarke, V. (2006). Using thematic analysis in psychology. *Qualitative Research in Psychology, 3,* 77–101.

Brough, P. (2019). *Advanced Research Methods for Applied Psychology: Design, Analysis and Reporting.* London, New York: Routledge.

Cook, C., Schouten, V., Henrickson, M., & McDonald, S. (2017). Ethics, intimacy and sexuality in aged care. *Journal of Advanced Nursing,* 73(12), 16 July, 3017–27. http://doi.org/10.1111/jan.13361

Cope, V., Jones, B., & Hendricks, J. (2016). Why nurses chose to remain in the workforce: Portraits of resilience. *Collegian,* 23, 87–95. http://dx.doi.org/10.1016/j.colegn.2014.12.00

Creswell, J., & Creswell, D. (2018). *Research Design: Qualitative, Quantitative, and Mixed Method Approaches* (5th edn). Sage.

Emden, C. (1998). Conducting a narrative analysis. *Collegian, 5*(3), 34–9.

Evans, A., Pereira, D., & Parker, J. (2008). Discourses of anxiety in nursing practice: A psychoanalytic case study of the change-of-shift handover ritual. *Nursing Inquiry, 15*(1), 40–8.

Flanagan, B., Lord, B., Reed, R., & Crimmins, G. (2019). Listening to women's voices: The experience of giving birth with paramedic care in Queensland, Australia. *BMC Pregnancy and Childbirth, 19*(1), December. http://doi.org/10.1186/s12884-019-2613-z

Flick, U. (2018). *An Introduction to Qualitative Research* (6th edn). Sage.

Foucault, M. (1965). *Madness and Civilization: A History of Insanity in the Age of Reason*. New York, NY: Pantheon.

Foucault, M. (1972). *The Archaeology of Knowledge*. London: Tavistock.

Foucault, M. (1975). *The Birth of the Clinic* (A. M. Sheridan-Smith, trans.). New York, NY: Vintage/Random House, originally published 1973.

Foucault, M. (1978). *The History of Sexuality – Part 1: An Introduction* (R. Hurley, trans.). New York, NY: Vintage/Random House, originally published 1976.

Foucault, M. (1979). *Discipline and Punish* (A. M. Sheridan-Smith, trans.). New York, NY: Vintage/Random House, originally published 1975.

Foucault, M. (1980). *Michel Foucault – Power/knowledge: Selected Interviews and Other Writings*. Brighton, UK: Harvester Press.

Foucault, M. (1981). The order of discourse. In R. Young (ed.). *Untying the Text* (pp. 48–78). Boston, MA: Routledge and Kegan Paul.

Foucault, M. (1991). Orders of discourse. *Social Science Information, 10*(2), 7–30.

Gould, G. S., Bovill, M., Clarke, M. J., Gruppetta, M., Cadet-James, Y., & Bonevski, B. (2017). Chronological narratives from smoking initiation through to pregnancy of Indigenous Australian women: A qualitative study. *Midwifery, 52*, September, 27–33. http://doi.org/10.1016/j.midw.2017.05.010

Lawler, J. (1991). *Behind the Screens: Nursing, Somology and the Problem of the Body*. Melbourne: Churchill-Livingstone.

Marsh, C. A., Browne, J., Taylor, J., & David, D. (2019). Making the hidden seen: A narrative analysis of the experiences of assumption of care at birth. *Women and Birth, 32*(1), February, e1–11. http://doi.org/10.1016/j.wombi.2018.04.009

McClosky, R. (2008). A guide to discourse analysis. *Nurse Researcher, 16*(1): 34–5.

Meyer, M., & Wodak, R. (2016). *Methods of Critical Discourse Studies*. Sage.

Nowell, L. S., Norris, J. M., White, D. E., & Moules, N. J. (2017). Thematic analysis. *International Journal of Qualitative Methods, 16*(1), 2 October, p160940691773384. http://doi.org/10.1177/1609406917733847

Petty, J., Jarvis, J., & Thomas, R. (2018). Core story creation: Analysing narratives to construct stories for learning. *Nurse Researcher, 25*(4), 16 March, 47–51. http://doi.org/10.7748/nr.2018.e1533

Pilkington, L., Haig, M. M., Durey, A., Katzenellenbogen, J. M., & Thompson, S. C. (2017). Perspectives of Aboriginal women on participation in mammographic screening: A step towards improving services. *BMC Public Health, 17*(1), 11 September. http://doi.org/10.1186/s12889-017-4701-1

Richardson-Tench, M. (2007). Technician or nurturer: Discourses within the operating room. *ACORN Journal, 20*(3), 12–15.

Richardson-Tench, M. (2008). The scrub nurse: Basking in reflected glory. *Journal of Advanced Perioperative Practice, 3*(4), 125–34.

Richardson-Tench, M. (2012). Power, discourse, subjectivity: A Foucauldian application to operating room nursing practice. *ACORN Journal, 25*(3), 36–7.

Saldana, J. (2021). *The Coding Manual for Qualitative Researchers* (4th edn). Thousand Oaks California: Sage.

Skjott Linneberg, M., & Korsgaard, S. (2019). Coding qualitative data: A synthesis guiding the novice. *Qualitative Research Journal, 19*(3), 8 May, 259–70. http://doi.org/10.1108/qrj-12-2018-0012

Springer, R. A., & Clinton, M. (2015). Doing Foucault: Inquiring into knowledge with Foucauldian discourse analysis. *Nursing Philosophy, 16*, 87–97.

Tobler-Ammann, B. C., Weise, A., Knols, R. H., Watson, M. J., Sieben, J. M., de Bie, R. A., & de Bruin, E. D. (2020). Patients' experiences of unilateral spatial neglect between stroke onset and discharge from inpatient rehabilitation: A thematic analysis of qualitative interviews. *Disability and Rehabilitation*, 22 November, 1–10, http://doi.org/10.1080/09638288.2018.1531150

Tucakovic, M. (2005). *Nursing as an Aesthetic Praxis*. Bloomington, IN: AuthorHouse.

FURTHER READING

Billings, D. M. (2016). Storytelling: A strategy for providing context for learning. *Journal of Continuing Education in Nursing, 47*(3), 109–10.

9 MIXED METHODS

Chapter learning objectives

The material presented in this chapter will assist you to:

1 define mixed methods research
2 describe the reasons for using a mixed methods design
3 design a mixed methods study
4 discuss ethical issues in mixed methods research
5 describe the different types of mixed methods designs
6 outline the strengths and limitations of mixed methods research
7 discuss rigour in mixed methods research
8 understand how to critique a mixed methods study.

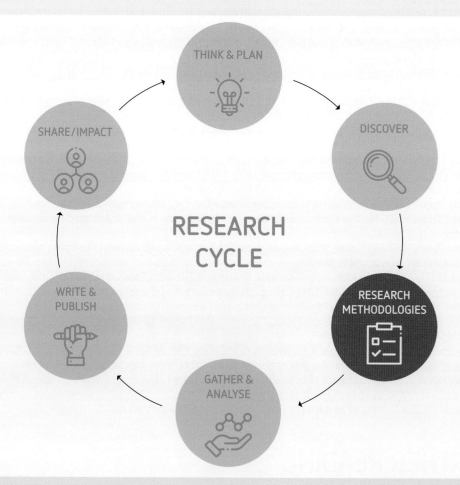

Research cycle

The primary focus of this chapter is on mixed methods research. This is a key component of research methodologies, as highlighted in the research cycle above.

Introduction

Earlier in this text the two main research designs – quantitative and qualitative – were introduced. Every so often, debate rages about which of these designs is the best, or about the differences between them (though not the apparent similarities). Any such argument about which is superior is flawed because neither is the best. Instead, each serves a specific purpose or function and the researcher chooses one based on the aims of their study.

Every research project also has limitations, which could be a reflection of the research design. A quantitative design might, for example, be used to determine the incidence of multiple sclerosis (MS) but it cannot uncover how someone feels about receiving such a diagnosis. Similarly, a qualitative design can describe how it feels to be a paraplegic but not the risk of injury when drink driving.

What is mixed methods research?

There is some debate in the literature as to the correct for research that combines two studies to complete the project. The term **mixed methods design** is used throughout this chapter to refer to research that combines two methods of data collection.

Morse (2017) argues that the correct term is mixed method as the design consists of one complete project, that could be publishable by itself, called the core component. Additionally, there is a supplemental project consisting of a different data type that enables an extra question to be answered – either qualitative or quantitative – but which does not demand the structure of a complete second project.

While a mixed method design enables the researcher to explore quantitative and qualitative data, it also does so much more. As its name implies, it involves mixing two methodological approaches within the one study. The two methodological approaches used are typically quantitative and qualitative, though they could be just one of these (Morse, 2017), with the mixing coming from data collection and analysis or the interpretation phases of the study. Some researchers who use mixed methods are actually referring to two research methods conducted simultaneously or sequentially, and although they use the same name (mixed methods), they are actually conducting multiple methods (Morse, 2017). It is important to distinguish a mixed methods design from a **multimethod design**. These two designs are sometimes incorrectly referred to interchangeably.

FOR EXAMPLE

MULTIMETHOD RESEARCH

Stefana and colleagues (2018) used a multimethod approach of ethnographic observation, semi-structured interviews with fathers, a self-report questionnaire and clinical information between September 2015 and March 2017 to investigate fathers' emotional experiences of their infant's preterm birth and subsequent stay in a neonatal intensive care unit. The authors said that the research design approach was chosen to provide a rich understanding of fathers' experiences and to develop a conceptual framework which could be informative to nursing practice and psychological support.

RELEVANCE TO PRACTICE

The authors argued that the results of this study could be used to develop guidelines to support fathers' emotional experience and for the development of nursing guidelines and standards of care should be developed, specifically aimed at facilitating and supporting paternal involvement in their infant's care.

Mixing research methods enables the researcher to achieve a greater depth of understanding of the phenomenon under investigation than through using either approach alone. It also allows them to challenge the 'either/or' debate. Some researchers believe that mixed methods studies produce new knowledge, not through the complementarity of different data types and analysis techniques, but through the integration of different methods at the analytical, interpretive or epistemological levels (Creswell & Plano Clark, 2018; Grove, 2020; Morse, 2017).

Why might a researcher want to mix research methods? Consider the example of a nurse performing a patient assessment. The nurse can collect qualitative data by asking how a patient is feeling, and quantitative data by taking a patient's pulse, blood pressure and temperature. By itself, each piece of assessment datum is insignificant, but when the qualitative and quantitative data are collated, the nurse can reach rigorous conclusions about the patient's condition (e.g. hypovolaemia, shock) that are far more sound and that the nurse can have confidence in. The same can be said for conclusions arising from a mixed methods study.

Mixed methods research typically involves integrating quantitative and qualitative data collection and/or analysis in a single study or program of inquiry. The emphasis must be on integration, as simply adding a quantitative phase to a qualitative study (or vice versa) is not a new concept and does not constitute a mixed methods approach (Creswell & Plano Clark, 2018). Newer conceptualisations of mixed methods research acknowledge that a study is not considered mixed if there is no integration across research stages (Creswell & Plano Clark, 2018; Brough, 2019). Nevertheless, the process of mixing different components of the study can be quite challenging.

Mixed methods research is not a new research design. Denzin (1978), for example, described mixed methods research more than three decades ago. Furthermore, many research topics have been rigorously examined within nursing and outside the health professions using this approach.

Philosophical basis

Researchers are expected to position their research within a selected research paradigm. A research paradigm is a way of looking at natural phenomena that encompasses a set of philosophical assumptions and that guides one's approach to inquiry (Polit & Beck, 2018). Examples of paradigms include **pragmatism**, constructivism and postpositivism. Research paradigms are sometimes referred to as 'world views' or as a 'theoretical lens'. Quantitative research is influenced by the positivist paradigm, while qualitative research is influenced by the naturalistic or constructivist paradigms. These differing paradigms tend to imply that quantitative and qualitative research are not compatible. However, the researcher undertaking a mixed methods study is not trying to make them compatible but rather to benefit from the strengths of each method while minimising their inherent limitations.

A number of world views (paradigms) can be assumed by the research that uses a mixed methods design. Creswell and Plano Clark (2018) highlight the three philosophical stances on mixed methods research.

1   There is one paradigm that best fits mixed methods research.
2   Researchers who use a mixed methods approach can use multiple paradigms.
3   World views relate to the type of mixed methods design and vary depending on the type of design.

The researcher using a mixed methods approach may find themselves in a conundrum because of the differing world views associated with qualitative and quantitative research.

TIP

Just because a quantitative phase and a qualitative phase were used within the one study, do not consider that study to be a mixed study. It is the interpretation of the results of both quantitative and qualitative phases.

Polit and Beck (2018) argue that the research question is of prime importance, more so than the method or philosophical underpinnings of the method. This is consistent with the pragmatism paradigm. Researchers using this approach ask what works to determine the best method for answering a research question, a method that rejects the 'either/or' approach of the postpositive and constructivist paradigms (Mertens, 2019). As such, the values or beliefs of the researcher may have a significant influence on how the study is conducted or the data interpreted. Pragmatism has a number of other characteristics:

- a lack of commitment to any one philosophy or view of the world
- valuing both subjective and objective knowledge
- the belief that knowledge is constructed by and based on the reality of the world one experiences and lives in
- the problem (and its solution) is of prime importance
- methods for solving the problem are of lesser importance.

A researcher who uses mixed methods research is using a research design based on philosophical assumptions as well as methods of inquiry. As a methodology, it involves philosophical assumptions that guide the direction of collecting, analysing and mixing qualitative and quantitative approaches in many phases in the research process. As a method, it focuses on collecting, analysing and mixing both quantitative and qualitative data in a single study or series of studies (Creswell & Plano Clark, 2018; Grove, 2020).

Method or methodology?

Methods and methodology are important parts of any study. These terms are sometimes used interchangeably; however, they do not refer to the same concept. The *method* (or methods) of a study refers to the tools the researcher uses to complete the study (i.e. to collect and analyse data), which could involve the use of a survey, interviews with participants or a software program (e.g. SPSS) for data analysis. The choice of methods could also take into account issues regarding time frames, financial support or other resources. There are no rules about which tools should or should not be used, but a justifiable reason for their choice must be evident; for example, that people's opinions may be acquired more easily through an interview than a questionnaire, provided the researcher has enough time to conduct one.

Methodology refers to the theoretical assumptions and values that underpin a particular research approach (Giddings & Grant, 2007). Consider, by way of analogy, how different religions view issues such as birth, death and illness. None of these views are right or wrong, they are just opinions or beliefs that dictate how believers of the particular religion live their lives. The same could be said of a methodology in that it dictates how each part of the study is conducted because methodologies contain assumptions about knowledge; for example, whether it is generated inductively or deductively. Methods of data collection and analysis are often chosen based on the assumptions the overriding methodology makes about the nature of knowledge generation and validation (for a further discussion of this, see Chapters 5 and 7). Hence, the methodology has the greatest influence on the conduct of the study.

Some authors view mixed methods research as a methodology because of its focus on collecting, analysing and interpreting qualitative and quantitative data (Bharmal et al., 2018). Those who view mixed methods research as a methodology argue that a method cannot stand alone or separate itself from the other parts of the research process, such as the philosophical assumptions and data collection strategies (Polit & Beck, 2018). Irrespective of the researcher's view, clear and transparent decisions need to be made about the methods used in the study and it must be obvious which theoretical assumptions are guiding it.

Why use a mixed methods approach?

There are a variety of reasons for using a mixed methods design, but it should not be assumed that using a mixed methods design is inherently a better choice than a single method. Some of the common reasons for using a mixed methods design include that it:

- enables the researcher to acquire a much greater understanding of the problem under investigation than could be acquired by a single method alone
- is a way of capitalising on the strengths of quantitative and qualitative methods while minimising the limitations of each single approach
- is a way of adding strength to any study and of increasing rigour in the research process (Morse, 2017)
- enables the researcher to answer important questions, such as: 'What is happening?' (quantitative data) and 'Why is it happening?' (qualitative data), within the one study so that any conclusions reached are based on these two types of data rather than just one.

The main assumption underpinning mixed methods research is that using quantitative and qualitative approaches in the same study results in complementary strengths. Furthermore, the limitations of one approach may be corrected or balanced by the other approach. The philosophy of pragmatism advances the notion that the consequences are more important than the process and therefore the end justifies the means (Creswell & Plano Clark, 2018). So even though each method's strengths might complement one another, it is what this combination produces that is of greatest benefit.

Why might a nurse researcher want to conduct a mixed methods study? Over the last two decades, nurses have increasingly been expected to engage in evidence-based practice (EBP). While randomised controlled trials are considered by many to be the best form of evidence, the context and experience of providing nursing care unfortunately do not lend themselves to be easily evaluated by such a trial (Flemming, 2007). It has even been argued that the knowledge generated by these trials merely serves to restrict or devalue other forms of knowledge and ultimately stifle nursing scholarship (Rolfe, 2009). A mixed methods design enables the researcher to evaluate nursing care using quantitative and qualitative methods, thereby creating a greater depth of understanding than could a randomised controlled trial alone.

In summary, mixed methods designs are usually used in the following circumstances (Morse, 2017):

- when the research question does not completely encompass the phenomena of interest
- when, during the course of inquiry, interesting or unexpected phenomena are revealed, in which case a mixed methods design allows the researcher to incorporate the new phenomena into the study while the present one is ongoing
- when unexpected findings are revealed in a quantitatively driven study, in which case a mixed methods design allows the researchers to qualitatively explore quantitative data which is puzzling.

TIP

Using more than one method does not by itself make a study more rigorous or the results more significant.

Designing a mixed methods study

Obtaining an accurate answer to the research question, one that the researcher has confidence in, is the ultimate goal or outcome of the study. The accuracy of the answer can be influenced by many variables during the course of the study, such as the amount of time or financial support the researcher has or the willingness of the subjects to be interviewed.

Because answering the research question is the primary focus, the question strongly determines the method that the researcher will use. The following suggestions for writing research questions for a mixed methods study may be helpful (Creswell & Plano Clark, 2018).

- Write separate quantitative and qualitative questions followed by an explicit mixed method question.
- Write an overarching mixed research question which is later broken down into separate quantitative and qualitative sub-questions to answer in each strand or phase of the study.
- Write research questions for each phase of a study as the study evolves.

ACTIVITY

Discuss what the basic characteristics of qualitative and quantitative research questions are and how they differ. How might mixed methods questions differ from qualitative and quantitative research questions?

Decisions about the method need to be given careful consideration before data collection commences, although this is not always easy. For example, a nurse might decide to survey all the wards of a hospital to determine the number of patients who experience an adverse event, such as a fall. If one ward is found to have a much higher incidence of the event than other wards, the researcher might want to identify the reasons why. But, if staff know their ward has a much higher incidence of an adverse event, they might provide false or misleading answers when interviewed by the researcher (i.e. the Hawthorne effect). If the quantitative data (incidence of adverse events) and qualitative data (staff opinions of the causes of adverse events) were collected concurrently, staff might provide more truthful and honest answers, particularly if they are blinded to the quantitative results.

Also decide which phase (qualitative or quantitative) is exploratory and which is confirmatory. Is the purpose of the study to confirm what is already known or suspected (that adverse events occur or how many)? Or is it to identify what has previously not been known (e.g. nurses' opinions of the causes of adverse events)? In a mixed methods study, the qualitative phase is typically exploratory and the quantitative phase is confirmatory, but the researcher must decide the role of each phase of their study.

Perhaps the most important decision to be made is how the qualitative and quantitative phases of the study will be mixed, because if no mixing occurs, a mixed methods study has not been conducted. This tends to be the greatest challenge facing researchers: many may struggle to articulate exactly how their study is mixed. This problem might exist because of the debate about what actually constitutes a mixed methods study. Again, there are no right or wrong answers, but researchers must be able to justify the decisions they made about their study.

Different kinds of **research objectives** lend themselves to being addressed by a mixed methods design. Some common objectives are (Creswell & Plano Clark, 2018):

- to develop conclusions that are well substantiated by quantitative and qualitative data
- to validate quantitative data (e.g. collected via survey)
- to generate and test hypotheses
- to build, test and refine theories
- to enhance an experimental design
- to test the efficacy and effectiveness of nursing interventions
- to understand why specific relationships exist within a correlational design
- to explain certain aspects of quantitative results (i.e. explication)
- to select participants for an in-depth qualitative study
- to help develop a quantitative data collection tool (i.e. instrumentation)
- to help generalise qualitative findings with quantitative data.

Figure 9.1 provides some guidelines for integrating quantitative and qualitative results.

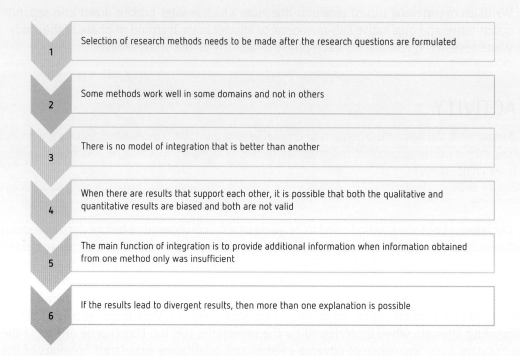

1	Selection of research methods needs to be made after the research questions are formulated
2	Some methods work well in some domains and not in others
3	There is no model of integration that is better than another
4	When there are results that support each other, it is possible that both the qualitative and quantitative results are biased and both are not valid
5	The main function of integration is to provide additional information when information obtained from one method only was insufficient
6	If the results lead to divergent results, then more than one explanation is possible

▸ **Figure 9.1** Guidelines for integrating quantitative and qualitative results

Source: Wurtz, K. (n.d.). Using mixed methods research to analyze surveys. Chaffey College. http://www.chaffey.edu/research/IR PDF Files/Presentations/Other/0809-MixedMethods.pdf

In their latest work, Creswell and Plano Clark (2018) posit that integration is the point in the research procedures where qualitative interfaces with quantitative research. They further state that integration is central to mixed method research and differs depending on the type of mixed methods design. The authors suggest the following considerations:

- integration intent – conveys why researchers integrate in a study
- integration data analysis procedures – reflects key steps used to accomplish the integration intended and describes what the researcher actually does to achieve integration
- the representation of the integration results – concerns how the findings are reported
- the interpretation of the integration results – means the researcher makes inferences from the combined results.

Another important decision the researcher needs to make is how each phase of the study is weighted. Are the qualitative and quantitative phases weighted equally so they play an equal role in answering the research question, or does one phase have greater weighting and thus more influence on the research process?

Other issues also need to be considered, such as if the phases are given equal weighting or more resources (time, financial support) (Creswell & Plano Clark, 2018). If the research is being conducted for a masters or doctoral thesis, then the resources available could influence the weighting decision far more than any other factors. The choice of weighting might also reflect the researcher's experience or expertise in one method (Creswell & Plano Clark, 2018). The dominant method may be the one that the researcher has the greater understanding of and experience using.

Finally, the researcher may need to consider the target audience (Creswell & Plano Clark, 2018). A quantitative research journal with little history of publishing mixed methods studies may be less willing to publish a study where the qualitative method was dominant. Similarly, a thesis examiner with a qualitative background might look more favourably upon a mixed methods thesis in which the qualitative phase was dominant.

Ethical issues in mixed methods research

Obtaining ethics approval for a mixed methods study can pose unique challenges. Although ethics committees are familiar with qualitative and quantitative research, they may not be familiar with the concept of mixed methods due to it being a relatively recently developed research method.

Ethics

There are several issues that need consideration when submitting an application for ethics approval, including the following.

- Has the way in which the mixing will occur been stated?
- Has a rationale for the design been included in the application (including strengths and limitations)?
- Have the ethical issues created by the particular mixed methods design been addressed?
- Should the ethical issues arising from each phase of the study be addressed separately in the application?
- Have the ethical issues for the participants been stated, such as consent, privacy and level of risk (including how these issues will be addressed)?

ACTIVITY

Identify a mixed methods study of interest to you and consider how, if you had to conduct this study, you would address the following practical issues as suggested by Halcomb (2018) in her editorial.

- Time: _____

_____

- Financial cost: _____

_____

- Skill: _____

_____

- Supervision: _____

_____

- Managing more than one dataset: _____

_____

- Ethics approval: _____

_____

Types of mixed methods approaches

The mixed methods approach to research offers a variety of designs or frameworks, rather than a single approach (Grove, 2020). There are also differing schools of thought about the types or classification of mixed methods designs. Creswell and Plano Clark (2018) suggest there are three mixed methods designs: convergent design, explanatory sequential design and exploratory sequential design. There are variants within each of these designs and it is not the intention of this chapter to provide an overview of each of them, particularly as they have much in common (for an explanation of each of these, see the cited references). The shared theme of the different classifications is the collection of data either sequentially or concurrently. Morse (2017) suggests that the researcher has three choices.

1   Collect quantitative and qualitative data at the same time.
2   Collect quantitative data first and then collect qualitative data.
3   Collect qualitative data first and then collect quantitative data.

FOR EXAMPLE

MIXED METHODS RESEARCH

Thompson and colleagues (2019) conducted a mixed methods intervention research project to explore nurses' attitudes towards management of clinical aggression. Pre-post surveys were used followed by semi-structured interviews and an educational program of simulated scenarios of clinical aggression as the intervention.

Concurrent or convergent mixed methods design

Concurrent or convergent mixed methods design (also referred to as 'mixed methods simultaneous design') (Morse, 2017) is so-called because the qualitative and quantitative methods are used at the same time (see **Figure 9.2**), which means that careful planning is needed at the start of the study before data collection commences. The intent of this mixed method approach is to seek information from different levels and to collect quantitative and qualitative data simultaneously (Murdolo et al., 2017). Findings from each method are integrated in the interpretation phase of the study.

A concurrent/convergent design may be considered by the researcher if, during the planning phase of a study, the research question or problem is considered rather complex. Morse and Niehaus (2009) suggest that a concurrent design could be used when:

- a study has multiple groups of participants
- a study has several types of variables that do not fit well together in the analytical scheme
- the phenomenon under investigation changes over time
- different components of interest require different types of data to be collected
- complex concepts are combined with concrete phenomena
- a theory has various concepts and different types of outcome variables
- there is a broad, encompassing question rather than a narrow, targeted question.

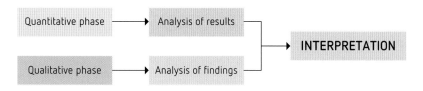

▶ **Figure 9.2** Concurrent mixed methods design

FOR EXAMPLE

CONCURRENT MIXED METHODS RESEARCH

Pighills and colleagues (2019) conducted a concurrent mixed methods study to identify factors that support the local adoption of best practice environmental assessment for falls prevention by occupational therapists within a rural health service. The qualitative and quantitative data were collected simultaneously but analysed separately and then merged to develop a comprehensive understanding of the research question.

Concurrent embedded design

The concurrent embedded design (also referred to as the 'embedded experimental model' or 'concurrent nested design' or convergent embedded) involves collecting quantitative and qualitative data at the same time, but one is dominant and guides the study (mixing occurs at the design phase of the study). The second, less-dominant method is embedded (nested) within the dominant method. Typically, the dominant method is quantitative and the less-dominant method is qualitative.

This nesting means that the embedded method can address different questions or seek information from different participants. Within this design, the qualitative and quantitative data sets can first be analysed separately and the findings then integrated in a final analysis or interpretation stage. The embedded design simultaneously provides the opportunity to look for consistency in findings between the two methods used, and at the same time to identify any inconsistencies. The qualitative findings can be used to explain the quantitative result.

One of the advantages of using an embedded mixed methods design is that it enables the researcher to use a research method they are familiar with as the dominant method, so the researcher does not have to spend vast amounts of time developing expertise in a less familiar method (as it is less dominant). The challenge, as with any mixed methods study, is that competence in a new method still needs to be developed.

FOR EXAMPLE

CONCURRENT EMBEDDED DESIGN

Eskola and colleagues (2017) undertook research to understand parents' experiences and needs during a child's end-of-life care at home. A concurrent embedded mixed method design with a dominant qualitative component was used. Quantitative data were embedded in the qualitative data generated from semi-structured parental interviews.

Concurrent triangulation design

Triangulation typically involves the use of two methods (data collection), methodologies, theoretical frameworks or data analysis techniques within the one study. Triangulation may be used to overcome some of the intrinsic weaknesses of a method or methodology and provides the researcher with a different perspective on the data than does a single method alone.

The concurrent triangulation mixed methods approach involves the use of a qualitative and quantitative phase to confirm, cross-validate or corroborate findings within the one study (Creswell & Plano Clark, 2018). The qualitative and quantitative data are collected concurrently. Each phase may be given equal priority or one phase may dominate. The findings of each phase are integrated during the interpretation phase. There are four variants of a triangulation design (Creswell & Plano Clark, 2018):

- the convergence model
- the data transformation model
- the validating quantitative data model
- the multilevel model.

A strength of the concurrent triangulation design when compared with a sequential design is that less data collection time may be needed.

FOR EXAMPLE

CONVERGENT EMBEDDED MIXED METHODS RESEARCH

Liu and colleagues (2019) used a convergent embedded mixed methods design to research how health education received by patients with acute coronary syndrome and type 2 diabetes mellitus influenced patients' self-efficacy and self-management following hospital discharge. A survey and patient healthcare review record comprised quantitative data collection; interviews were used for qualitative data.

CONCURRENT TRIANGULATION MIXED METHODS RESEARCH

du Toit and Buchanan (2018) undertook an occupational therapy study to identify best-practice scenarios for supporting older adults with moderate to advanced dementia from culturally and linguistically diverse backgrounds who lived in care facilities. The researchers used a mixed methods concurrent triangulation strategy to enable quantitative and qualitative data to be collected concurrently and then compared them to determine if there was divergence, differences or some combination. The researchers' data collection comprised the following: 'two levels of data were collected: a workshop using an appreciative inquiry technique, and a consensus process with adapted Delphi technique that consisted of two rounds' (p. 2).

Sequential mixed methods design

Sequential mixed methods design is so-called because the qualitative and quantitative methods are used in a sequence or linear approach (see Figure 9.3). The purpose of this approach is for the data from one method to build on the other (Creswell & Plano Clark, 2018). Data analysis occurs after each phase but interpretation does not occur until the end of the study. Typically, results from the first phase of the study inform the design of the second.

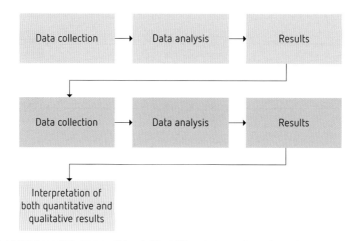

▶ **Figure 9.3**   Sequential mixed methods research design

Source: Adapted from Creswell, J. W., & Plano Clark, V. L. (2018). Designing and Conducting Mixed Methods Research (3rd edn). Thousand Oaks, CA: SAGE.

EVIDENCE FOR BEST PRACTICE

USING A SEQUENTIAL MIXED METHODS APPROACH

Tarling and colleagues (2017) used a fully mixed, sequential, equal status, mixed methods design conducted in two phases to explore the potential sources of variation and understand the meaning of safety climate for nursing practice in acute hospital settings in the United Kingdom. Data was collected by cross-sectional survey and focus group interviews. Results from the survey and thematic analysis were then compared and synthesised.

The strength of a sequential design is that it is a relatively simple method for the researcher to implement. This may be an advantage for novice researchers. The simplicity of the method also makes it easier to report or describe the study. The main limitation of this design is that, as the phases do not occur concurrently, a lot of time may be needed for data collection, particularly if the phases are assigned equal weighting. There are three types of sequential designs: exploratory, explanatory and sequential embedded. (See Figure 9.4.)

Exploratory design

The purpose of an exploratory mixed methods design is to explore a phenomenon about which little is known. To do so involves conducting a qualitative study followed by a quantitative study. The qualitative data is then translated into an approach or tool that is tested quantitatively. This means the approach or tool is grounded in the views of the participants. Creswell and Plano Clark (2018) emphasised that the data are mixed through being connected between qualitative data analysis and the quantitative data collection.

Exploratory mixed methods research has two main variants:
1   the instrument development model
2   the taxonomy development model.

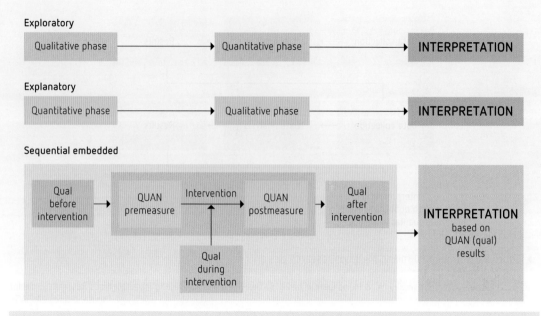

▶ **Figure 9.4** Exploratory, explanatory and sequential embedded mixed methods design

The former is used when researchers want to develop a quantitative research instrument based on qualitative findings (Creswell & Plano Clark, 2018). The latter is used when a qualitative study is necessary to identify variables or to develop a classification system or an emergent theory that is then tested quantitatively.

EVIDENCE FOR BEST PRACTICE

SEQUENTIAL EXPLORATORY MIXED METHODS RESEARCH

Mackie, Marshall and Mitchell (2017) used a sequential exploratory mixed method design to explore the beliefs, attitudes and perceptions of nurses regarding family participation and collaboration in the care of hospitalised adult relative. Observer-as-participant observation data and semi-structured interviews were undertaken. Following separate analysis, data were triangulated. Two contrasting categories emerged: enacting family participation and hindering family participation. These findings can be used to make informed evidence-based changes to the way nurses practice and communicate with families to ensure fundamental care is delivered.

Explanatory design

Previously called the 'sequential explanatory mixed methods design', the main aim of the explanatory mixed methods design is to explore a phenomenon. To do so involves the initial collection and analysis of quantitative data, the results of which feed the second, qualitative phase of the study. The qualitative findings assist in the interpretation of the quantitative results by examining them in greater detail. Greater weight or attention is typically given to the quantitative data as they are collected first. This design may be preferred by researchers who favour quantitative designs (Creswell & Plano Clark, 2018).

Performing the qualitative phase second enables the researcher to examine in more detail unexpected or unusual results from the quantitative phase. Another strength of this approach is that it is easy to implement because of its simple nature, which also makes it easy to describe the method and report the results. The explanatory design also readily lends itself to multiphase investigations and single mixed methods studies (Creswell & Plano Clark, 2018). Challenges faced by the researcher include having to decide how and when to connect the quantitative and qualitative phases of the study and how to integrate the results of these phases to answer the research question.

EVIDENCE FOR BEST PRACTICE

SEQUENTIAL EXPLANATORY MIXED METHODS RESEARCH

Zugai, Stein-Parbury and Roche (2017) undertook two-phase explanatory sequential mixed methods design research to understand the context of the inpatient setting for the treatment of anorexia nervosa and the implications for the therapeutic alliance between nurses and consumers. Descriptive statistics from phase one informed phase two interviews. Phase two date were analysed through thematic analysis.

Sequential embedded design

The sequential embedded design usually involves the collection of qualitative data before or after an intervention. Creswell and Plano Clark (2018) note that, when collected before the intervention, qualitative data can be used to:
- help recruit participants
- help test the treatment before the actual experiment
- select participants who are best suited to the experimental or control conditions.

When collected after the intervention, the qualitative data can be used to help explain why different outcomes occurred (Creswell & Plano Clark, 2018).

Mixed methods designs classification and characteristic summary

The varying classifications of mixed methods designs are presented in **Table 9.1**, and the characteristics of mixed methods designs are presented in **Table 9.2**.

▶**Table 9.1** Classifications of mixed methods designs

Sequential	**Sequential**
• Explanatory • Exploratory • Transformative	• Explanatory • Exploratory • Sequential embedded
Concurrent	**Concurrent**
• Triangulation • Nested • Transformative	• Triangulation • Concurrent embedded

Concurrent	Simultaneous
• qual + quant • qual + quant • quant + qual	• qual + quant • qual + qual • quant + quant • quant + qual
Sequential • quant → qual • qual → quant • qual → quant • qual → quant • quant → qual • quant → qual	**Sequential** • quant → qual • qual → qual • qual → quant • quant → quant

Sources: Creswell, J., et al. (2003). Advanced mixed methods research design. In A. Tashakkori & C. Teddlie (eds), *Handbook on Mixed Methods in the Behavioral and Social Sciences.* Thousand Oaks, CA: SAGE, 209–40; Creswell, J., & Plano Clark, V. (2011). *Designing and Conducting Mixed Methods Research,* Thousand Oaks, CA: SAGE; Martin-Misener et al. (2014). A mixed methods study of the work patterns of full-time nurse practitioners in nursing homes. *Journal of Clinical Nursing, 24*: 1327–37. Morse, J., & Niehaus, L. (2009). *Mixed Method Design: Principles and Procedures.* San Francisco: Left Coast Press, 28–9.

▸ **Table 9.2** Characteristics of mixed methods designs

Design	Characteristics
Embedded	• A concurrent quantitative/qualitative data collection phase within which one dominant method guides the project • The second, less-dominant method is embedded, or nested, within the dominant method
Triangulation	• Qualitative and quantitative phases are implemented at the same time and given equal weighting
Exploratory	• Qualitative data are collected first • Quantitative data are collected to provide a greater understanding of the qualitative findings • Often used for a research problem about which little is known
Explanatory	• Quantitative data are collected first and may be used as a sampling frame or for coding of qualitative data • Qualitative data are collected to provide a greater understanding of the quantitative results

Regardless of how the designs are classified, decide which is most appropriate for your study based on the study's aims and the chosen method's strengths and weaknesses. Also decide whether the two research methods will be used to collect data concurrently or sequentially.

Strengths and limitations of mixed methods research

Strengths of mixed methods research

The strengths and benefits of combining research methods are widely described (Creswell & Plano Clark, 2018; Denzin & Lincoln, 2017; Morse, 2017; Mertens, 2019). Some of the main strengths include the following.

- Qualitative and quantitative research methods have innate strengths and weaknesses. Mixing two research methods enables the researcher to use one method to offset or balance the weaknesses of the other. Doing so adds to the rigour of the study's findings by limiting the impact of one method's weaknesses on the research process.
- Mixed methods enable the researcher to simultaneously ask confirmatory and exploratory questions and thereby verify and generate theory in the same program of inquiry.
- Using a mixed methods approach enables the researcher to explore the data more deeply to acquire a greater understanding of the phenomenon under investigation.
- Using quantitative and qualitative data enables the researcher to simultaneously generalise results from a sample to a population and gain a deeper understanding of the phenomenon of interest.
- Using mixed methods creates the ability to be inclusive of multiple approaches to a problem so there is more certainty in the results.
- Using mixed methods enables researchers to use all possible methods to explore research questions. Doing so produces a better, more complete understanding of the problem under investigation than would looking at the problem from only one perspective.
- The validity of a study's conclusions is enhanced if the conclusions have been confirmed by more than one dataset or method.

Limitations of mixed methods research

There are numerous limitations to combining research methods within a single study.

- Combining two methods requires a lot of time to complete both data collection phases, even if the phases are conducted concurrently.
- Mixed methods research can be more resource or labour intensive and require greater financial support.
- There are possible unintentional effects of combining data collection methods in a single study. A limitation or weakness of one of the methods could be enhanced as opposed to enhancing the strengths of both methods.
- Using two methods creates twice the amount of data as a single method and so requires even more time for analysis and interpretation.
- Sound knowledge of each method is needed.
- If the results of both phases of the study are published together, the journal in which they are to be published must be willing to accept a manuscript that could be much lengthier than their recommended guidelines. If they are not willing to do so, the researcher might be tempted to slice their study, but doing so fails to present the integrated whole and the reader may not have the opportunity to comprehend the significance of the study.

TIP

In exploring and answering the research question, the goal is to make sure that the different methods complement each other.

Rigour in mixed methods research

Every researcher is expected to provide evidence that their findings are accurate and represent the truth. In quantitative research this is known as reliability and validity, while in qualitative research it is called *trustworthiness*. Four criteria can be used to determine the trustworthiness of a study: credibility, dependability, confirmability and transferability (Polit & Beck, 2018).

These concepts differ because of the varying paradigms the two methods are associated with. Debates have been, and continue to be, conducted over the use and application of these terms. Although mixed methods research is a relatively new way of collecting the truth, researchers using this method are not exempt from providing evidence that their results are genuine and credible.

In quantitative research, establishing the truth can be much easier than in qualitative research. Quantitative researchers can provide their data for independent analysis; numbers are entered into an equation giving an indisputable answer. Although rigour in quantitative research is a bit more complex than this, it can be even more challenging in qualitative research. After all, how can you demonstrate that a participant's opinions represent the truth? How can a researcher make generalisations from a sample of only three or four participants?

Rigour is initially established by the researcher providing sound justification for choosing to use a mixed methods approach. As mentioned earlier, a mixed methods design should not be used simply because it can provide a deeper level of understanding than the use of a single method. The research problem under investigation must lend itself to quantitative and qualitative examination within the one study.

Consider the example of a nurse who wants to know how effective a new wound-care product is. Such a problem could be addressed quantitatively. A qualitative question could be to ask patients how they feel about having a pressure ulcer, but this question does not flow logically from the first. A more appropriate question for a mixed methods study would be to ask patients if their pain increased when using the new product, because if the new product increases patients' pain, then it should be considered ineffective. Or nurses could be asked if using the new product increased the amount of time they spent performing wound dressings, as this limitation might outweigh any obvious benefits.

Critiquing a mixed methods study

As a mixed methods approach to research has only recently become popular, research students might struggle to determine the best way to critique studies that have used it. While numerous guidelines exist for critiquing quantitative and qualitative studies (Grove, 2020; Polit & Beck, 2018), these guidelines cannot simply be combined and used as a tool for evaluating mixed methods studies. Other factors must be considered. Some of these criteria could be used to evaluate a qualitative or quantitative study, but a mixed methods approach must have a distinct and justifiable mixing of research methods.

Mertens (2019) suggests the guidelines shown in **Figure 9.5** for critiquing the rigour of mixed methods research.

Creswell and Plano Clark (2018) propose additional evaluation standards:

- Does the study meet the common definition of a mixed methods study?
- Does the study demonstrate purposeful and intentional collection of both qualitative and quantitative data?
- Do the researchers report the specific type of mixed methods design used?
- Does the study demonstrate an awareness of the challenges and limitations of the chosen design?

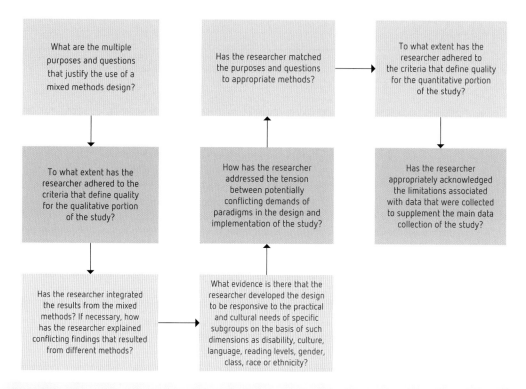

▶ **Figure 9.5**   Guidelines for critiquing the rigour of mixed methods research

Source: Adapted from Mertens, D. (2019). *Research and Evaluation in Education and Psychology: Integrating Diversity with Quantitative, Qualitative and Mixed Methods* (5th edn). Thousand Oaks, CA: SAGE.

ACTIVITY

Identify a qualitative or quantitative study of interest to you. Based on its findings, use a mixed methods approach to consider what other research questions might be worth exploring (if the study is qualitative, try to conceptualise a study using a quantitative approach and vice versa). Which of the main mixed methods approaches would be most suitable for your study? Why?

SUMMARY

This chapter has discussed the meaning of mixed methods research, and outlined the types of mixed methods designs and their associated characteristics.

1	Define mixed methods research	• Involves mixing two methodological approaches within the one study
2	Describe the reasons for using a mixed methods design	• When the research question does not completely encompass the phenomena of interest • When, during the course of inquiry, interesting or unexpected phenomena are revealed – a mixed methods design would allow the researcher to incorporate the new phenomena into the study while the present one is ongoing • When unexpected findings are revealed in a quantitatively driven study – a mixed methods design would allow the researchers to qualitatively explore quantitative data that is puzzling
3	Design a mixed methods study	• There are many factors to consider, including how mixing will occur and whether data will be collected sequentially or concurrently
4	Discuss ethical issues in mixed methods research	• Has the way in which the mixing will occur been stated? • Has a rationale for the design been included in the application (including strengths and limitations)? • Have the ethical issues created by the particular mixed methods design been addressed? • Should the ethical issues arising from each phase of the study be addressed separately in the application? • Have the ethical issues for the participants been stated, such as consent, privacy and level of risk (including how these issues will be addressed)?
5	Describe the different types of mixed methods designs	• There are two main mixed methods designs: sequential and concurrent • Within each of these designs, there are different types
6	Outline the strengths and limitations of mixed methods research	• Mixed methods research has inherent strengths and limitations. The researcher needs to consider these before deciding to use this method
7	Discuss rigour in mixed methods research	• Sound justification must be provided for choosing to use a mixed methods approach • The research problem under investigation must lend itself to quantitative and qualitative examination within the one study
8	Understand how to critique a mixed methods study	• The justification for the choice of method must be provided • How the methods were mixed should be stated

REVIEW QUESTIONS

1   What is the difference between mixed methods research and triangulation?
2   What is the difference between a method and a methodology?
3   List three benefits of using a mixed methods approach.
4   List three limitations of a mixed methods approach. How might these be avoided or minimised?

CHALLENGING REVIEW QUESTIONS

1   What are the philosophical assumptions that underpin a mixed methods approach to research?
2   What criteria can be used to critique a mixed methods study?
3   How do each of the mixed methods designs differ and in which circumstances would they be used.

CASE STUDY 1

Katie, an experienced registered nurse with a master qualification, works in the dementia ward in a large aged-care facility. Katie has observed that some dementia patients have a positive response to music being played in the ward.

This observation led Katie to undertake a literature search for any current research that might help in the care of these residents. While she found research on the use of music as a treatment to improve cognitive function in people with dementia, there was a lack of standardised methods for music therapy interventions and the effect on quality of life was inconclusive. Katie has decided to undertake some research herself on music therapy interventions to see if these have any effect on the quality of life for residents with dementia.

She wants to collect both quantitative data and qualitative data and has heard that mixed methods studies are becoming more commonly used. What should you tell Katie in relation to:

1   using a mixed methods design
2   factors to consider in using this design
3   the benefits of using a mixed methods design
4   the limitations of using a mixed methods design?

CASE STUDY 2

Pamela is a clinical midwife working in a regional hospital whose role includes identifying quality of care issues and undertaking quality improvement research projects to improve midwifery care. Pamela and her midwifery team have identified that an increasing number of women receiving care in the birthing unit seem uncertain of the natural and pharmacological pain relief options available to them in labour. Pamela and her team want to understand why this might be occurring to determine how they can improve the quality of antenatal education and support women's preparation for labour and birth.

Pamela decides that a mixed methods approach would be appropriate to explore women's knowledge of pain relief options in labour, and their experiences of antenatal education and use of pain relief in labour. She designs an online survey for women who had given birth in the last six months to identify the level, type and timing of pain relief information during pregnancy, how well informed they felt prior to labour to make pain relief decisions, and their subsequent use of pain relief during labour. Pamela plans to invite 10 to 15 women who have completed the survey to then participate in semi-structured, in-depth interviews. The interview questions will enable women to share their perceptions of antenatal pain relief education and related preparation for labour, and the positive or negative impacts this had on their labour and birthing experience. Pamela will also ask women to provide their insights and recommendations on how midwives can better support women to make informed decisions regarding pain relief in labour.

1   What are the benefits of Pamela using mixed methods research to meet her quality improvement research project aim? Explain your answer.

2   Pamela has planned an explanatory mixed methods design, where the quantitative phase is followed by the qualitative phase of the study. Why is this an appropriate design for this study?

3   What are two strengths and two limitations of mixed methods research?

REFERENCES

Bharmal, M., Guillemin, I., Marrel, R., Arnold, B., Lambert, J., Hennessy, M., & Fofana, F. (2018). How to address the challenge of evaluating treatment benefits-risks in rare diseases? A convergent mixed methods approach applied within a Merkel cell carcinoma phase 2 clinical trial. *Orphanet Journal of Rare Diseases*, 13:95 https://doi.org/10.1186/s13023-018-0835-1

Brough, P. (2019). *Advanced Research Methods for Applied Psychology: Design, Analysis and Reporting*. Routledge.

Creswell, J. W., & Plano Clark, V. L. (2018). *Designing and Conducting Mixed Methods Research* (3rd edn). Thousand Oaks, CA: SAGE.

Denzin, N. (1978). *The Research Act: A Theoretical Introduction to Sociological Methods* (2nd edn). New York: McGraw-Hill.

Denzin, N., & Lincoln, Y. (2017). *The SAGE Handbook of Qualitative Research* (5th edn.). Thousand Oaks, CA: SAGE.

du Toit, S. H. J., & Buchanan, H. (2018). Embracing cultural diversity: Meaningful engagement for older adults with advanced dementia in a residential care setting. *American Journal of Occupational Therapy*, 72(6), 7206205090p1. https://doi.org/10.5014/ajot.2018.027292

Eskola, K., Bergstraesser, E., Zimmermann, K., & Cignacco, E. (2017). Maintaining family life balance while facing a child's imminent death – a mixed methods study. *Journal of Advanced Nursing*, 73(10), 2462–72. https://doi.org/10.1111/jan.13304

Flemming, K. (2007). The knowledge base for evidence-based nursing: A role for mixed methods research? *Advances in Nursing Science*, 30(1), 41–51.

Giddings, L., & Grant, B. (2007). A Trojan horse for positivism? A critique of mixed methods research. *Advances in Nursing Science*, 30(1), 52–60.

Grove, J. R. (2020). *Burns and Grove's The Practice of Nursing Research: Appraisal, Synthesis, and Generation of Evidence*. Elsevier Health Science.

Halcomb, E. J. (2018). Mixed methods research: The issues beyond combining methods. *Journal of Advanced Nursing*, 75(3), 499–501. https://doi.org/10.1111/jan.13877

Liu, X., Willis, K., Wu, C., Fulbrook, P., Shi, Y., & Johnson, M. (2019). Preparing Chinese patients with comorbid heart disease and diabetes for home management: A mixed methods study. *BMJ Open*, 19(9), 1–13. http://doi.org/10.1136/bmjopen-2019-029816

Mackie, B. R., Marshall, A., & Mitchell, M. (2017). Acute care nurses' views on family participation and collaboration in fundamental care. *Journal of Clinical Nursing*, 27(11–12), 2346–59. https://doi.org/10.1111/jocn.14185

Mertens, D. M. (2019). *Research and Evaluation in Education and Psychology: Integrating Diversity with Quantitative, Qualitative, and Mixed Methods*. (5th edn). Thousand Oaks, CA: SAGE.

Morse, J. M. (2017). *Essentials of Qualitatively-Driven Mixed-Method Designs*. Routledge.

Morse, J., & Niehaus, L. (2009). *Mixed Method Design: Principles and Procedures*. San Francisco, CA: Left Coast Press.

Murdolo, Y., Brown, T., Fielding, L., Elliott, S., & Castles, E. (2017). Stroke survivors' experiences of using the Graded Repetitive Arm Supplementary Program (GRASP) in an Australian acute hospital setting: A mixed-methods pilot study. *Australian Occupational Therapy Journal*, 64(4), 305–13. https://doi.org/10.1111/1440-1630.12363

Pighills, A., Tynan, A., Furness, L., & Rawle, M. (2019). Occupational therapist led environmental assessment and modification to prevent falls: Review of current practice in an Australian rural health service. *Australian Occupational Therapy Journal*, 66(3), 347–61. https://doi.org/10.1111/1440-1630.12560

Polit, D. F., & Beck, C. T. (2018). *Essentials of Nursing Research: Appraising Evidence for Nursing Practice.* (9th edn) Wolters Kluwer.

Rolfe, G. (2009). Writing-up and writing-as: Rediscovering nursing scholarship. *Nurse Education Today, 29*(8), 816–20.

Stefana, A., Padovani, E. M., Biban, P., & Lavelli, M. (2018). Fathers' experiences with their preterm babies admitted to neonatal intensive care unit: A multi-method study. *Journal of Advanced Nursing, 74*(5), 1090–8. https://doi.org/10.1111/jan.13527

Tarling, M., Jones, A., Murrells, T., & McCutcheon, H. (2017). Comparing safety climate for nurses working in operating theatres, critical care and ward areas in the UK: A mixed methods study. *BMJ Open, 7*(10), e016977. https://doi.org/10.1136/bmjopen-2017-016977

Thompson, R., Thomson, H., Gaskin, C., & Plummer, V. (2019). Nurses' attitudes toward management of clinical aggression: A mixed methods study using actor-based simulation. *MEDSURGNursing, 28*(4).

Zugai, J. S., Stein-Parbury, J., & Roche, M. (2017). Therapeutic alliance, anorexia nervosa and the inpatient setting: A mixed methods study. *Journal of Advanced Nursing, 74*(2), 443–53. https://doi.org/10.1111/jan.13410

FURTHER READING

Green, J. (2007). *Mixed Methods in Social Inquiry.* San Francisco, CA: Jossey-Bass.

Hesse-Biber, S. (2009). *Mixed Methods Research: Merging Theory with Practice.* New York, NY: Guilford Press.

Ingham-Broomfield, R. (2016). A nurses' guide to mixed methods research [online]. *Australian Journal of Advanced Nursing, 33*(4), 46–52. http://search.informit.com.au/documentSummary;dn=269785235073075;res=IELHEA> ISSN: 0813-0531

Jordan, S., Philpin, S., Warring, J., Cheung, W., & Williams, J. (2006). Percutaneous endoscopic gastrostomies: The burden of treatment from a patient perspective. *Journal of Advanced Nursing, 56*(3), 270–81.

Myors, K. A., Johnson, M., Cleary, M., & Schmied, V. (2014). Engaging women at risk for poor perinatal mental health outcomes: A mixed-methods study. *International Journal of Mental Health Nursing, 24*(3), 241–52. https://doi.org/10.1111/inm.12109

Ridenour, C., & Newman, I. (2008). *Mixed Methods Research: Exploring the Interactive Continuum* (2nd edn). Carbondale, IL: Southern Illinois University Press.

Stoller, E. P., Webster, N. J., Blixen, C. E., McCormick, R. A., Hund, A. J., Perzynski, A. T., Kanuch, S. W., Thomas, C. L., Kercher, K., & Dawson, N. V. (2009). Alcohol consumption decisions among non-abusing drinkers diagnosed with hepatitis C: An exploratory sequential mixed methods study. *Journal of Mixed Methods Research, 3*(1), 65–86.

10 INTERPRETATIONS OF RESEARCH FINDINGS

Chapter learning objectives

The material presented in this chapter will assist you to:

1 interpret quantitative relationship findings
2 distinguish between causal and non-causal relationships
3 distinguish between statistically significant and non-significant findings, and between statistically and clinically significant findings
4 differentiate between analysis and interpretation in qualitative analysis
5 relate varieties of findings to specific methodological approaches
6 understand the process for synthesising results.

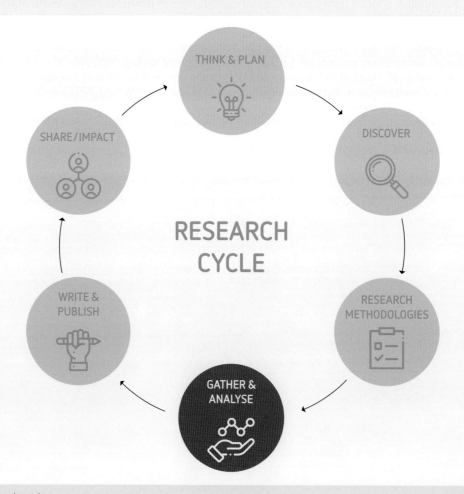

Research cycle

The primary focus of this chapter is interpreting quantitative and qualitative research results. This is a key component of gathering and analysing data, as highlighted in the research cycle above.

Introduction

You have collected and analysed your data. Now you are about to enter another phase of the research process: interpreting the results to make a coherent, meaningful interpretation of the findings. As a researcher, you are responsible for interpreting your findings. You will describe the findings, search for their meaning, draw conclusions from them, determine implications for practice and make recommendations for implementing any significant findings.

If you have been doing interpretation while undertaking the data analysis, then this process has already begun. Indeed, the processes of data analysis and interpretation are somewhat iterative. Some findings need immediate interpretation, while others will take you back to do more data analysis to answer questions that emerge from the initial analysis.

This chapter discusses the interpretation of both quantitative and qualitative research findings. It commences with a description of the process for interpreting quantitative research. It then introduces some of the ways that the analysis phase of qualitative research leads to interpretation and theories, results, findings, insights, recommendations or implications. Although the processes for interpreting analysed information vary according to research methodologies, for ease of reference and the sake of continuity, this chapter will distinguish between them under the categories of interpretive qualitative research and critical qualitative research. In addition, some discussion of postmodern influences on interpretation is offered as another perspective on research.

Interpreting quantitative relationship findings

You are sitting at your desk with what will probably seem like an impossible amount of computer printout to analyse. Where to start? First, make sure that you are confident about the accuracy of the data input. This point is emphasised again because the value of your findings and the interpretation of the findings rest on the accuracy of your data analysis, which in turn rests upon the accuracy of the data and their input into the computer.

Organise the material into logical groupings so that they can be tackled one section at a time. Each project will suggest its own groupings. It is best to start with the purely descriptive data analysis output and then work up to the more complex analyses grouped according to the conceptual framework, hypotheses or questions. Some people like to keep track of their findings on a spreadsheet so that they can easily see the overall picture. Transforming the findings into graphs also makes interpretation easier. This can be done with a statistical analysis program such as SPSS.

It is advisable to commence documenting the interpretation of the data analysis findings, which will then serve as a preliminary draft of a research report.

An overview of quantitative results with examples is shown in Table 10.1.

Data reduction and summaries

One of the first things to do with a large pool of data is to reduce the data to smaller and more useable summary statistics. Produce a set of simple descriptive statistics that includes for each variable a frequency table, and a mean and (where appropriate) standard deviation. It is sometimes useful to generate cross-tabulation tables for any key variables you might want to compare as well.

▶ **Table 10.1** Examples of quantitative results

Interpretive descriptive findings	• Age • Gender
Findings of association and difference	• Between males and females • Control and experimental groups • Pretest and post-test

Causal relationships	• Exposure
	  – outcome relationships
	  – Risk factors to develop coronary disease
	• Treatment
	  – outcome relationship
	  – Is diet and exercise effective in reducing coronary disease?

Non-significant	• Lack of difference may be important
Significant	• Question the validity
Confidence intervals	• Provide a range of likely estimates for an effect
Odds ratio	• Ratio between the incidence of lung cancer in people who smoke and people who do not smoke
Risk calculations	• Relative risk: the prevalence of lung cancer in smokers compared to non-smokers • Attributable risk: the degree of risk of acquiring lung cancer by smoking

Reducing your data into simple summaries enables you to look over it and make decisions about more complex levels of data analysis that may follow.

Interpreting descriptive findings

It is easier to start with the purely descriptive data analysis. In looking at the descriptive statistics, first examine the results for your general descriptive variables such as age, sex and so forth, which will give you a profile of your sample, and then compare your sample with the known characteristics of the population to see how typical it was. This will reinforce the earlier point that it is important to plan your data analysis so that when you come to compare it with the population, you have the correct data for the comparison.

If your sample matches the population reasonably well on the major variables of interest in the study, it is fairly safe to generalise about the external validity of your results. Large samples tend to be less risky in terms of matching the population, but careful sampling and good participation rates can produce representative samples. If your sample is not similar to the population or if it does not match on any one major variable of interest, you do not claim that your findings are valid for any group other than your sample. If, for example, you collected data on participants only from urban areas, it would not be legitimate to claim that your results were typical of all clients in the country or, indeed, the state or territory.

Once the descriptive data about the characteristics of the sample have been looked at, explore the descriptive data analysis of the variables being investigated. For example, if the researcher is relating the variable 'amount of alcohol consumption' to demographic data, they would look first at the descriptive information about the smoking. This will give them a picture of the sample in relation to the major variables. They would then compare this picture with that of the population to look for its representativeness.

TIP

In generalising your findings, it is always better to err on the side of caution.

> **TIP**   If you have created a questionnaire in which you have identified your first-round responders from your follow-ups, it is useful to compare them against the various variables to see whether they are the same. If so, you can treat them as one group for the rest of the interpretation. If they are different, you will need to account for that in your interpretation of the findings.
>
>   If you are doing a clinical study or one that requires more than one data-collection point, it is also useful to compare your dropouts with your persisters on the demographic variables. This will tell you if your study has been affected by participant mortality.

FOR EXAMPLE

DESCRIPTIVE AND INFERENTIAL STATISTICS

Yeo and colleagues (2018) undertook a descriptive cross-sectional study to examine factors influencing women having pap smears in Singapore. Descriptive and inferential statistics were used by the authors to analyse data obtained from a questionnaire given to 350 participants at a local maternity hospital.

Findings of association and difference

If your hypotheses have expressed associations between variables or possible differences between groups, these hypotheses will require testing for such associations and differences. Common differences that are examined are between:
- males and females
- control and experimental groups
- pretest and post-test groups.

    You may or may not find differences in the dependent variable for the different groups. Sometimes you will want to compare the pretest values for a control and experimental group to see if they were the same before the experiment. If not, the results of the experiment could be in doubt. Again, you need to look at the p value to decide whether to reject the null hypothesis (see Chapter 12 for details of the null hypothesis).

    You also need to check that the results are not due to an intervening variable. Suppose that you found, say, that there was a higher rate of domestic violence in one racial group than another. The violence might not be related to the race but to an increased alcohol intake in that group.

    A correlational study looks for an association between variables within one group. It can be positive (a high level of one variable with a high level of the other) or it can be negative (a high level of one variable accompanied by a low level of the other). You may also find that there is no association. To determine whether a relationship is statistically significant, it is necessary to determine whether the probability level is above or below the level of confidence you set. Usually, if the p value is below 0.05, the result is statistically significant at any rate.

    In interpreting findings, it is very important not to go beyond what the findings actually tell you. If you find a relationship between two variables, it means only that where you find one, you find the other. It is very important not to assume that because one thing is related to another it is caused by the other. For example, both of the variables might be related to a third variable that may or may not cause the effect. You may have found that there is an increase in body malfunction in people who live in a district that has a high-power transformer. It would be premature to conclude that power lines cause the malfunction. Perhaps the area is a low-socioeconomic-status area where there is poor nutrition. It might, then, be the nutritional status of the people that underlies the malfunction, not the emissions of the transformer. Relationships such as these require further investigation before causality can be concluded.

Also, just because one thing is statistically related to another, there is not necessarily any meaningful relationship between the factors. If you looked at the census data, you might find all sorts of correlations that were present but not meaningful.

Causal and non-causal relationships

Causal relationships

In health research, the two most important forms of evidence we are looking for are as follows.

- *Exposure–outcome relationships*: how different types of exposures result in different types of health problems; for example, which risk factors are most important in the development of type 2 diabetes.
- *Treatment–outcome relationships*: how different types of treatment or intervention result in different types of health outcomes; for example, whether exercise and diet are effective in reducing the risk of type 2 diabetes.

There are relatively few health problems for which a direct cause-and-effect relationship can be seen. Microbial infections, poisoning and accidents are the best examples. Modern lifestyle diseases have multiple risk factors that combine in different ways for different people. So, it is not a simple cause-and-effect relationship between one factor and one outcome. It is possible to estimate the strength of the effect of each factor from well-designed research studies. In such cases, it may be possible to estimate which factors have the strongest effect and which are not so strong.

Discuss **causal relationships** only if it is certain that the one variable causes the other. In order for one thing to cause another:

- *the causative factor must precede the effect*, such as how nicotine is a causative factor in lung cancer
- *the two variables must be specifically and strongly related to each other*; for example, a microorganism and a disease – when you have a patient with meningococcal meningitis, you will always find the organism Neisseria meningitidis in the body
- *the relationship should be reasonable*; if you found that two things were related but it did not seem logical that one caused the other, you would probably conclude that the relationship was correlational rather than causal.

Usually, causal relationships can be demonstrated only by an experiment in which a change in the independent variable can be shown to result in a corresponding change in the dependent variable. Even then, the experiment should be so highly controlled that the independent variable is the only factor that could have caused the result.

It is normally through experimentation that scientists have built up knowledge about causes of diseases. Sometimes, though, if a statistical relationship is very strong and the other criteria are satisfied, we can assume causality if it is not possible to experiment. Sometimes, a particular disease in humans (AIDS, for example) is always linked to a specific microorganism (the HIV virus) that has been demonstrated to cause the disease in other primates. It would be reasonable, then, to assume that the microorganism causes the disease despite the fact that you cannot, for ethical reasons, do an experiment on humans.

If your results suggest a causal relationship, be suspicious of a placebo effect and be very cautious in your interpretation of it. It pays to use a placebo-controlled design to allow for the placebo effect.

TIP A causal relationship will almost always require the examination of differences between a pretest and a post-test on the same group to see if the manipulation of the independent variable resulted in a change in the dependent variable.

FOR EXAMPLE

CAUSAL RELATIONSHIP RESEARCH FINDING

Qualitative research undertaken by Liu (2018) explored factors influencing the coping styles of elderly Chinese oncology patients with their levels of distress. Results support a causal relationship between these factors. For example, the 'confrontation' and 'resignation' coping styles were related to less distress and more 'benefit findings' (such as positive reframing and religious activity as coping mechanisms), which improved the long-term quality of life and health outcomes too.

Non-causal relationships

Not all relationships are causal. In non-causal relationships, the relationship that is evident between the two variables is not completely the result of one variable directly affecting the other. In the most extreme case two variables can be related to each other without either variable directly affecting the values of the other.

Significance of findings: statistical versus clinical

The findings from any research study can be presented and interpreted in several ways. For instance, the study might have profound healthcare implications, but it might not have achieved **statistical significance** simply because of a small sample size. Likewise, a huge sample size may have achieved a slight level of statistical significance. How is sense made of these findings?

Interpreting or making sense of findings is the most important phase of the research process. It is at this stage of the process that an attempt is made to apply the findings to clinical practice or to the theory that the study emerged from. Research is the link between theory and practice, and it is at the point of interpretation that these links must be demonstrated.

Non-significant findings

First, examine the findings to see whether they are significant. If they do not meet the criterion set previously for significance (usually $p < 0.05$), then the findings are not significant and the null hypothesis is not rejected. Then an explanation has to be made as to why they are not significant. Before reporting non-significant findings, an alternative explanation for them is looked for. Perhaps they can be explained by an inadequate or biased sample, incorrect methodology, a design flaw, errors in measurement, data collection or analysis, or even by some unforeseen event that affected participants. Results that are statistically non-significant may still be important if they add to our knowledge because the lack of difference is important.

Significant findings

If the findings are statistically significant, there are questions still to be answered.

Are the findings pointing in the direction that was predicted?

It is possible to have findings that are significant but that are the opposite of what was expected. Now an explanation must be made. The whole study must be critiqued to see if an explanation can be made. Data entry and analysis must be checked to see whether they were correctly carried out. An incorrect recoding step, for instance, such as omitting to recode a variable in the opposite direction, could explain the results. If so, the mistake can be fixed and the corrected data analysis can be reinterpreted. If not, an explanation has to be made as to why the results didn't meet expectations. If the study was well designed and the methods appropriate and carried out correctly, then a conclusion may be that the theory is wrong.

The findings might be statistically significant, but are they valid?

It is necessary to be cautious in the interpretation of statistically significant findings. Be sure that there is continuity between the problem, theoretical framework, methodology, methods and findings. Also, be certain that the findings have not been affected by any of the threats to validity. Consider whether they could be accounted for by another explanation, such as a very large sample resulting in very small differences being statistically significant. Be careful not to mistake statistical significance for meaningful differences.

Indeed, a critique of the study needs to be done so that the validity of the findings can be evaluated and defended against colleagues' criticism. If the study problem, conceptual framework, design, data-collection methods and data analysis were adequate, then the findings are likely to have internal validity. It is easier to see the flaws in the study in hindsight, and some events cannot be predicted, so the adequacy of every part of the study must be reviewed.

ACTIVITY

You have completed a study of student health among Year 12 students at a local high school. You measured the body mass index (BMI) of all students and found the following results.

- Female students: mean BMI = 27.2; standard deviation = 4.2.
- Male students: mean BMI = 25.1; standard deviation = 3.4.
- t-test of mean BMI between males and females, $p = 0.02$.
  What do these findings mean?

Difference between statistical and clinical significance

In interpreting research results, it is important to distinguish between statistical significance and **clinical significance**. Statistical significance is a difference in groups that is related to testing a hypothesis. It says only that the results probably could not have happened by chance alone. A small difference may turn out to be statistically significant, particularly if there are many participants. Clinical significance is the strength of the effect in your study. The effect could be what happens when someone is exposed to a risk factor, or it could be the actual effect of a treatment on an existing condition.

There are several techniques used in epidemiology that help clinicians determine the clinical significance of their findings. They include confidence intervals, odds ratios and risk calculations.

Confidence intervals

Confidence intervals are often used in health research to demonstrate the level of confidence that a finding is true and not the result of a sampling error. While p values tell us the probability that the result is a true estimate of the given statistic in the real population, they can vary according to the sample size and the actual effect size being measured (the size or strength of difference or association between two sets of measurements). Health research is more concerned with the real strength of an effect, not so much with the sample size needed to make it statistically significant. This refers to the clinical significance of an effect.

Confidence intervals provide the range of likely estimates for an effect. Point values are provided in p, which tell us about the significance of a single point of measurement. The difficulty of relying on p values in clinical research is that they may obscure the clinical significance of a finding by relying totally on the statistical significance of a single point. A real health benefit or health problem may be ignored because the sample size was small, while a clinically insignificant result may be considered important simply because an extremely large sample produced a statistically significant result based on a small effect level.

Confidence intervals are a way of discriminating between statistical significance based purely on p values and the actual clinical significance of a result. A 95 per cent confidence interval will tell us where 95 per cent of the likely results would fall from all possible samples used.

When calculating confidence intervals, upper and lower limits are calculated to demonstrate 95 per cent confidence in the result, and these are then added and deducted from the mean to give the 95 per cent confidence interval.

Formulae for confidence intervals:

$$\text{lower} = (\text{mean} + [1.96 \times \text{standard deviation}]) \div \sqrt{n}$$
$$\text{upper} = (\text{mean} + [1.96 \times \text{standard deviation}]) \div \sqrt{n}$$

(The number 1.96 in these formulae corresponds to a z score of 1.96 either side of the mean, which covers 95 per cent of the area under the normal curve; n is the size of the sample.)

Odds ratios

An *odds ratio* refers to the ratio between the incidence of a health problem in a group of people exposed to a risk factor compared with the incidence of a health problem in a group of people not exposed to a risk factor. An example is the rate of lung cancer in smokers compared with the rate of lung cancer in non-smokers. Imagine if a hypothetical study of cigarette smoking and lung cancer produced the data summary shown in Table 10.2.

▶ Table 10.2   Smoking survey data summary

	Smoker	Non-smoker
Lung cancer	12	2
No lung cancer	88	98

Using the data in this contingency table, you could make the following calculations,
- The odds of getting lung cancer if a smoker = $(12 \div 100) \div (88 \div 100) = 12 \div 88$.
- The odds of getting lung cancer if a non-smoker = $(2 \div 100) \div (98 \div 100) = 2 \div 98$.
- The odds ratio related to the risk of smoking and lung cancer = $(12 \div 88) \div (2 \div 98) = 6.68$.

Risk calculations

Risk and cause are not the same thing. Many modern lifestyle diseases, such as coronary heart disease, do not have a single cause. They are acquired by exposure to multiple risk factors, including genetic predisposition, diet, exercise and cigarette smoking. No one risk factor causes these types of disease, but some are more influential than others.

Understanding the importance of various risk factors in disease has become a significant part of epidemiological research. Risk can be measured in two ways.

1 *Relative risk*: the rate at which disease occurs in people who are exposed to a particular risk compared with the rate among those who are not so exposed; for example, the prevalence of lung cancer in smokers compared with the prevalence of lung cancer in non-smokers. From Table 10.2, this would be $12 \div 2 = 6.0$, which means that lung cancer is six times more likely in smokers than non-smokers.

2 *Attributable risk*: the difference between the rates at which a disease occurs in exposed people and the rates at which it occurs in non-exposed people; for example, the degree of risk of acquiring lung cancer simply by smoking cigarettes. In other words, having subtracted the overall likelihood of getting lung cancer in the non-smoking population, how much risk can be attributed to cigarette smoking alone? From Table 10.2, this would be $12 - 2 = 10.0$, which means that of all the deaths caused by lung cancer, 10 out of 12 can be directly attributed to cigarette smoking.

ACTIVITY

From your earlier study of student health among Year 12 students at the local high school, you produced the following results.

FEMALE STUDENTS

- Mean BMI = 27.2
- Standard deviation = 4.2
- Number of females in the group = 37
  What is the 95 per cent confidence interval for these data?

Mixed findings

Mixed findings occur when some null hypotheses and not others have been rejected, or some findings are in the direction of the hypotheses and some are not. It is important to consider each finding carefully in light of the methodology and the theoretical framework. It may be that the different findings reflect different methods of measurement, different data collectors or a faulty theory.

Serendipitous findings

Serendipitous findings are those that are unexpected. On the majority of projects, most researchers cannot resist doing extra analyses if they have the data, just to find out what might be there. Sometimes, this will result in a finding that you were not expecting. Some of these findings can be useful and some not. Serendipitous findings can go either for or against the hypotheses, or they might be totally unrelated to the study but noticed by chance. A classic example is the story of the discovery of penicillin, which resulted when Alexander Fleming noticed that a culture plate contaminated with Penicillium notatum mould showed no growth around the bacteria. He concluded that the mould contained a bacteriostatic agent and thus penicillin was born.

An unexpected finding needs to be considered very carefully as to how this could have happened – whether it is a spurious finding that occurred because of an error or whether it is genuine. If it is thought to be genuine, an explanation for this finding needs to be found. Also, the finding should be considered in light of the theoretical framework. Serendipitous findings will usually need to be investigated further to determine whether they are valid, and another method may be more appropriate for a research project arising out of a serendipitous finding.

Searching for meaning within the study

Within the study findings, it is important when searching for meaning to look at the patterns and connections in the total picture as well as in the individual parts. Often, individual variables produce data, but when compared with one another or clustered into groups for comparison, they can yield insights that were not evident when examining the individual variables.

TIP When attempting to interpret patterns in the findings, particularly if it is a complex set of findings, it can be useful to have a whiteboard or large notebook on hand on which to make notes.

It is important to go beyond a description of the findings and ask why something did or did not occur. Any competent researcher can look at and describe findings, but to make a meaningful commentary they need to go beyond documentation or narration of the results and ask what it means. This involves interpreting for the research consumer the real difference that these findings make, which is a difficult step because it requires much thought and reasoning, and sometimes intuitive leaps. The process of relating your findings is outlined in Figure 10.1.

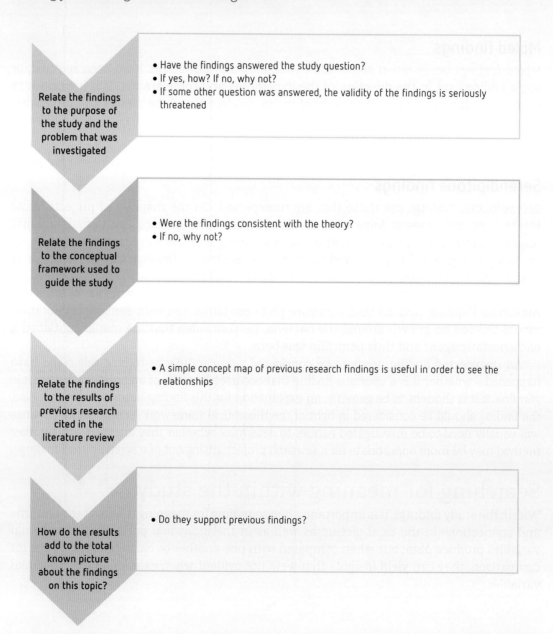

| Relate the findings to the purpose of the study and the problem that was investigated | • Have the findings answered the study question?
 • If yes, how? If no, why not?
 • If some other question was answered, the validity of the findings is seriously threatened |

| Relate the findings to the conceptual framework used to guide the study | • Were the findings consistent with the theory?
 • If no, why not? |

| Relate the findings to the results of previous research cited in the literature review | • A simple concept map of previous research findings is useful in order to see the relationships |

| How do the results add to the total known picture about the findings on this topic? | • Do they support previous findings? |

▶ **Figure 10.1**   Relating your findings: The process

Again, it is useful to group the previous findings according to an individual question or topic rather than on a study-by-study basis.

Searching for meaning beyond the study

It is important to evaluate your study in terms of its implications for further theoretical development. Your findings may confirm the theory or part of it, they may reject the theory, or they may make no difference either way if they are not significant. Similarly, they may help to develop the theory further or help to critique it.

It is also important to evaluate your findings in terms of the implications for future research. It is rare for a study not to give rise to other questions that need to be researched further.

FOR EXAMPLE

RESEARCH STUDY THAT RAISED FURTHER QUESTIONS

Richardson-Tench and colleagues (2012) undertook research in a day surgery centre in Melbourne to evaluate which preadmission care intervention was more effective in enhancing the physical preparedness of patients undergoing day surgery: preadmission telephone screening or preadmission clinic assessment. There was no statistically significant difference between the groups. However, the authors recommended research of the differences within Australia's large multicultural and multilingual population, as well as where clients find further information and the impact this may or may not have on their experiences.

It is also important to evaluate the findings for the implications for practice, assuming they are clinically significant. If they are, how can clinicians improve practice on the basis of your findings? What would be the outcomes for clients or their families if the practice was changed? What would be the cost in poorer client outcomes if the changes were not made?

EVIDENCE FOR BEST PRACTICE

RESEARCH FINDINGS WITH IMPLICATIONS FOR PRACTICE

A study undertaken by Wallin and colleagues (2020) employed a descriptive qualitative study to highlight preceptors' experiences of supervising students on clinical placement in the ambulance service (emergency medical service in Sweden). Using individual interviews, the researchers found that the preceptor role in this unique and ever-changing environment had multiple challenges and provided implications for future practice. Preceptors develop the ability to promote the independence of their students via reflexivity in their work; for those with additional academic training this was an easier task. The role was also found to involve varying degrees of loneliness, which has implications for the non-standard levels of support given by universities and colleagues. Lack of continuity with their students and the variance in day-to-day workload made providing learning opportunities and assessment of competence difficult.

When the implications have been addressed, what conclusions can be drawn from the findings? Conclusions may be tentative or firm, depending on the certainty about the external and internal validity of the findings.

Consider what recommendations would be made based on the findings, implications and conclusions derived from any significant and meaningful results. They can be for research, practice, theoretical development or testing, or education. These recommendations will follow naturally from the implications. Recommendations are very important because they are one of the major products of the research.

Differentiation between analysis and interpretation in qualitative research

It is important to draw a distinction between analysis and interpretation; even though they are related, they are separate processes. To be able to make **interpretations**, data must be analysed thoroughly. Qualitative researchers may find it difficult to explicate the actual methods and processes they use when they analyse and interpret research data. The conundrum of qualitative analysis interpretation is in contrast to quantitative approaches, in which confidence is placed in valid and reliable instruments that produce objective results as mathematical relationships. Even given the difficulty of working with words and language, qualitative researchers must attempt to set out the analytic and interpretive phases of the project for readers of the research.

ACTIVITY

Locate two qualitative research reports published in peer-reviewed journals. Read the articles and examine the extent to which the researchers have described what they did in their respective projects to analyse and interpret the data.

Defining analysis and interpretation

Analysis

Analysis involves systematically reviewing research data with the intention of sorting and classifying them into representational groups and patterns. After analysis, the data are organised from their raw state as words and images (alone or in combination) into groupings and symbolic forms that require explanation to ensure that the meaning is as clear as it can be.

Interpretation

Interpretation involves taking the forms of analysed information to another level or levels of abstraction, so that statements can be made about what they mean in light of the intentions, methods and processes of the research. This basically means that the analysed words and/or images are refined into more words and/or images that make the research outcomes more meaningful. In qualitative research, if the interpretations and explanations of the analysed data are not given, readers are left to infer their own conclusions.

Qualitative research findings can be left open to multiple interpretations in line with the context-dependent and relative features of qualitative research approaches. Qualitative researchers and participants, having been actively involved in the project, may place their unique interpretations on the data. Readers of the research may not necessarily agree with the researchers' and participants' interpretations, or they may posit other possible conclusions about the findings. This freedom to interpret or to leave interpretations open does not relieve qualitative researchers of their fundamental responsibility to be open and transparent in their methods and processes. Readers of the research need to be able to trace the methods and processes that were used in a project so that they can audit the researcher's activities and/or have a sound rationale for their differing interpretations.

Analysis generally precedes interpretation

Generally speaking, analysis precedes interpretation, although some qualitative researchers, such as those using phenomenological writing, having focused on the data so closely and thoroughly, describe an intuitive grasp of the data. Also, some qualitative researchers who use participatory research methods and processes with participants as co-researchers may experience spiralling and integrative processes in which analysis and interpretation blend and seem to become indivisible. Bearing in mind these and other possible exceptions to the rule, the approach taken here will to be to assume that interpretation occurs after a period of analysis, however protracted and by whatever means.

Interpretation requires immersion in the text

Although images and numbers can also be part of qualitative analysis and interpretation, words are the main symbols from which meaning is derived. Text may be, among other things:

- interview transcripts
- field notes
- historical documents
- journal entries
- summaries
- audio recordings of group discussions.

Invariably, qualitative interpretations of words and language require protracted time with the text to ensure that meaning is found and that it is as clear as possible to convey to other people. Therefore, qualitative interpretation is generally not a matter of putting data through a computer system to come up with statistical relationships for interpretation. Rather, analysis is usually done through reading and rereading text by manual or computer-assisted means. Interpretation follows further reflection and validation by people such as other researchers, co-researchers, participants and peers.

Interpretations as relative truth

Qualitative researchers agree that there is no way of guaranteeing absolute truth because truth is relative, subjective, context-dependent and elusive. The idea that truth is relative may appear to leave open the whole issue of whether qualitative interpretations can be relied on as having some foundation for adding to knowledge. But even though truth is regarded as being relative, it is still considered important to reveal it in its various forms. The main difference between qualitative and quantitative assumptions about knowledge in this regard is that the former does not seek to generate absolute, indisputable truths and facts because they agree that the changing and complex nature of human existence does not permit research approaches to guarantee this kind of knowledge. Even so, qualitative researchers use various means of demonstrating the worthiness of their projects. For example, measures for ensuring validity may involve asking the participants to confirm that the interpretations are truthful for them.

Interpretations by other names

Various words are used synonymously to mean 'interpretations'. Qualitative research reports use words such as 'theories', 'findings', 'results', 'insights', 'strategies', 'implications', 'examples of reflective awareness', 'changed practice' and so on. The words used may have been selected specifically to reflect the assumptions and intentions of the research methodology, because qualitative research is set up in different ways to fulfil different purposes.

FOR EXAMPLE

METHODOLOGY EXAMPLES

Methodology	Interpretations	Example
Grounded theory	Middle-range theories	Sala Defilippis et al. (2020)
Phenomenological	Insights or essences	Olano-Lizarraga et al. (2020)
Feminist	Themes	Armour-Burton & Etland (2020)
Action research	Reflective awareness	Afshar et al. (2020)
Critical ethnography	Changed practice	Laging et al. (2018)

Most qualitative research approaches do not claim to generate interpretations that can be considered to be generalisable to the wider population.

An exception to this is grounded theory, which sets out to make general statements in the form of middle-range theories about what might be expected in similar circumstances.

It might typically be expected that interpretations resulting from phenomenological approaches that provide insights will be useful to those people with whom they resonate. In other words, if readers of the research find it is relevant to them, then it has scope for also being informative to them.

Action research approaches reporting examples of reflective awareness and changed practice have scope for local theories of practice. This means that the people who have participated in the project have realised local, personal truths that are relevant for them. The scope of the interpretations is broader when the people involved in the research influence other people, policies and practices in the wider setting.

Qualitative findings in relation to methodological approaches

Qualitative findings will differ according to the underlying theoretical assumptions of the approach and the intentions of the research. There are many ways of categorising methodological approaches in qualitative research. A very simple and comprehensive way of thinking about kinds of qualitative research is to categorise them according to interpretive and critical forms and differences as presented in previous chapters. Although categorisations of this kind have their shortcomings, they are useful for students who are trying to plot their way through a wide and deep range of ideas about research.

Qualitative interpretive methodologies

Qualitative interpretive methodologies intend mainly to generate meaning by exploring, explaining and describing things of interest in order to make sense out of them. Examples of these methodologies are historical research, grounded theory, ethnography and phenomenology. These methodologies are described in Chapter 7.

Qualitative critical methodologies

Qualitative critical methodologies aim to bring about change in the status quo by questioning aspects that are taken for granted. Through systematic political critique, these methodologies attempt to expose factors of control, oppression, power and domination, and they also cause raised awareness and change activities. Examples of these methodologies are critical ethnography, feminisms, interpretive interactionism and action research.

Similarities and differences

The major difference between interpretive and critical qualitative research lies in the main intention of what those responsible hope to achieve through the research process. Interpretive forms are involved mainly with generating meaning, whereas critical forms concern themselves with change. Even though they both can bring about change, they differ in the intensity of their intentions and their choice of methods to do this. Critical methodologies are most intense in bringing about change because they have an up-front change agenda and tend to use participatory research processes to realise change intentions.

Qualitative interpretive and critical categories

The process for interpretation may differ according to what kind of qualitative research it can be considered to be; that is, whether it is essentially an interpretive (concerned mainly with meaning) or critical (concerned mainly with change) project. Some researchers argue that they have combined methodologies across the interpretive and critical categories. In this case, they may need to use a combination of interpretive processes appropriate to the assumptions, aims, objectives, methods and processes of the project.

Clarifying some preconditions for qualitative interpretation

A researcher may have made a clear decision as to the placement of a project in either the interpretive or critical methodology categories. Alternatively, the project may be placed in a combination of methodologies. In some cases, a project may defy categorisation into methodological groupings altogether; for example, postmodern research. Regardless of the nature of the project, there are some general necessary preconditions for interpretation of which qualitative researchers are advised to be aware.

The need for congruency

Congruency in qualitative research means the fit or correspondence between foundational ideas and the activity phases of the research. Even though the phases of a project may be carefully planned from the outset, parts of the overall project may change over the course of the research. Therefore, before embarking on making sense of the analysed data, it may be useful to take some time to reorient to the overall project. This will involve you asking yourself some questions to check on the congruency of the project's assumptions, aims, objectives, methods and processes. See Figure 10.2 for some questions that may be posed.

Reasons for asking questions

The reasons for asking certain questions at the transition from analysis to interpretation are to reorient to the overall project; to check on the degree of congruency between the

Assumptions
- What ideas underlie this project concerning the nature of knowledge and how it is verified?
- What choices were made about selecting a paradigm in which the project would fit most appropriately?
- If no paradigm category was chosen then, does it matter now?

Aims and objectives
- What did I intend to research?
- Why did I want to research these things?
- At this stage, to what extent has the project fulfilled its stated purposes?

Methods
- What methods were chosen to gather the information?
- To what extent do the methods appear to be a good fit with the assumptions, aims and objectives of the research?
- To what extent did the methods gather the information required?

Processes
- How was the research undertaken in terms of the researcher–participant relationships?
- How was the research undertaken in terms of the overall management of the project?
- To what extent did the processes appear to be a good fit with the assumptions, aims, objectives and methods of the research?

▶ **Figure 10.2** Questions for checking congruency

assumptions, aims, objectives, methods and processes; and to prepare for the process of interpretation.

Reorienting to the overall project

In reorienting to the overall project, the researcher's memory is refreshed and an assessment can be made as to whether the project has progressed as anticipated to this point. If it has not gone as expected, it might be helpful to look at the ways in which it has differed and locate the reasons for this. It may be necessary to have this in mind when beginning the interpretation, as this will help to sort out twists and turns in the data that otherwise may be confusing.

Checking on the degree of congruency

Congruency may not be an issue for some qualitative researchers, but it is worth bearing in mind that most qualitative research provides a theoretical basis for its choice of methodological approach, methods and processes (Atkinson et al., 2007; Denzin & Lincoln, 2007; Flick, 2009; Polit & Beck, 2017). However, just because there are many qualitative approaches from which to choose, this does not mean they all have the same assumptions about what constitutes knowledge and how to go about finding and verifying it. Supporters of having a theoretical basis might argue that researchers need to be clear about the degree of congruency within and between all the research phases. This is because it helps them prepare for interpretation and will provide a strong rationale for readers of the research as to what has been done, why it has been done and how it has been done.

Preparing for the process of interpretation

When it comes time to move from analysis to interpretation, using the questions outlined in Figure 10.2 may help determine the degree of congruency in the research to date. It will help you to focus thoroughly on the data. This intense focus can help you to extract meaning that is congruent with the assumptions, aims, objectives, methods and processes of the research. It will also mean that some time will elapse between the analysis and interpretation phases of the research, which will not only give you time for thinking, but will also permit time for reading and rereading so that there is deeper and deeper immersion in the data in preparation for making sense out of it.

Processes for synthesising results

The processes for synthesising qualitative interpretive and critical interpretations happen as cognitive activities within the researcher. This interpretation process must happen for the researcher to make sense of the analysed data.

From analysis to interpretation

Being able to describe interpretation is tantamount to being able to describe cognitive processes, such as making intellectual leaps, connections, intuitive grasps and so on. This makes interpretation a very difficult thing to describe on the biochemical and psychological levels. In tackling the vexed problem of what it is inquirers do when they interpret, philosophers have taken different approaches to addressing various forms of hermeneutics (Gadamer, 1975; Habermas, 1981).

Hans-Georg Gadamer was a philosopher in the phenomenological tradition. Gadamer asserted that the key to understanding existence is through language. He also contended that it is the task of hermeneutics to make distinctions between true and false prejudices by a process of effective historical consciousness. By this, he was advocating the need to be open to and be surprised by what may emerge through interpretation.

For Jurgen Habermas, interpretation is more a matter of realising that knowledge is socially constructed through human interaction, and that interpretation involves social, cultural, economic, political and personal dimensions. Habermas links truthful interpretation to the idea of rational consensus gained through discourse, which means that people have the potential to create their own interpretations through non-coercive and non-manipulative rationality. He considers that people orient towards finding truth through daily communicative acts of speaking, and that ideal speech situations involve comprehensibility of the utterance, truth of the content, rightness of the performative content and veracity of the speaker.

The next section will attempt to break through the lack of direction to give clues as to ways in which interpretation might be made by raising some questions and suggesting some tentative answers. The assumptions underlying the listing of these suggested processes relate to differences in research relationships between researchers and participants. Qualitative interpretive methodologies involve participants by working *with* them in research processes, rather than by doing research *to* them. Qualitative interpretive methodologies are not as mindful of group participatory processes or co-researcher status for participants.

Qualitative interpretive methodology process

Interpretation subsumes all the phases in the research that have gone before. The products of the analysis are incomplete in themselves. They only have fullest meaning when they have been described and explained through interpretation.

Figure 10.3 outlines the steps in the qualitative interpretive methodology process.

ACTIVITY

Use the interpretation steps described in Figure 10.3 to move from analysis to interpretation in your story or a series of stories about an experience in your life that was of great significance to you. How does your analysis of the story differ from your interpretation?

Qualitative critical methodology process

The following should be considered when undertaking the qualitative critical methodology process.

- Given that critical methodologies have an emancipatory intent for groups of oppressed or otherwise disenfranchised people, the interpretive processes can often be shared by the people involved.
  - Go through the exercise as a group, asking each other the questions listed in this chapter as preconditions for qualitative interpretation.

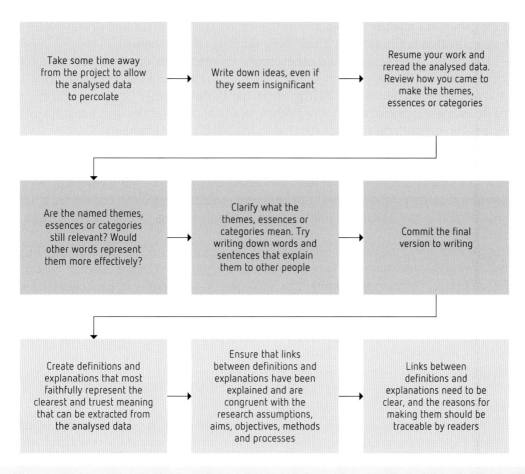

▶ **Figure 10.3** Qualitative interpretive methodology process

- Acknowledge the potential of group members to make a collective interpretation of the information based on their active involvement in the collaborative project.
- Give group members the option of taking some time away from the intensity of the project. This can be negotiated, depending on the time you have available to complete the project and on factors the members may raise as being important.
- If the members decide to take time away from the project, suggest that during the time away they notice any ideas that come to mind.
  - Ask them to write these down, even if they seem insignificant, so that they can be shared with others in the group.
  - Resume or continue group meetings and decide on a way of reviewing the analysed data. Review how you came to make the decisions you made at the time of analysis.
- Multiple interpretations of competing discourses are possible. There may be no easy answers to complex sociopolitical questions that have been raised by the research, but the group may be able to identify some tentative connections and interpretations related to interpersonal and institutional power relationships. The interpretations subsume all the phases in the research that have gone before.
- The products of the analysis are incomplete in themselves. They only have fullest meaning when they have been described and explained through critical appraisal and interpretation.

- If the group has already named any of the issues, themes, ideas and action cycles that were generated in the analysis phase, why did they choose them?
  - Are they still relevant? Would other issues, themes, ideas or action cycles represent them more effectively now in light of further critiques and new information?
- In an open group discussion, clarify what the issues, themes, ideas or action cycles mean. Ask group members to write down words and sentences and explain them to each other; invite them to share them with the other group members.
- It may be useful to have an audio recorder operating during the sharing of interpretations so you can play back and expose the interpretations to critique. Try to reach consensus on a shared and agreed set of statements about the interpretations. Note any possible alternative interpretations in light of the unique social, historical, economic, political, cultural and personal determinants of the research setting, intentions, processes and methods.
- Suggest that group members work in pairs to discuss individual interpretations. Suggest that they speak spontaneously about what the analysed data might mean in light of the overall project. Encourage members to make the clearest possible explication of what they want to say. Suggest that they raise questions about interpretations and seek other possible explanations and conclusions. These are then shared with the whole group.
- As a group, create statements and explanations that most faithfully represent the multiple discourses that can be extracted from the analysed data.
- Ensure that you have created and explained links between the multiple discourses that are congruent with the assumptions, aims, objectives, methods and processes of the research.
- Links between the multiple discourses need to be as clear as possible and the linking argued carefully for the benefit of the participants and readers of the research.
- Ensure that the final version of the overall interpretations represents what all the group intended them to mean after full discussion and critical appraisal of the social, historical, economic, political, cultural and personal determinants operating in the research. Commit the final version to writing.

How will the interpretations look?

There are various ways in which interpretations may be viewed.
- Interpretations will not look alike and will differ according to the ways in which they were extracted from the data.
- Interpretations will bear a resemblance to the language of the methodologies that guided them.
- Interpretations can be represented as diversely as words, phrases, sentences, models, theories, action strategies, group summaries and so on.
- Interpretations can be put forward to readers of the research as theoretical propositions, findings, results, insights, strategies, implications, and examples of reflective awareness, changed practice, multiple discourses and so on.

ACTIVITY

Given that interpretations look different, would you describe the interpretations of your story as theoretical propositions, findings, results, insights, strategies, implications, examples of reflective awareness, changed practice, multiple discourses or something else? Explain your answer.

How will I know if the interpretations are relevant?

- Interpretations will have a high chance of being relevant if they can demonstrate **methodological congruency**. This means that they show that they are related directly to the analysed data, which in turn are related to the assumptions, methods and processes of the research.
- Interpretations have meaning only in terms of the research because they are specific to the research.
- Interpretations are context-dependent; that is, they are relative to the total set of circumstances that make up the research.
- Ways of checking relevance differ according to the methodological approach. The tests of relevance that are applied are particular to the approach taken.

Interpreting the text considering the literature

The need to do a research project may be based on revisiting the literature review and confirming knowledge gaps or conflicting results. In contrast, if a researcher is interested in taking an inductive approach, such as that taken in grounded theory, the literature review may be delayed until during or after the data collection. Even so, at some point, qualitative researchers will go to the literature to see what it contains on an area of interest.

Interpretations are compared or contrasted with the results of other studies. Research reports might include a section in which the connections are spelled out clearly. If connections are found between the newly interpreted data and those already in the literature, qualitative researchers would not necessarily use this discovery to make a claim for the truthfulness of the interpretations. Rather, the similarities would be documented in the research report as a point of interest.

The other reason for consulting the literature is to provide a firm grounding for the interpretations in the methodological tradition of choice. A phenomenological project may, for example, use certain concepts to show readers that the assumptions underlying the choice of methods and processes relate to the project, while a feminist project will be guided by the literature relating to feminisms and feminist research processes, and a critical ethnography may cite references derived from critical social science to augment its questioning approach to the research interest. In each of these cases, the aim is to present the key ideas of the methodology to show the kind of knowledge it is capable of generating in research projects. Research reflecting postmodern influences could stand outside methodological categorisation on the basis that it represents grand narratives. Even so, researchers who are reflecting postmodern influences may appeal to literature that affirms key ideas, such as multiple voices, difference, fragmentation and deconstruction.

SUMMARY

1	Interpret quantitative research findings	• Researchers are responsible for accurately and objectively interpreting their data to convey to the audience a coherent, meaningful interpretation of the findings
2	Distinguish between causal and non-causal relationships	• A causal relationship should only be inferred from an experiment, not stated as definitive • In non-causal relationships, the relationship that is evident between the two variables is not completely the result of one variable directly affecting the other
3	Distinguish between statistically significant and non-significant findings, and between statistically and clinically significant findings	• Statistically significant findings may not be clinically significant • Clinically significant findings can be used to influence practice
4	Differentiate between analysis and interpretation in qualitative analysis	• Analysis involves systematically reviewing research data with the intention of sorting and classifying them into representational groups and patterns • Interpretation involves working with the forms of analysed information so that statements can be made about what they mean in light of the intentions, methods and processes of the research • The processes for interpretation may differ according to what kind of qualitative research it can be considered to be
5	Relate varieties of findings to specific methodological approaches	• Consider findings in the context of implications for further research, theory development and practice
6	Understand the process for synthesising results	• The process for synthesising research occurs as a cognitive activity within the researcher

REVIEW QUESTIONS

1 Discuss the difference between causal and non-causal relationships.
2 How do statistically significant and non-significant findings differ?
3 Describe two indicators of clinical significance.
4 Why is it important to search for the meaning behind the findings and the relationships between the findings?

CHALLENGING REVIEW QUESTIONS

1 Explain why qualitative analysis usually precedes interpretation.
2 Discuss why qualitative interpretation is connected to assumptions about truth.
3 Describe the nature of qualitative critical interpretations.
4 Discuss how affirmative postmodern approaches influence research interpretations.

CASE STUDY 1

Prisha is an undergraduate nursing student beginning third year. Prisha is considering her options for a graduate position after she completes her course. As a student nurse Prisha is aware that stress and burnout are important considerations for hospital nurses and would like to ensure she is fully prepared.

In her investigation of appropriate strategies for a healthy working environment Prisha found a research article (Freeman et al., 2020) that describes meditation. Prisha wants to understand what the quantitative research findings describe and determine the implications for her as a student nurse. Would it be in Prisha's interest to undertake meditation practice?

1   What are some examples of descriptive statistical variables used for quantitative data analysis?
2   Would you consider a causal relationship if a pretest post-test method was used?
3   When considering the significance of the research, what are the important factors you should keep in mind?

CASE STUDY 2

As the midwifery unit manager of a busy regional antenatal clinic, Sue is concerned about the decline in pregnant women receiving the flu vaccine in her region. Sue believes the decline may be related to changes in the provision of antenatal care and the resulting move to refer women to online educational materials regarding vaccination recommendations rather than providing face to face advice.

After gaining hospital ethics approval, Sue undertakes a quantitative research study surveying woman who have received antenatal care through the clinic in the last year since the service changes occurred. The survey includes questions asking women if they were vaccinated against the flu in their previous pregnancy, if they received information about the vaccine verbally by their midwife, through the online information page, or a combination of both. The survey also asked questions to ascertain women's knowledge of flu vaccination.

1   Sue surveyed 980 women who had received antenatal care through her regional health service. Can she generalise the external validity of her results?
2   Sue wants to establish a definitive 'causal relationship' between flu vaccination rates and online antenatal education. Is this possible given her research method? Justify your answer.
3   Sue's study determined that women who received verbal education from a midwife during antenatal visits were slightly more likely to have the flu vaccine during pregnancy than if they gained their information only through the online information page. However, unexpectedly, women who received information from both sources were far less likely to be vaccinated during pregnancy. What measures should Sue take regarding these serendipitous findings?

REFERENCES

Afshar, M., Sadeghi-Gandomani, H., & Masoudi Alavi, N. (2020). A study on improving nursing clinical competencies in a surgical department: A participatory action research. *Nursing Open*, 7(4), 1052–59. https://doi.org/10.1002/nop2.485

Armour-Burton, T., & Etland, C. (2020). Black feminist thought: A paradigm to examine breast cancer disparities. *Nursing Research*, 69(4), 272–9. https://doi.org/10.1097/NNR.0000000000000426

Atkinson, P., Coffey, A., Delamont, S., Lofland, J., & Lofland, L. (eds). (2007). *Handbook of Ethnography*. Thousand Oaks, CA: SAGE.

Denzin, N., & Lincoln, Y. (eds). (2007). *Handbook of Qualitative Research* (3rd edn). Thousand Oaks, CA: SAGE.

Flick, U. (2009). *An Introduction to Qualitative Research* (4th edn). Thousand Oaks, CA: SAGE.

Freeman, R. C., Sukuan, N., Tota, N. M., Bell, S. M., Harris, A. G., & Wang, H-L. (2020). Promoting spiritual healing by stress reduction through meditation for employees at a veterans hospital: A CDC framework-based program evaluation. *Workplace Health and Safety*, 68(4), 161–70. https://doi:10.1177/2165079919874795

Gadamer, H.-G. (1975). *Truth and Method* (G. Barden & J. Cumming, trans. and eds). New York, NY: Seabury.

Habermas, J. (1981). *The Theory of Communicative Action: Reason and the Rationalization of Society*. Boston, MA: Beacon.

Laging, B., Kenny, A., Bauer, M., & Nay, R. (2018). Recognition and assessment of resident' deterioration in the nursing home setting: A critical ethnography. *Journal of Clinical Nursing*, 27(7–8), 1452–63. https://doi.org/10.1111/jocn.14292

Liu, Z., Zhang, L., Cao, Y., Xia, W., & Zhang, L. (2018). The relationship between coping styles and benefit finding of Chinese cancer patients: The mediating role of distress. *European Journal of Oncology Nursing*, 34, 15–20. https://doi.org/10.1016/j.ejon.2018.03.001

Olano-Lizarraga, M., Zaragoza-Salcedo, A., Martin-Martin, J., & Saracibar-Razquin, M. (2020). Redefining a 'new normality': A hermeneutic phenomenological study of the experiences of patients with chronic heart failure. *Journal of Advanced Nursing*, 76(1), 275–286. https://doi.org/10.1111/jan.14237

Polit, D., & Beck, C. (2017). *Nursing Research: Generating and Assessing Evidence for Nursing Practice* (10th edn). Philadelphia, PA: Lippincott.

Richardson-Tench, M., Rabach, J., Kerr, D., Adams, W., & Brown, S. (2012). Comparison of preparedness after preadmission telephone screening or clinic assessment in patients undergoing endoscopic surgery by day surgery procedure: A pilot study. *Ambulatory Surgery*, 17(4), 74–8.

Sala Defilippis, T., Curtis, K., & Gallagher, A. (2020). Moral resilience through harmonised connectedness in intensive care nursing: A grounded theory study. *Intensive & Critical Care Nursing*, 57, 102785. https://doi.org/10.1016/j.iccn.2019.102785

Wallin, K., Hörberg, U., Harstäde, C. W., Elmqvist, C., & Bremer, A. (2020). Preceptors' experiences of student supervision in the emergency medical services: A qualitative interview study. *Nurse Education Today*, 84, 104223. https://doi.org/10.1016/j.nedt.2019.104223

Yeo, C., Fang, H., Thilagamangai, S., Koh, S. & Shorey, S. (2018). Factors affecting Pap smear uptake in a maternity hospital: A descriptive cross-sectional study. *Journal of Advanced Nursing*. 74(11), 2533–43.

FURTHER READING

Atefi, N., Abdullah, K. L., Wong, L. P., & Mazlom, R. (2014). Factors influencing registered nurses' perception of their overall job satisfaction: A qualitative study. *International Nursing Review*, 61(3) 352–60.

Delany, C., Edwards, I., & Fryer, C. (2018). How physiotherapists perceive, interpret, and respond to the ethical dimensions of practice: A qualitative study. *Physiotherapy Theory and Practice*, 35(7), 663–76. https://doi.org/10.1080/09593985.2018.1456583

Flanagan, B., Lord, B., Reed, R., & Crimmins, G. (2019). Listening to women's voices: The experience of giving birth with paramedic care in Queensland, Australia. *BMC Pregnancy and Childbirth*, 19(1). https://doi.org/10.1186/s12884-019-2613-z

Hickey, S., Kildea, S., Couchman, K., Watego-Ivory, K., West, R., Kruske, S., Blackman, R., Watego, S., & Roe, Y. L. (2019). Establishing teams aiming to provide culturally safe maternity care for Indigenous families. *Women and Birth*, 32(5), 449–59. https://doi.org/10.1016/j.wombi.2019.06.019

Mize, D. (2017). The meaning of patient-nurse interaction for older women in healthcare settings: A qualitative descriptive study. *International Journal of Older People Nursing, 13*(1), e12167. https://doi.org/10.1111/opn.12167

Moorley, C., & Cathala, X. (2019). How to appraise mixed methods research. *Evidence Based Nursing, 22*(2), 38–41. https://doi.org/10.1136/ebnurs-2019-103076

Munns, A., Toye, C., Hegney, D., Kickett, M., Marriott, R., & Walker, R. (2018). Aboriginal parent support: A partnership approach. *Journal of Clinical Nursing, 27*(3–4). https://doi.org/10.1111/jocn.13979

11 DEVELOPING THE RESEARCH PROPOSAL

Chapter learning objectives

The material presented in this chapter will assist you to:

1. understand the purpose of writing a research proposal
2. identify the process of preparing a research proposal
3. discuss the ethical considerations of a research project
4. describe the structure and content of a research proposal
5. understand how to style, format and present a research proposal
6. discuss how informal approval for a research proposal is attained
7. discuss how appropriate funding opportunities are identified.

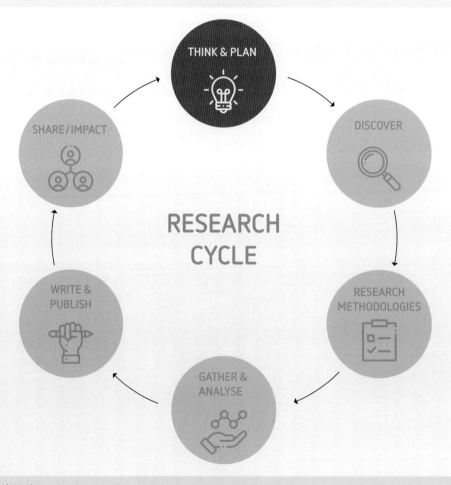

Research cycle

The primary focus of this chapter is developing a research proposal, which relates to thinking about and planning the project. This is highlighted in the research framework diagram above.

Introduction

Writing a **research proposal** is an important step when developing a research project as it provides an outline of the project, explaining what will be done, as well as providing a justification for why the research project should be undertaken (Denscombe, 2012). A well-constructed proposal provides a blueprint for the research project (Denscombe, 2012; Sudheesh, Duggappa & Nethra, 2016), describing the scope and significance of the research, as well as the proposed **methodology** and chosen **research design** (Sudheesh, Duggappa & Nethra, 2016). The purpose and process of writing a research proposal will be discussed in this chapter.

There are a number of reasons why a research proposal is developed, with several particularly noteworthy in healthcare. The first reason is as an assessment unit requirement in undergraduate and postgraduate research modules, or as part of a dissertation that is intended to identify the academic potential of the research idea (Denscombe, 2012; Harper, 2007; Hollins Martin & Fleming, 2010; Juni, 2014). Applying for ethics approval will require a clear and reasoned explanation of the research project to be developed, with securing research funding another reason for developing a research proposal (Denscombe, 2012).

Developing novel ideas is the cornerstone of scientific research, which often requires funding for the study to be completed (Jackowski & Leggett, 2015; Singh, Cameron & Duff, 2005). Securing funding for research projects is a competitive process with only a minority of research proposals successful (Inouye & Fiellin, 2005). Although proposal writing is one of the most challenging parts of the research process, it is considered a fundamental skill for a researcher (Hollins Martin & Fleming, 2010).

Regardless of the purpose, there are common principles that should be followed when developing a research proposal. A research proposal not only communicates what the researchers are aiming to achieve, it follows a set of sequential steps that detail the structure of the proposed study (Hollins Martin & Fleming, 2010; Juni, 2014). It also provides a sound argument for funders to consider whether the study is feasible, well designed and worthy of financial support (Boyle, 2019; Harper 2007; Jackowski & Leggett, 2015; Jonker & Marshall, 2010; Juni, 2014; Singh, Cameron & Duff, 2005). Denscombe (2012) describes a logic to research proposals that include seven sequenced questions when deliberating about whether a proposal is feasible and whether it is worthwhile. These are displayed in Figure 11.1.

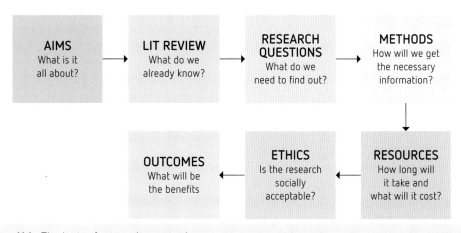

▸ **Figure 11.1** The logic of research proposals

Source: Denscombe, M. 2012. *Research proposals: A practical guide.* Open University Press, p. 6.

The purpose of writing a research proposal

A research proposal is a written account of the plan for the research project. The purpose section presents:

- an argument as to why a particular problem should be investigated
- the appropriate research design to investigate it
- what the researcher intends to do (how, why, where, when)
- the significance of the study
- the cost of the project
- the researchers' ability to complete the proposed study (Boyle, 2019; Harper, 2007; Juni, 2014; Proctor et al., 2012.).

The process of preparing a research proposal

Writing a strong research proposal requires a good understanding of the research process. It also requires an extensive literature review to be undertaken, a research question to be developed, an appropriate methodology to be selected and an understanding of the ethical implications of the proposed research to be demonstrated (Boyle, 2019; Denscombe, 2012; Hollins Martin & Fleming, 2010; Jonker & Marshall, 2010; Juni, 2014).

A **research plan** enables a researcher to:

- identify the relationships between parts of the proposal, such as the purpose, research design and expected outcomes (Inouye & Fiellin, 2005)
- identify potential problems during the planning phase
- receive constructive objective feedback and suggestions from colleagues for improvement (Boyle, 2019; Inouye & Fiellin, 2005).

Many organisations and committees provide guidelines and application forms that are required to be used when submitting a research proposal. Guidelines, consistent with the aims and priorities of the organisation, are developed to expedite the process and to help the reviewers reach a decision about the proposal. Therefore, before writing the research proposal, a copy of the relevant guidelines should be accessed from every committee or agency that will be approached for approval.

Guidelines include the format of the proposal, word limit and submission details, and should therefore be followed exactly as detailed in the document. Research proposals that do not meet the guidelines are often returned without being reviewed or not funded if it does not fit the brief of the organisation (Boyle, 2019). Where the process is competitive, such as for scholarships or funding, committees often have a points system for scoring proposals (Devine, 2009). Therefore, when submitting a proposal under such conditions, it is wise to direct attention to where the most points can be scored.

The audience that the proposal is aimed towards (usually committees or organisations who have the power to approve or reject the proposal) should be identified. This may require additional research to be done to identify the nature and type of services provided by the organisation so that only proposals directly related to their cause are submitted. For example, if the organisation only supports cardiac-related proposals, it is a waste of time submitting a proposal that includes a study on post-operative joint pain. All committees will be concerned with the quality of the proposal, but different committees have specific concerns, as outlined in Table 11.1.

▶ Table 11.1   Research committees

Committee type	Main concerns
Human research ethics committees (HREC)	• Protection of the population recruited into the study (e.g. confidentiality and anonymity) • Scientific rigour of the research project • Ethical standards
Research committees	• Adequacy of the research design • Budgetary aspects • Adding to or enhancing current professional knowledge
Clinical research committees or gatekeepers	• Impact on the institution, such as how the proposed project will affect other projects and if it will interfere with the agency's routine
Funding bodies	• That the proposal is consistent with their identified objectives and priorities • That the proposed budget is appropriate

Any items that require clarification should be followed up before and during the research proposal writing process (Harper, 2007; Inouye & Fiellin, 2005), which may only involve a telephone call or an email to the Secretary of the human research ethics committee or funding body. Generally, university approval is required prior to submitting the documents to other organisations, therefore any errors are addressed in-house before the proposal is submitted to external committees for review. Student projects should be assessed and approved by a supervisor before being submitted to the appropriate university committee, followed by the external committees. It can take up to 6 to 12 months to develop a proposal and get all the necessary approvals, depending on the complexity of the project. The chance for success will be maximised by allowing enough time to revise the proposal in response to feedback provided during the review process (Boyle, 2019; Inouye & Fiellin, 2005).

ACTIVITY

Explain the importance of providing a detailed explanation of the research design in a research proposal.

Ethical considerations

It is almost always necessary to write a proposal for any intended research project because approval to carry out the research must be obtained from the appropriate authorities, such as a university research committee, a **human research ethics committee (HREC)** or a funding body (National Health and Medical Research Council [NHMRC], 2007, updated 2018). This mechanism protects the researcher in the event of any repercussions from the research, such as a lawsuit, in which case the researcher can show that they have gained the appropriate approval. The committees that approved the study would have to take some of the responsibility in the form of legal liability. Obtaining approvals also protects participants as they are assured of anonymity, **confidentiality** and privacy.

All research projects under the auspices of a university will require the approval of the relevant university HREC. Projects in the clinical field must have the approval of the relevant HREC committees in the clinical facility where data collection is planned. Approval will have to be granted by each clinical facility involved, unless there are joint committees operating, as most funding bodies will require a letter of approval from all the relevant committees when submitting an application for funding.

It is important to find out the relevant HREC committees' approval process and meeting schedules and deadlines for submission of proposals. Meetings in some organisations are scheduled four to six weeks apart, even longer over the summer holidays or midyear break. Most committees require submission at least 10 days before the meeting to allow time to circulate the papers to members. Each proposal undergoes a preliminary screening by the secretariat of the HREC to confirm that the necessary documentation has been submitted. If the ethics application is complete the secretariat will forward the documents to members of the HREC for review. Therefore, an important consideration is to submit the application on time, or even early, as the secretariat do not take kindly to sending a proposal out separately because it has been submitted late.

The ethical conduct of research is a responsibility shared by the researcher(s) who conducts and designs the research, those employed by the researcher, those employing the researcher (e.g. a university or hospital), the ethics committee(s) charged with ensuring that ethical standards are met, and all the other organisations or personnel involved (NHMRC, 2007, updated 2018).

In Australia, the guiding value for conducting research 'includes respect for human beings, research merit and **integrity**, justice, and beneficence to help shape the relationship as one of trust, mutual responsibility and ethical equality' (NHMRC, 2007, updated 2018, p. 9). Inexperienced researchers should become familiar with the *National Statement on Ethical Conduct in Human Research* prior to conducting research' (NHMRC, 2007, updated 2018).

A brief overview of the important National Statements include the following.

Ethics

> Research that has merit is … designed to ensure that respect for the participants is not compromised by the aims of the research, by the way it is carried out, or by the results (National Statement 1.1 d, p. 10).

> Research that is conducted with integrity is carried out by researchers with a commitment to: … following recognised principles of research conduct; conducting research honestly; and disseminating and communicating results, whether favourable or unfavourable, in ways that permit scrutiny and contribute to public knowledge and understanding (National Statement 1.3 b, c, d, p. 10)

> In research that is just: … the process of recruiting participants is fair; there is no unfair burden of participation in research on particular groups; and there is no exploitation of participants in the conduct of research (National Statement 1.4 b, c, e, p. 10).

> The likely benefit of the research must justify any risks of harm or discomfort to participants. The likely benefit may be to the participants, to the wider community, or to both (National Statement 1.6, p. 10).

TIP

If the deadline cannot be met, it is better to wait for the next meeting rather than submit an incomplete ethics application that wastes the HREC's time.

Where the risks to participants are no longer justified by the potential benefits of the research, the research must be suspended to allow time to consider whether it should be discontinued or at least modified. ... The review body must be notified promptly of such suspension, and of any decisions following it (National Statement 1.9, p.11).

Respect for human beings is a recognition of their intrinsic value. In human research, this recognition includes abiding by the values of research merit and integrity, justice and beneficence. Respect also requires having due regard for the welfare, beliefs, perceptions, customs and cultural heritage, both individual and collective, of those involved in research (National Statement 1.10, p. 11).

Researchers and their institutions should respect the privacy, confidentiality and cultural sensitivities of the participants and, where relevant, of their communities (National Statement 1.11, p. 11).

Respect for human beings involves giving due scope, throughout the research process, to the capacity of human beings to make their own decisions (National Statement 1.12, p. 11);

Where participants are unable to make their own decisions or have diminished capacity to do so, respect for them involves empowering them where possible and providing for their protection as necessary (National Statement, 1.13, p. 11).

FOR EXAMPLE

ETHICAL CONDUCT OF RESEARCH

Unfortunately, there have been instances in the past where researchers have taken advantage of participants and acted unethically. Gibbs and Lowton (2012) provided an example of a study into untreated syphilis in the 'negro male', which began in 1932 and lasted four decades. The study did not contribute any treatment; no new drugs were tested and the efficacy of old treatment modalities was neither confirmed nor refuted to the participants. Walker (2009) critiqued this study, which although it began in the 1930s was only identified as being unethical in 1997. Both critiques, Gibbs and Lowton (2012) and Walker (2009), highlight the reasons why values and principles of ethical conduct are so important.

ACTIVITY

Consider a type of research inquiry that could unintentionally harm a participant, and identify which sections of the community would be vulnerable.

A model for writing a research proposal

The primary element of a successful proposal includes a significant and innovative research question (Boyle, 2019; Proctor et al., 2012). Prior to writing the proposal, regardless of the format required, a **research question** should be developed (Hollins & Fleming, 2010). The plan for addressing the aims or purpose of the study, and how the **hypothesis** will be tested using a review of the literature as a foundation, is also included (Engberg & Bliss, 2005). Following a review of the literature, the research design, a critical component of a research proposal, is identified and detailed. Justification for the selection of the study design should also be succinctly explained (Engberg & Bliss, 2005). For quantitative research, the research proposal is like a blueprint for a building in that it assists the researcher to follow a process that has been laid down. For qualitative research, the research proposal is much more flexible because the method tends to evolve with the research.

Content of a research proposal

While the overall structure of a research proposal is fairly standard, there may be additional content required. Research proposals begin with the title, followed by an abstract or summary, an introduction and a methods and procedures section. References and appendices are included at the end of the proposal. A logical flow of ideas for the proposal, from problem to budget, should be developed and then presented in the correct order. The preferred order is sometimes set by the committee or agency reviewing the proposal. **Figure 11.2** shows a sample format for a standard research proposal.

A 15-step model to writing a research proposal	
Step 1	Give the research proposal a title.
Step 2	Provide relevant personal and professional details.
Step 3	Provide a short abstract or summary of around 300 words.
Step 4	Supply five keywords to describe the research proposal.
Step 5	Construct an introduction that contains a rationale and relevant literature review.
Step 6	State the aim, research question, sub-questions and hypotheses/null hypotheses of the proposed research study.
Step 7	Outline the research method.
Step 8	Select setting, participants, sampling method, inclusion/exclusion criteria and method of recruitment.
Step 9	Describe data collection instruments.
Step 10	Detail intended data processing and analysis.
Step 11	Declare any ethical considerations and outline data protection procedures.
Step 12	Produce a timetable and consider potential problems that may occur.
Step 13	Estimate resources that may be required.
Step 14	Append relevant additional material.
Step 15	Append key references

▶ **Figure 11.2** Sample format of a research proposal

Source: Used with permission of *British Journal of Midwifery*, from 'A 15-Step Model for Writing a Research Proposal', Hollins Martin, C. J., & Fleming, V., 18/12, 2010; permission conveyed through Copyright Clearance Center, Inc.

Elements of a quantitative research proposal

In this section, to illustrate the elements of a quantitative research proposal, the impact of perioperative factors on medication compliance for chronic conditions has been detailed.

Preliminaries

The preliminaries are the first part of the proposal, and precede the body of the proposal. These (as shown in Figure 11.3) comprise a title and title page, an abstract and the details of the research team.

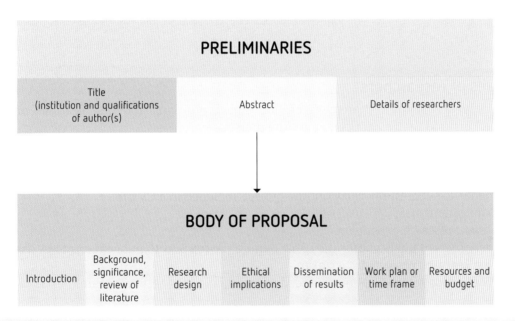

▸ **Figure 11.3** The elements of a research proposal

Title

The title should convey the intention of the proposal. This can be achieved by using keywords, but no more than 20. Some agencies require long (full) and short (subtitles) titles.

An example of a suitable title for a quantitative proposal is: 'The impact of perioperative factors on medication compliance for chronic conditions'.

As well as the title of the proposal, the title page should include:

- name, position, affiliated institution and qualifications of the author/s
- telephone numbers
- postal and email addresses of the author(s).

The date of submission is included on the page, traditionally presented as a header or a footer.

Abstract

The abstract is a brief summary of the proposal that gives the reader an overview of the project. Major themes or threads of the project are included with a focus on the objectives and design of the project. This section should be concise, with a limit of 250 to 300 words.

FOR EXAMPLE

ABSTRACT

This study will include a retrospective, exploratory cohort design to identify the impact of perioperative factors on compliance with medication for chronic conditions. The relationship between medical compliance and the risk of postoperative complications will also be explored.

Source: Nicholson, P., Manias, E., & Kusljic, S. (2016). Unpublished research proposal.

Details of researchers

This section requires a statement of the names, positions and qualifications of the researchers, and the contact person for the project.

For proposals other than classroom projects the curricula vitae (CVs) of the researchers involved in the project may also be required to be submitted. CVs are included so that the person evaluating the proposal can judge whether the applicants have the relevant experience to successfully carry out the project. Included in a CV are:

- qualifications
- relevant research experience
- a list of recent publications (may only require the top 5 to 10 publications to be listed)
- other research projects undertaken
- any previous research grants awarded to members of the research team.

Body of the proposal

Introduction

The body of the proposal begins with the introduction, with the following information presented:

- the problem or issue that the study will be investigating
- the specific aims of the study
- the research question
- the hypotheses (if it is an experimental or quasi-experimental study).

FOR EXAMPLE

PURPOSE STATEMENT

A typical purpose statement might state the following aims.
>   The aim of this study is to:
> - examine the impact of perioperative factors on medication compliance for chronic conditions;
> - the incidence of postoperative complications;
> - the association between postoperative complications and medication compliance.

Source: Nicholson, P., Manias, E., & Kusljic, S. (2016). Unpublished research proposal.

Background, significance and review of the literature

The background to the study begins by orienting the reviewer to previous key research in the area or key theoretical issues. It shows how the problem was identified, key theoretical issues are alluded to and how the proposed research builds on what has already been done in the area is demonstrated. Furthermore, it establishes the rationale for doing the study and shows why the outcome will provide a solution to the problem, for reasons that could include the following:

- previous research left questions unanswered
- new evidence has been discovered that supports further research
- a theory suggests such a line of inquiry
- there is a new line of inquiry that may be justified by logical argument.

FOR EXAMPLE

BACKGROUND AND REVIEW OF THE LITERATURE

> Although adverse drug events are a major cause of morbidity and mortality in hospital practice, with an estimated 15% to 59% of these adverse drug events acknowledged as being preventable, there is little focus in the literature on surgical patients. This is despite numerous factors in the perioperative period that may adversely impact the ongoing administration of medications for surgical patients. … Perioperative fasting may affect preoperative medication intake and route of administration resulting in changes to prescribed medications. Of equal importance is the mechanism of action of the drug, which may result in unanticipated postoperative complications, and as a consequence medications may be ceased for a certain period of time pre-operatively.

Source: Nicholson, P., Manias, E., & Kusljic, S. (2016). Unpublished research proposal.

The statement of the study's significance follows the discussion of background and rationale, and demonstrates why this study is worth doing. It answers the question 'So what?' by indicating how the results of this study could advance knowledge or practice in healthcare. Relevant statistics about the incidence, prevalence, distribution, relevance to health and impact on morbidity or mortality related to the problem is included to support the argument.

FOR EXAMPLE

SIGNIFICANCE OF THE STUDY

This study will obtain critical information about different medications that increase the risk of complications following major surgery in an Australian context. Nurses are involved in assessing and evaluating the therapeutic and unwanted effects of medications, therefore the findings of this study could be used to develop strategies to improve nursing practice in both preoperative and postoperative settings.

Source: Nicholson, P., Manias, E., & Kusljic, S. (2016). Unpublished research proposal.

A review of the literature completes the introduction. An effective way of organising the review, particularly if there are several independent variables, is according to the independent variables or questions being asked. Findings about each variable are explained, with a summary presented at the end. The literature review should lead into the specific research question. References used in this section should be included in the reference list (see Chapter 2 for information on literature reviews).

Research design

The research design section describes in detail the framework for the study and asks:

- On whom?
- How?
- When?
- Where?

The design that is chosen depends entirely on the research question that has been developed (Ingham-Broomfield, 2008; Proctor et al., 2012; Ratan, Anand & Ratan, 2019). In healthcare, the question of cause and effect is crucial; for example, whether exposure to a certain element causes health problems or whether treatments cause certain health outcomes. Different quantitative designs answer these cause-and-effect questions in different ways and with different levels of veracity. The reasons for choosing an approach must be explained; that is, why it is appropriate to the research question. If it is a complex design, a diagram or flowchart could assist the reader to better understand the design (Harper, 2007). In deciding how much detail to provide in the design of the study section, consider the level of the question. If it is a descriptive design, less detail will be required than for an experimental design. Enough detail should be provided to enable the reviewer to understand how the research question is intended to be answered.

Table 11.2 lists the elements of a research design, which are discussed in detail in Chapters 5 and 7.

An instrument is any tool, including a questionnaire, that is used to collect the data. Where possible an instrument that has already been developed and validated should be used. If a tool is being developed for the study it should be noted why no existing instrument meets the needs of the research project.

▸ Table 11.2   Research design

Elements	Information provided

Design of the study	• Experimental or quasi-experimental:
	  — requires a statement of the hypothesis, stated as a description of the anticipated outcomes, presented as well-defined, logical, clear and necessary to answer the research question
	  — the relationship between the variables is stated in measurable terms
	  — the independent and dependent variables are identified and, where possible, stated in measurable terms
	• Correlational
	• Descriptive
	• Comparative

The setting	• Agency details • Participant numbers available

The participants	• Characteristics of the group from which they will be selected and where they will be recruited
	• Rationale for selecting this particular group of participants
	• Sample size, including justification for size
	• Participant attrition and extra participants built in: approximately 10%
	• Type of sample:
	  — a random sample or stratified random sample
	  — how the sample was drawn from the population
	  — convenience sample; for example, they were the first 50 patients treated in a clinic etc. (types of samples are discussed in Chapter 5)
	• Criteria for participant selection and the rationale for the criteria
	• Recruitment details; for example, by letter, telephone or personal contact
	• Describe number of groups, number of participants in each group, how they will be allocated to the groups, and special procedures, such as matching participants on criteria

The instruments	• Describe the instrument or materials that will be used to collect data • Explain any unconventional techniques, tests or instruments • Describe any questionnaires included in the proposal and refer the reader to an appendix where a full copy of the questionnaire should be included • If the questionnaire is subject to copyright, permission from the author should be obtained prior to it being used in a research project • Name the physical instrument if it is well known (e.g. a sphygmomanometer) or describe it if it is unusual or new • Describe how the instrument is scored or measured; for example, on a Likert scale or in millimetres of mercury. Diagrams or photographs of an instrument can be used to avoid a long description • Include a brief discussion of how, according to the literature, the instrument has been used previously • Justify the choice of instrument in terms of its appropriateness to the research question or design • Discuss the strengths and limitations of each instrument in terms of its reliability and validity (these concepts are discussed in Chapter 5)

Elements	Information provided
The procedures	• Describe how an experimental treatment will be applied • State how, when and where the data will be collected. This information should be given in enough detail to enable someone else to replicate the process • Describe the procedures for collecting the data in terms of what the participants will be required to do. This will include procedures such as observing subjects or participants, administering a questionnaire, applying an instrument or administering an experimental treatment. Any lengthy instructions to the participants may be included in the appendix but summarised here • Describe any calibration of the instruments or training to be provided for the data collectors • Provide timelines for the procedures (when the procedures will be carried out and how long they will take) so that each participant's time commitment is clear. If there is a particular time of day, week, month or year involved, details should be clearly noted. If the timing is complex, a diagram or flowchart might be helpful • State how the data will be recorded • Include a sample data roster as an appendix

Managing the data	• Includes:
	  – coordination of data management if multiple sites are involved
	  – data entry into the computer
	  – storage of original data, including how, where and for how long it will be stored
	  – consideration of the ethical aspects of data management, including confidentiality of the data
	  – addressing the aspects of data coding: Who will do it and how will it be done? Provision should be made for checking the data for errors in data entry
	  – demonstration of a strong, clear and rigorous program for analysing the data; the methods of data analysis should follow from the research question, research design and hypotheses.
	• State if the data will be analysed by hand or computer, and if the latter, cite which data analysis package will be used
	• Justify the data analysis by detailing the tests that will be used to describe the variables and check the validity of each hypothesis, including a restatement of the hypothesis. This enables the reader to assess the appropriateness of the data analysis in terms of the hypotheses and research questions. If the data analysis is complex, including a flowchart will assist the reader in understanding data analysis processes to be followed
	• If a pilot study is being planned, details of the study should be included. If the pilot study has already been done, an outline of the methods and results should be included. Such an outline gives the reader confidence in the expertise of the team and provides an indication of the feasibility of the study

FOR EXAMPLE

RESEARCH DESIGN SECTION

Design

The design is a low-risk retrospective, exploratory cohort study that will use a specifically designed retrospective audit tool to collect data.

Setting

This study will be conducted at a surgical unit in a major tertiary hospital.

Participants

Patients who underwent intermediate to major surgery (surgery longer than 2 hours), with at least one comorbidity, will be included in the study.

Methods and procedures

1   Surgical patients identified on the surgical register who have attended a pre-anaesthetic clinic and underwent major surgery will be included in the study.
2   An equal number of patients will be selected from those who did not attend the pre-anaesthetic clinic.
3   Identifiable patient data will be replaced with a unique identification code during data collection ensuring confidentiality of all patients.
4   Descriptive statistical analysis will be performed on patients' demographics using SPSS. Chi-squared tests will be used to examine the association between each of the explanatory categorical preoperative factors and each of the postoperative factors. P-values for the hypothesis test with null hypothesis of no association will be reported.

Source: Nicholson, P., Manias, E., & Kusljic, S. (2016). Unpublished research proposal.

Ethical implications

An ethics committee will examine the general design of the study, not only to assess its scientific merit but also to determine the ethical implications of the study.

Ethics

Once the reader understands how the study is going to be carried out, it is appropriate to discuss the ethical implications inherent in the procedures (see Figure 11.4). The proposed procedures should be stated so that ethics approval from university and/or clinical HREC committees can be arranged.

There are some special considerations that may have to be dealt with in certain studies. If special populations are included in the study, a justification must be provided for their inclusion (NHMRC, 2007, updated 2018; Smith, 2008); this comprises:

- describing the procedures that will be put in place to protect participants' rights
- details of the person who will be approached to give consent on their behalf if the participant is unable to.

If participants are going to be observed without their express individual consent, a justification must be provided for why this method has been selected and how the cost, in terms of potential invasion of privacy, are less than the potential benefits of such a study.

At the end of the research design section, it is customary to acknowledge any limitations of the approach selected. It should be remembered that the reader may be an experienced and distinguished scientist who will spot flaws in the design. It is therefore better to acknowledge the flaws in the design and the threats to validity and explain how these will be dealt with, rather than to try to gloss over them and hope no-one will notice.

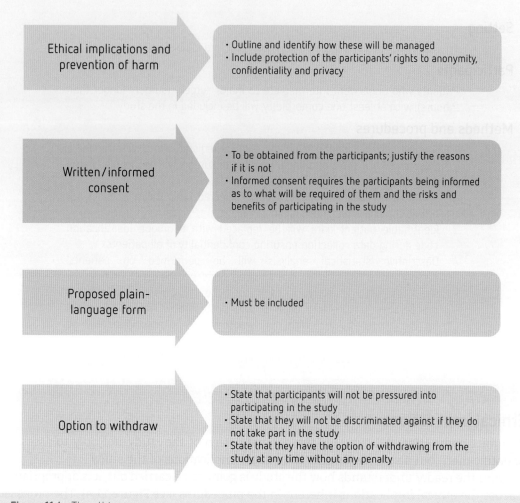

Ethical implications and prevention of harm
- Outline and identify how these will be managed
- Include protection of the participants' rights to anonymity, confidentiality and privacy

Written/informed consent
- To be obtained from the participants; justify the reasons if it is not
- Informed consent requires the participants being informed as to what will be required of them and the risks and benefits of participating in the study

Proposed plain-language form
- Must be included

Option to withdraw
- State that participants will not be pressured into participating in the study
- State that they will not be discriminated against if they do not take part in the study
- State that they have the option of withdrawing from the study at any time without any penalty

▶ **Figure 11.4** The ethics process

FOR EXAMPLE

A TYPICAL ETHICS STATEMENT

The study will be conducted according to the NHMRC National Statement on Ethical Conduct in Human Research 2007 (and updates). This study is a retrospective audit of patient medical records therefore a waiver of consent will be sought from the Human Research and Ethics Committee. All data will be de-identified and analysed in a coded form. Individual patients will not be identifiable from the presented or published material.

Source: Nicholson, P., Manias, E., & Kusljic, S. (2016). Unpublished research proposal.

Dissemination of results

A plan for the dissemination of results should be included in the proposal as well as the implementation of the findings. It could, for example, be stated that the results of the study and/or a written report will be presented to the institution, or will be presented as a paper at a conference, or be submitted for publication in a journal.

Work plan or time frame

An overall description of the sequence and duration of tasks to be carried out should be presented. It indicates to the reader how realistic the research plan is and how thorough the researcher has been in taking into consideration all that is required to complete the project. The work plan incorporates the tasks, personnel requirements, estimate of time required to carry out each part of the project and the date by which each part will be completed. It is often shown as a schedule or a flowchart (see the following section: 'Elements of a qualitative research proposal').

Resources and budget

A good research proposal shows that the physical and human resources available are sufficient to carry out the project. Granting agencies and universities require a section on the background of the researcher and the physical resources and budget needed to complete the project. In the budget, the costs for all the materials, personnel and equipment required to successfully complete the project should be included. The major cost components are direct costs, which are costs that are specific to the project, and indirect costs, which are infrastructure costs that are incurred by the institution as a result of supporting the project.

Direct costs are usually broken down into the following categories.

- *Salary costs*, which might include:
  - salaries of administration assistants, research assistants, the researcher and clinicians involved in collecting data
  - a component for on-costs such as annual leave, payroll tax
  - costs for work carried out by non-salaried personnel such as keyboard operators, consultants and data-entry/transcription personnel.
- *Costs for equipment, materials and procedures*, which might include:
  - any instruments, computer software, equipment such as video cameras or digital recorders, and the purchase or rental of computers
  - stationery, DVDs, postage and costs for report preparation and dissemination
  - printing, photocopying and laboratory analysis of data
  - travel and other incidental costs, such as flight costs and accommodation (if data collection involves travel).

Indirect costs are usually referred to as 'infrastructure costs'. These include telephone, internet, office, computing time and other such costs. Students carrying out projects for a qualification will usually not have to include infrastructure costs in a proposal because it is taken for granted that the university supplies these facilities as a part of the student's educational package. Proposals from outside the institution will normally need to include an infrastructure component in the budget. Infrastructure costs are usually calculated using a formula devised by the institution, which should be used to calculate any such costs (see the sample budget statement in the 'For example' box titled 'Justification of the budget' on page 294).

ACTIVITY

Think of a research project you are interested in doing that involves collecting data in numeric form, and answer the following questions related to such a project.

- What is your research question?
- Why is this a worthwhile question to ask?
- Who would you recruit into the study?
- Where would you collect the data?
- How could you gather the data you need?
- Who would you need to get support and/or approval from to do this project?

Elements of a qualitative research proposal

To some extent, there are similarities between quantitative and qualitative research proposals in that the preliminary pages are much the same and the introduction has a similar structure. However, the body of a qualitative proposal may be substantially different from that of a quantitative proposal. Qualitative proposals may also differ from one another depending on the kind of approach taken (Klopper, 2008; Vivar, 2007).

Qualitative proposals have to be scrutinised by academic departments, health agency organisations, funding bodies and ethics committees, which are often composed of people who have backgrounds in quantitative research, so qualitative proposals must conform to some extent with these people's expectations of what constitutes a 'proper' research proposal. Too much creativity at this stage of the research may result in obstruction from the outset. It is important, then, that qualitative proposals are written carefully, clearly and with a sound rationale for the proposed research (Vivar, 2007).

Examples from the successful research proposal submitted by Richardson-Tench and Brookes (2006) will be used in the following sections.

Title

The title should clarify the research approach, what the research is about and the people and setting involved; for example: 'Understanding the experience of managing pain in patients with hip and knee osteoarthritis'.

Summary

Sometimes called an abstract, the research summary provides an overview of what the project aims to achieve, as well as when and how it will be achieved. It is important to be concise.

FOR EXAMPLE

SUMMARY

Nurses' role in negotiating consent with patients warrants exploration to develop theory to inform and guide practice and identify processes that facilitate the consent process. Current nursing ethics theory offers little to nurses when faced with negotiating consent with patients whose capacity to consent is impaired. The project will investigate the efficacy of categories for defining consent (implied, informed, voluntary, competent, valid) with two groups: psychogeriatric acute care patients and perioperative patients. The project will make a significant contribution to normative ethics and understanding of the nurse—patient relationship.

Source: Richardson-Tench, M., & Brookes, A. (2006). Unpublished research proposal.

Significance, aims and objectives

At this point, a statement may be made about the significance of the project. Such statements inform readers why this research is worthwhile. Aims are overall intentions and objectives are specific subsets of the intentions.

FOR EXAMPLE

SIGNIFICANCE, AIM AND OBJECTIVES

Significance

Consent is a concept that is inherent in any nurse—patient relationship. While it is more common for theories of nursing ethics to be developed in response to the more dramatic or invasive interactions between patients and the health system, for most patients less dramatic interactions form their day to day experiences of consent-giving. While it is necessary for consent to be understood in relation to surgery, participation in research, etc., more mundane interactions must also be recognised as important arenas of ethical decision making. It is the daily tasks of nursing that constitute the greatest number of actions and interactions in the health system dependent upon the consent of patients. In addition, nurses' role in negotiating consent on behalf of other health practitioners warrants exploration and recognition.

Aim

The aim of this project is to explore the ethical and professional challenges of the consent process with compromised patients.

Objectives

To raise critical awareness of practice problems RNs face every day, to work systematically through problem-solving processes to uncover constraints against effective nursing care, and to improve the quality of care given by hospital nurses in light of the identified constraints and possibilities.

Source: Richardson-Tench, M., & Brookes, A. (2006). Unpublished research proposal.

Research questions

Specific questions related to the research objectives may be posed at this point. These questions will indicate the problem focus taken in the research. Questions of this nature may not be appropriate to all qualitative proposals, as some critical approaches may involve participatory processes in which the participants work collaboratively to raise questions as the research moves through cycles and group processes. If questions are posed in a proposal, they may resemble the following examples:

- 'What are current and emerging trends impacting on the paramedic workforce?'
- 'What factors influence healthy eating habits among adolescents?'
- 'How, considering the identified constraints, can the quality of nursing care provided in nursing homes be improved?'

Background and literature review

Although the reasons for the literature review are similar to those already outlined in this chapter in the earlier section 'Elements of a quantitative research proposal', there are some areas that need to be highlighted in a general approach to writing a literature review for qualitative proposals.

First, there may not be much empirical literature in a highly unusual area of interest, as is the case with many qualitative projects that try to push the boundaries of what can be known about phenomena. In this case, the literature may need to be linked indirectly to the main ideas in the research. Allied, non-specific information can be shown through the proposed methods and processes to be related to and informative for the research interest.

Second, some approaches, such as grounded theory, may claim that the inductive style suggests that literature should not be amassed at this stage, which is a good enough stance if it can be substantiated. With these disclaimers in mind, the rules of a thorough literature review still apply just as much to qualitative proposals as they do to quantitative proposals.

Research plan

A research plan is roughly equivalent to the methodology section of a quantitative proposal in that it includes information about the study setting, participants and methods to be used. But there are differences that relate mainly to the use of specific language. Generally, when qualitative researchers refer to methodology, they are referring to the theoretical assumptions underlying the choice of methods. This means that in the proposal, under the word 'methodology', there will appear a brief description of the theoretical tradition informing the project.

FOR EXAMPLE

METHODOLOGY

This is a post-positivist study and will employ critical incident technique (CIT) interviewing. The critical incident for this project is defined as commonplace consent episodes negotiated by nurses.

Source: Richardson-Tench, M., & Brookes, A. (2006). Unpublished research proposal.

Methods and processes

Qualitative research often differentiates between the ways of organising the research and collecting and analysing the information (methods), and the interpersonal processes that are used in accessing, informing, maintaining and closing relationships with participants throughout the research (processes).

ACTIVITY

Explain the differences between methods and processes in qualitative research. Discuss the importance of proposing particular methods and processes rather than simply letting them evolve during the project.

It may be necessary to provide a rationale for the number of participants, especially if the proposal is likely to be judged against empirico-analytical criteria. Committee members may not be aware of the assumptions of the nature of knowledge generated and validated through qualitative research. It is important to provide a sound set of reasons for what could be construed by some commentators as a small sample size. A justification for the sampling methods should also be provided; that is, how participants will be accessed. The details should be clearly provided in the statement; for example: 'This research approach is interested in accessing participants who work with the specified patient population. They have been sought intentionally for their ability to inform the research from their personal perspectives'.

Data collection

Include all the points about what data will be collected and how. Examples of the questions that may be asked should also be provided, even if they are open-ended. For a collaborative project, it may not be possible to predict questions that could arise from group processes. This needs to be explained so that people who are uninformed about the particular methodology will be able to understand why the questions are not included in the proposal.

Ethical requirements

Ethics

It is necessary to provide a full account of ethical considerations to be communicated to participants, including **informed consent** to ensure their privacy and anonymity, and the assurance that they can choose to withdraw from the research at any time without penalty. Full ethical approval will need to be sought from participating institutions. It is usual to submit a full research plan, including ethical statements, a plain-language statement and a consent form for each category of participants.

Analysis and interpretation

The analysis and interpretation of the data should be clearly set out so that the committee members judging the merits of the proposal can consider whether the plans for this phase are reasonable in relation to the rest of the project. This is a main area whereby the project will be judged as being trustworthy.

Disseminating findings

The proposal should contain a plan for the dissemination of findings. This provides an indication of how the research will be rendered meaningless if the results are not shared with the people who may benefit from them. Detail should include a presentation describing findings at a staff seminar and/or a conference and submission of an article for publication.

Time frame and time management

The funding body and/or the organisation will want details to be provided about the time frame, including what will be done and when, so that they can be assured about the project being completed on time. Using a Gantt chart provides a visual representation of the project's timelines and activities, as well as their interdependence (commonly referred to as a project schedule). A bar chart displays the start and end dates, showing the progress of the project, as well as the duration required for each task to be completed. Although there are some disadvantages to using a Gantt chart, including having to update it regularly, Gantt charts enable teams to improve overall efficiency and accountability in terms of meeting set timelines. A number of great videos can be accessed via YouTube (youtube.com) with explanations about how to develop a Gantt chart, such as the following:

- 'Gantt Chart Excel Tutorial - How to make a Basic Gantt Chart in Microsoft Excel 2016'
- 'TECH-005 - Create a quick and simple Time Line (Gantt Chart) in Excel'.

Further examples on developing a Gantt chart for three-year projects can be accessed by searching for 'Gantt Chart For 3 Years With Proposal Research Analysis And Project Design' at https://www.slideteam.net.

Managing the project, including its timelines, is important. Friedman (2017) details practical strategies to avoid distractions and to become more productive, including the following.

1 Devoting the first 10 minutes of your day to prioritise your work so that you can feel a sense of achievement at the end of the day.
2 Scheduling work to your strengths by identifying 'high-potential' hours (points during the day when you are most energetic).

3   Chunking activities: Look for similar activities that can be chunked together (e.g. answering emails) and schedule them for a single session.
4   Scheduling intermissions on your calendar twice a day (three when focused on a writing deadline) and devote the time to non-computer based.
5   Including exercise as part of your day and finding someone to share this with to keep you motivated.
6   Spending the last 10 minutes of your day by recording all night time activities to identify 'time sinks' that can be minimised to ensure you get enough sleep.

Figure 11.5 presents an example of such a time frame.

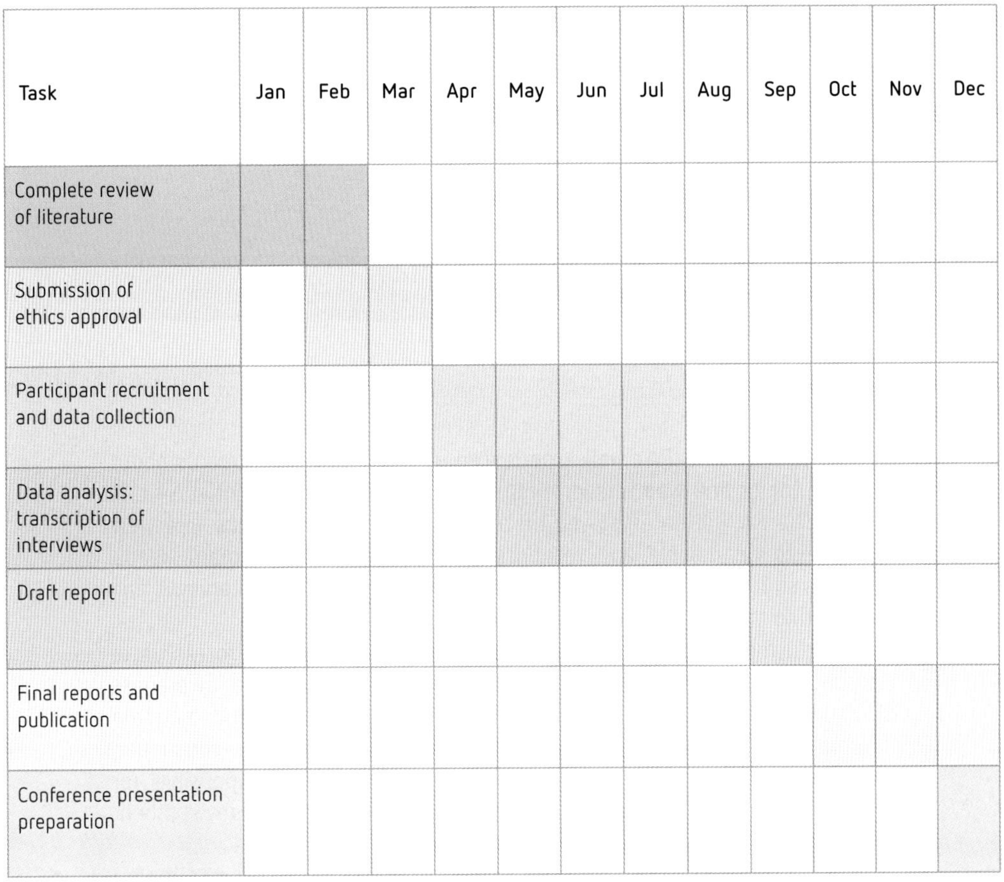

Task	Jan	Feb	Mar	Apr	May	Jun	Jul	Aug	Sep	Oct	Nov	Dec
Complete review of literature	▓	▓										
Submission of ethics approval		▓	▓									
Participant recruitment and data collection				▓	▓	▓						
Data analysis: transcription of interviews					▓	▓	▓	▓				
Draft report									▓			
Final reports and publication												
Conference presentation preparation												▓

▶ **Figure 11.5**   Proposed timing

ACTIVITY

Explain why it is important to predict a timeline for a project and why plans are proposed for the dissemination of the results.

Budget

If the proposal includes applying for a research grant to assist in completing the research, careful consideration should be given to the cost involved. Most funding bodies require a detailed budget that outlines costs for research personnel (research assistants, desktop publishers, clerical assistants), equipment (computer data analysis system, recording gear), travel at so many cents per kilometre, and other costs, such as photocopying and mailing. The application form will make it clear what the funding body will or will not fund, so this information should be read carefully.

The text in the following 'For example' box was submitted as part of a project funded internally by a university. It provides an example of what is expected in an itemised budget where justification is required for funds.

Funding bodies want to know about each item of research expenditure in the budget, to be convinced that funding the project is justified and that it will be used prudently. Therefore, this section should be as clear as possible about the actual costs involved (Devine, 2009).

FOR EXAMPLE

JUSTIFICATION OF THE BUDGET

Personnel

A research assistant (RA), well experienced in interviewing informants about sensitive topics and well versed in nursing ethics theory, is essential for this project. The RA will be employed on a casual basis to enable the interview schedule to be flexible and responsive to a variety of informant needs, including shift work. The RA will be responsible for conducting interviews and contributing to the database development.

The employment of an experienced administrator is essential for accurate transcription of interviews. This person's experience with and awareness of issues raised by research, such as the need to respect and maintain informant confidentiality, is paramount. In addition to the time-consuming task of interview transcription, the administrator will be responsible for printing and distribution of transcripts and reports, and the development and maintenance of a bibliographic database.

Compensation to hospitals for participants' time will facilitate recruitment by enabling nurses to participate within work hours.

Equipment and materials

A recorder will be used to record and store data as required by NHMRC guidelines for the conduct of research. There will be nominal stationery costs associated with the project.

Library fees and photocopying

Interlibrary loans will not only facilitate a speedy retrieval of literature, but also keep RA hours to a minimum. While the literature review has already begun, off-campus literature still requires accessing.

A typical budget

Budget information		
Detailed budget items for 2022 (include oncosts for personnel; see attached notes)	Priority A, B or C*	Amount requested ($)
Personnel	A	1754
Casual HEO2, 80 hours	A	1339
Casual Senior Research Assistant A, 40 hours	B1	518
Compensation to hospitals for participants' time:	B2	35
20 nurses, Div. 1 Grade 2, 1 hour each	C	25
Equipment and materials:	B3	600
20 cassette tapes @ $1.75	B4	150
Stationery		
Library fees and photocopying:		
Interlibrary loans (40 @ $15)		
Photocopying		
Total		4421
Minimum amount for project viability		3093

Source: Richardson-Tench, M., & Brookes, A. (2006). Unpublished research proposal.

Common final elements

The final pages of any research proposal include supporting materials, which is information that is relevant to the material included in the body of the proposal. Principally, these materials comprise a full reference list and any appendices containing additional material not central to the proposal, but which provide additional information and examples.

References

A list of references is included at the end of the proposal before the appendices. In-text references are cited in a consistent manner throughout the document. Each citation in the text refers to a reference in the reference list and each reference in the list is cited in the text; that is, they should match. The list of references is alphabetical by the first author's surname. Other references not cited in the text are listed in a bibliography. The referencing system stipulated by the funding body or university for the proposal should be used for the reference list.

Appendices

Appendices are included if it is necessary to provide material that is too cumbersome for the main text. Only material that supports or expands the information in the body of the text is included.

Examples of elements that are best put in an appendix are questionnaires, survey instruments or tests, diagrams of instruments, consent forms and letters of support. Each appendix should be presented on a new page and named alphabetically, for example: 'Appendix A (Survey Questionnaire)' and 'Appendix B (Demographic Data Collection Tool)'.

Writing style and format of a research proposal

Writing style

The writing style of a research proposal is fairly prescribed. In writing the research proposal, aim for:

- clarity
- coherence
- conciseness
- completeness.

Construct the proposal in a logical order (see Figure 11.6).

Avoid preaching or adopting a value-laden stance. You are supposed to be an objective researcher and bias is considered poor science.

Use good English, with short, crisp sentences. It is important to use language that can be understood by laypeople and/or members of other disciplines. Some of the people on the ethics committee will fall into that category.

Avoid jargon, especially that of your specialty. Where you must use specific terminology, clearly define the terms you use.

Use terms consistently and do not attempt to change terms to make your proposal read more like a novel.

Avoid sexist language: never use the pronoun 'he' to refer to everyone. Avoid the use of he/she and his/hers by using the plural rather than the singular; for example, 'Participants will have their blood pressure taken before and after the treatment'. It is acceptable to be specific about the gender of participants where it is relevant. If, for example, your study is going to be done only with females, then refer to them as 'the women', 'she' and so on.

Use the future tense for the parts of the proposal that state what you intend to do, past tense for the literature review and, if it has already been completed, the section on the pilot study.

Write statements of everyday knowledge in the present tense.

▶ **Figure 11.6** Writing style for proposals

There are specific books on writing research proposals and reports, such as *Assignment and Thesis Writing* (Anderson & Poole, 2001) or *Research Proposals: A Practical Guide* (Denscombe, 2012). A pro forma from the HREC or funding agencies may also set out instructions for guidance.

Using headings

Headings are mandatory in a research proposal. Use primary headings and subheadings generously to clarify the structure of the proposal and to prepare the reader for the text that is to come.

There are two major systems of headings. One uses differences in the physical appearance and the other uses a numbering system, with or without differences in physical appearance.

Physical appearance system

This system relies on differences in the appearance of the words being used. It uses a combination of lower- and upper-case letters, positions the headings on the left margin and uses italics or bold (heaviness) and type size for the typeface to differentiate the rank of heading. Another option is to use all upper-case letters for the main (A) headings, though this is less desirable. This system is suitable for four or five levels of headings in addition to the title. A simple example of a heading format using the physical appearance of lettering is demonstrated in the next 'For example' box. Under each heading the text in paragraphs, bullet points and points within bullet points are included.

> **TIP**
>
> Be succinct: reviewers are busy people who have to read many proposals.

FOR EXAMPLE

MAIN (OR CHAPTER/SECTION) HEADINGS

> # Major heading (A head)
> ## Second-rank heading (B head)
> ### *Third-rank heading (C head)*
> #### Fourth-rank heading (D head)
> ##### *Fifth-rank heading (E head)*

Numbering system

This system relies on sections being numbered and sometimes includes headings as well. It is more commonly used in large proposals. Each section is given a number that is used at the beginning of each heading in that section. Each rank of heading begins with the number '1'. For example, first-rank headings use 1, 2, 3 and so on. Second rank headings begin with the number of the section followed by the number of the point being made under that heading (1.1, 1.2, 1.3 and so on.). Third-rank headings follow on and show the number of the next rank of points being made, and so on. An example is shown in the next 'For example' box.

Notice that this system may also use physical characteristics. The space between the number and the text of the heading is called a 'gutter'. It is important to remember that with each rank down the scale, the numbers of the lesser headings are aligned with the text of the previous level of heading.

FOR EXAMPLE

NUMBERING

SECTION 2

METHODOLOGY

2.1   Setting

2.2   Participants

2.3   Instruments and Procedures

       2.3.1 Instruments

           2.3.1.1 The questionnaire

           2.3.1.2 The physical instrument

       2.3.2 Procedures for data collection

2.4   Data Analysis

Formatting the proposal

Accessing a copy of a successful proposal and one that was rejected will allow for a comparison to be made about the difference between the two before beginning writing a report.

The formatting of a research proposal should adhere to the guidelines provided. The guidelines will usually include expected spacing, font size and margin requirements. If there are no style guidelines to help with the formatting process, then the following are some general rules that apply.

- Double-space text unless it has to go on a pro forma with limited space, in which case 1.5 can be used.
- Make the margins wide.
- Print on good-quality white paper.
- Typeface should be no smaller than 12-point.
- Use a legible font such as Times New Roman and be aware of the differences between serif and sans-serif fonts and how this impacts readability.
- Number pages and include a header and footer.

Once the structure and content of the draft document has been completed, check grammar, punctuation and style while referring to books such as *The Elements of Style* (Strunk & White, 2008) or the *Publication Manual of the American Psychological Association: 7th Edition* (2020), and to the Australian Government's Style Manual website (https://www.stylemanual.gov.au/). All documents should be proofread, especially the final copy, to eliminate spelling and grammatical errors before the proposal is submitted.

Prior to submitting the document, check the submission for completeness and that it contains all the necessary pages, including appendices and references.

TIP

Remember: spell checking on the computer is not as precise as a manual proofread.

Submitting the proposal

Having completed the proposal, the next step is to submit it to the committee or agency. The exact number of photocopies should be submitted if hard copies are required; or if the application is submitted electronically, ensure a back-up copy is kept for future reference.

A written response can be expected from the committee, usually at least a fortnight after the meeting. Only if there is a time pressure in obtaining approval should the committee chair or secretary be contacted. An informal approval over the telephone enables the researcher to start making arrangements to carry out the study. Under no circumstances may data collection commence without written approval from the appropriate committees.

If the proposal is not successful, any feedback provided by the assessors of the application can be used to improve the proposal. Often the committee may require only minor modifications or they might stipulate that approval is granted subject to certain conditions. It is the responsibility of the researcher to respond in writing to the committee to explain how the conditions have been addressed. If in the committee's response they reject the entire proposal, redevelopment of the proposal may be necessary, taking into consideration the feedback. Members of the committee may be approached to clarify their points of concern if necessary.

Funding and approval

Funding

Frequently, the cost of a project makes it imperative to acquire funding from a source other than the researcher. For student projects, the researcher will have to bear the costs in excess of any funds granted by the institution. For graduate students, the university may provide a stipend, or a proposal for a grant from an outside body may be submitted. Some graduate students may do work that is funded by their supervisor's research grant. In addition, the university provides the infrastructure described earlier.

For clinicians, the sources of funding are from their own institution's research fund or from collaborative projects with university staff, who may be able to obtain a grant from the university. Alternatively, the other source of funding is from independent organisations, government or corporate bodies. The NHMRC controls government funds for clinical research, and the Australian Research Council (ARC) controls funding for non-clinical research such as disciplinary systems or education. The amount awarded by various bodies may vary from a few hundred dollars to thousands. Further details about funding sources can be provided by the research management unit at institutions supporting student researchers, or on the research website. Many professional bodies, such as the Australian College of Perioperative Nurses, provide scholarships for research projects.

When identifying a possible source of funds for research, it is important that the aims of the research project match those of the funding body, and that the amount of funding requested in the proposal is in line with the amount advertised by the funding body (Devine, 2009).

Obtaining informal approval

The formal approval granted by ethics and research committees for research projects provides entry to the institution for the purposes of the research project. In some states in Australia, such as Victoria, a proposal to the hospital ethics committee is also required in order to gain access to participants, and will need the approval of the staff concerned, such as the hospital ward staff. If patients of medical practitioners are going to be included in the study it is courteous to acquire the practitioner's approval prior to recruiting patients into the study. These people function as gatekeepers and it is important to involve them as well. Note, in particular, the following.

- Access to participants can be improved by gaining credibility within the institution and attending to the social amenities, which includes keeping key people informed of the progress of the study, acknowledging staff participation and behaving with professional courtesy at all times.
- Credibility is enhanced by promoting the benefits of the study to the staff, being visible in the clinical area during the course of the study and by minimising the intrusions and demands that the project makes on the daily operations of the site.

If the study is carried out over a long period of time, it is essential to implement strategies to ensure continued access to participants. If staff turnover is a problem, more than one briefing session may be required. Carrying out these strategies will help to ensure continued access. In addition, at the end of the project, the staff should be thanked more formally with a letter. Above all, don't forget to send the ward staff, as well as any other key people, a written summary of the findings. It is also appropriate to present the findings during an in-service training or education workshop.

If the research is being carried out at the university, key people should be briefed about the study, such as the head of nursing and academic staff. If a laboratory is used, organising access needs to be coordinated with whoever handles the bookings for its use. Liaise, too, with the laboratory technician, who may be able to help with setting up and returning the laboratory to its previous state.

These principles with regard to social amenities and feedback apply in the university setting as well as the clinical field.

SUMMARY

This chapter outlined the purpose and process of writing a research proposal, including the ethical requirements for submitting proposals. Key features of both quantitative and qualitative research have also been presented.

1	Understand the purpose of writing a research proposal	• Proposals are written to gain approval from funding bodies, university research committees, ethics committees and any other bodies from whom approval is required for the study to be completed
2	Identify the process of preparing a research proposal	• Identify the relationships between different parts of the proposal, such as the purpose, research design and expected outcomes • Identify potential problems during the planning phase • Receive constructive feedback and suggestions from colleagues for improvement as they will be more objective when reviewing the proposal
3	Discuss the ethical considerations of a research project	• Participants have the right to informed consent, anonymity, privacy, confidentiality, to not participate or to withdraw at any time and to not suffer harm

4	Describe the structure and content of a research proposal	• All proposals consist of:
		  – preliminary pages (title, researcher details)
		  – the body of the proposal and supporting materials
		  – the research problem identifying relevance gaps in the literature
		  – the research design and research questions
		  – all supporting documents (appendices)

5	Understand how to style, format and present a research proposal	• The style of a research proposal is fairly prescribed; therefore, when writing the research proposal aim for:
		  – clarity
		  – coherence
		  – concision
		  – completeness
		• Elements of a qualitative and quantitative research proposal include:
		  – Preliminaries:
		    Title and title page
		    Abstract
		    Details of the researchers
		  – Body of proposal:
		    Introduction
		    Research questions
		    Conceptual framework, theory, hypothesis
		    Research design
		    Significance of the study
		    Limitations
		    Ethical considerations: consent, access and participants' protection
		    Dissemination of results
		    Work plan
		    Budget
		    References
		    Appendices
		    (Headings may differ depending on the research design)

| 6 | Discuss how informal approval for a research proposal is attained | • Obtaining informal approval for a research proposal and gaining access to sites includes:
— formal ethics approval granted by ethics and research committees providing entry to the institution
— acquiring the practitioner's approval prior to recruiting patients into the study
— accessing participants by gaining credibility within the institution
— keeping key people informed of the progress of the study
— acknowledging staff participation and behaving with professional courtesy at all times
— promoting the benefits of the study to the staff
— being visible in the clinical area during the course of the study
— minimising the intrusions and demands that the project makes on the daily operations of the site
— implementing strategies to ensure continued access to participants if the study is conducted over a long period of time
— presenting more than one briefing session if there is a high turnover of staff
— thanking the staff formally with a letter, including a written summary of the findings
— presenting the findings at an in-service session |
| 7 | Discuss how appropriate funding opportunities are identified | • The university may provide a stipend to support student projects
• Funding may be provided by a supervisor's research grant if the work is linked to their project |

REVIEW QUESTIONS

1 Discuss why research proposals are developed prior to conducting a research project.
2 Explain what information is necessary before writing a research proposal.
3 Describe why it is necessary to demonstrate that all the ideas are linked when developing a research proposal.
4 Describe the differences between quantitative and qualitative research proposals. Explain how these differences are presented in a research proposal and provide a reason why it is important for this information to be included.

CHALLENGING REVIEW QUESTIONS

1 You are required to submit a research proposal to an organisation that is offering funding for up to $250,000. Explain the steps you will take when developing the research proposal so that you are successful in securing the funding required to complete this project.
2 Discuss the elements that should be included in the research proposal to explain the feasibility of the project.
3 Explain the key elements that should be included in the research proposal so that it is competitive when applying for funding.

CASE STUDY 1

In this case study we return to Katie to whom you were introduced in Case study 1 in Chapter 1. Katie, an experienced registered nurse with a master qualification, works in the dementia ward in a large aged-care facility. Katie has observed that some dementia patients have a positive response to music being played in the ward. Although a literature search included research on the use of music as a treatment to improve cognitive function in people with dementia, there was a lack of standardised methods for music therapy interventions and the effect on quality of life was inconclusive. Katie has enlisted the help of members of a multidisciplinary team in formulating a research topic, with the team deciding that they were all interested in exploring carers experiences of the impact of music therapy on quality of life for dementia patients.

Katie needs to write a research proposal. Although she realises that this project could be done using a mixed methodology (both quantitative and qualitative approaches), the group has decided to use a qualitative approach. It is proposed that 20 carers who work in the dementia ward and have assisted with music therapy will be interviewed. Katie is ready to develop the first draft of the proposal but there are several other details that need to be considered. She requests a meeting with you to help clarify the proposal writing process. What information would you provide in relation to the following questions?

1 How are the title, significance of the study, aims and objectives of the research developed?
2 When developing a research proposal, what literature should be included in the report?
3 How is the appropriate methodological approach selected for this study (e.g. grounded theory)?
4 How can Katie justify interviewing 20 carers in a qualitative project?

CASE STUDY 2

- Managers from a jurisdictional ambulance service are tasked with selecting an educational program in cultural competence and safety to be delivered to all paramedics employed with that service. There are two programs that they wish to consider.
- Program A is delivered by two facilitators who are considered experts in the field.
- Program B is delivered by two facilitators who are considered experts in the field, with targeted workshops delivered by representatives of multi-cultural communities and Aboriginal and Torres Strait Islander communities.

Both programs are of 2 days in duration and the content is delivered in a face to face setting. Sixty (60) participants can be randomly selected from the service's employees. The current program delivered by the service is an online 3 hour course. Researchers wish to assess participant understanding of and attitudes toward cultural competence before and after the programs.

1 Which research design/s could be used for this study? Refer to **Table 6.2** *Comparison of major research designs* and determine which design/s may be appropriate to study the programs and their outcomes.
2 Which design would be superior in the evidence hierarchy?
3 Identify major threats to internal and external validity.
4 What would be the major considerations for managing equipment and materials?

Table 6.2 Comparison of major research designs

	Simple descriptive	Comparative descriptive	Correctional	Experimental	Pre-experimental	Quasi experimental
Describes participants						
Compares groups						
Investigates cause-and-effect relationships						
Manipulates independent variables						
Has a control group						
Random assignment to groups						

REFERENCES

Anderson, D., & Poole, M. (2001). *Assignment and Thesis Writing* (4th edn). Milton, Qld: John Wiley & Sons.

American Psychological Association. (2019). *Publication Manual of the American Psychological Association: The Official Guide to APA Style* (7th edn). American Psychological Association.

Boyle, E. (2019). Writing a good research grant proposal. *Paediatrics and Child Health, 30*(2), 52–6.

Denscombe, M. (2012). *Research Proposals: A Practical Guide.* Open University Press.

Devine, E. (2009). The art of obtaining grants. *American Journal of Health-System Pharmacy, 66*, 580–7.

Engberg, S., & Bliss, D. (2005). Spotlight on research. Writing a grant proposal – Part 1: Research methods. *Journal of Wound, Ostomy & Continence Nursing, 32*(3), 157–62.

Freeman, R. (2017). How to boost your IQ. Practical strategies for performing at your best. https://ownyourworkday.com/wp-content/uploads/2018/12/HowtoBoostWorkIQ.pdf

Gibbs, C. L., & Lowton, K. (2012). The role of the clinical research nurse. *Nursing Standard, 26*(27), 37–40.

Harper, P. (2007). Writing research proposals: Five rules. *HIV Nursing, 8*(2), 15–17.

Hollins, M. C., & Fleming, V. (2010). A 15-step model for writing a research proposal. *British Journal of Midwifery, 18*(12), 791–8.

Ingham-Broomfield, R. (2008). A nurses' guide to the critical reading of research. *Australian Journal of Advanced Nursing, 26*(1), 102–9.

Inouye, S. K., & Fiellin, D. A. (2005). An evidence-based guide to writing grant proposals for clinical research. *Annals of Internal Medicine, 142*, 274–82.

Jackowski, M. B., & Leggett, T. (2015). Writing research proposals. *Radiologic Technology, 87*(2), 236–8.

Jonker, L., & Marshall, G. (2010). Writing a research grant proposal. *Synergy: Imaging & Therapy Practice*, 22–5.

Juni, M. (2014). Writing a research proposal. *International Journal of Public Health and Clinical Sciences, 1*(1), 229–40.

Klopper, H. (2008). The qualitative research proposal. *Curationis, 31*(4), 62–72.

National Health and Medical Research Council (NHMRC) (2007). *National Statement on Ethical Conduct in Human Research (Updated 2018)*. NHMRC.

Nicholson, P., Manias, E., & Kusljic, S. (2016). Unpublished research proposal.

Proctor, E. K., Powell, B. J., Baumann, A. A., Hamilton, A. M., & Santens, R. L. (2012). Writing implementation research grant proposals: Ten key ingredients. *Implementation Science, 7*(1), 96.

Ratan, S. K., Anand, T., & Ratan, J. (2010). Formulation of research question – stepwise approach. *Journal of Indian Association Pediatric Surgery, 24*(1), 15–20. doi: 10.4103/jiaps.JIAPS_76_18

Singh, M., Cameron, C., & Duff, D. (2005). Writing proposals for research funds. *Axon/L'axone, 26*(3), 26–30.

Smith, L. J. (2008). How ethical is ethical research? Recruiting marginalized, vulnerable groups into health services research. *Journal of Advanced Nursing, 62*(2), 248–57.

Strunk, W., & White, E. (2008). *The Elements of Style* (50th anniversary edition). Boston, MA: Allyn & Bacon.

Sudheesh, K., Duggappa, D. R., & Nethra, S. S. (2016). How to write a research proposal? *Indian Journal of Anaesthesia, 60*(9), 631–4. doi: 10.4103/0019-5049.190617: 10.4103/0019-5049.190617

Vivar, C. (2007). Getting started with qualitative research: Developing a research proposal. *Nurse Researcher, 14*(3), 60–73.

Walker, C. A. (2009). Lest we forget: The Tuskegee experiment. *Journal of Theory Construction & Testing, 13*(1), 5–6.

FURTHER READING

Bliss, D. (2005). Spotlight on research. Writing a grant proposal: Part 6: The budget, budget justification, and resource environment. *Journal of Wound, Ostomy & Continence Nursing, 32*(6), 365–7.

Bliss, D., & Savik, K. (2005). Writing a grant proposal – Part 2: Research methods – Part 2. *Journal of Wound, Ostomy & Continence Nursing, 32*(4), 226–9.

Broeder, J. L., & Donze, A. (2010). Evidence-based practice: The role of qualitative research in evidence-based practice. *Neonatal Network, 29*(3), 197–202.

Mitchell, M. (2011). A reflection on the emotional potential of qualitative interviewing. *British Journal of Midwifery, 19*(10), 653–7.

National Health and Medical Research Council (NHMRC). (2002). Human research ethics handbook: Commentary on the National Statement on Ethical Conduct in Research Involving Humans. https://www.nhmrc.gov.au/guidelines-publications/e42

National Health and Medical Research Council (NHMRC). (2011). Research integrity. http://www.nhmrc.gov.au/health-ethics/research-integrity

Osman, Z. (2016). Research Proposal Writing. *Current Therapeutic Research, 78*, S4. doi:10.1016/j.curtheres.2016.05.010.

12 DISSEMINATING RESEARCH FINDINGS

Chapter learning objectives

The material presented in this chapter will assist you to:

1 explain the purpose of preparing a research report
2 describe how to write a research report
3 identify the elements of a quantitative and qualitative research report
4 explain how to prepare and present a conference or seminar presentation
5 explain how to prepare and present a poster
6 describe how to write a journal article for publication
7 describe how to prepare monographs.

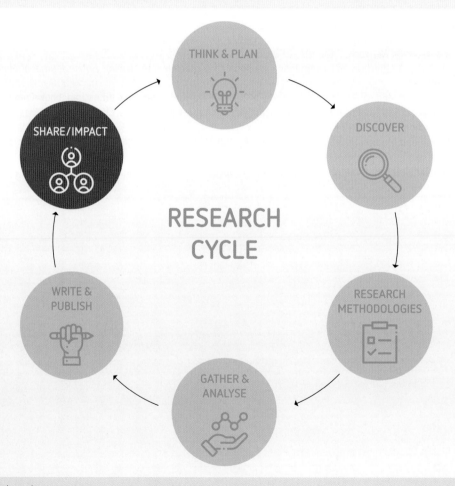

Research cycle

The primary focus of this chapter is dissemination of research findings, the share/impact part of the research cycle highlighted in the research framework above.

Introduction

A research report is a formal account of the research project, reporting the results of the study while contributing to the body of knowledge on a given topic. It is the major means by which essential information about the research project is disseminated. In fact, the results of research should be published so that it is accessible to other professionals, and potentially have an impact on the greater scientific community. There are multiple benefits, not only for clinicians but also patients, when research projects are published (Ketefian, 2018; Adams, Farrington & Cullen, 2012). Reporting research outcomes can be in written form, in which case it becomes a permanent record, or it can be an oral report to a group of colleagues at a seminar or conference. Although publications have the advantage of reaching a much larger audience, some clinicians may find the thought of preparing a manuscript for publication a daunting task (Hoogenboom & Manske, 2012; Adams, Farrington & Cullen, 2012), however, it is considered a critical step, especially if funding has been received for the project.

The research report

The value of a project is assessed through the research report as it may be the only tangible product of weeks, months or even years of work. The clarity, organisation and content is central to determining the quality and value of the report (Blake & Bly, 2000). Therefore, the most important purpose of publishing a research report is to communicate key aspects of the project to the research consumer. Clinicians read the report so that they can either replicate the study, include the article in a literature review, plan a new study or help find a solution for a clinical practice problem. In all these situations, readers will evaluate the study for validity and usefulness; therefore, in order for them to do this they will need to be able to determine how the study was conducted.

Research reports are presented in different media, have different word length requirements and serve different purposes. The scope and style of a research report will vary widely, depending on three key factors: the report's intended audience, the report's purpose and the type of information to be communicated. Depending on these factors, there are several different types of research reports.

- *Classroom project report and thesis or dissertation:* submitted as part of course requirements and are graded using specific marking criteria.
  - *Classroom research report:* usually submitted as an assignment of about 2000 to 4000 words.
  - *Thesis or dissertation:* a research thesis is submitted for an honours or master degree, with the purpose of testing the student's ability to demonstrate proficiency in the research process, whereas the dissertation completed by a doctoral student focuses on original research. A thesis for an honours or master degree may vary between 18000 and 30000 words, with a doctoral thesis equivalent to 100000 words.
- *Journal article:* disseminates the results of the research to a large target audience. It has the potential to reach the whole profession or a specialty group. Usually the word limit is between 3000 and 6000 words, depending on the journal.
- *Conference and seminar paper:* communicates work in progress or completed results to a specific target group of people. Communication about the work that has been completed is presented, with members of the audience offered the opportunity to ask questions.

- *Oral report:* such as a seminar report and conference paper, is an auditory and/or audiovisual experience that conveys information to an audience. Students completing a doctoral program are required to submit a written document and defend their work in an oral presentation to an expert panel of academics. Valuable feedback is provided by panel members who also assess the student's capability of completing the degree within the specified candidature time limit.
- **Poster**: includes a presentation on a poster board, usually at a conference, with the researcher in attendance to present the report and answer questions. While a poster presentation is visual, the information is supplemented by discussion between the presenter and the viewer. With the proliferation of research there has been an increasing tendency to use the poster as a medium for presenting research at conferences since many projects can be presented in one session. Posters also enable researchers to present work in progress, or work that has been completed.

Writing the research report

The target audience

Before beginning to write the report of a quantitative or qualitative project, the target audience should be considered. Depending on whether the report is being written for a lecturer, a thesis examiner or a journal editor, there will be expectations as to the structure and content of the report.

- A lecturer will be most interested in whether the student has demonstrated an understanding of the research process.
- A thesis examiner will be interested in whether the student has demonstrated proficiency in the subject, planning and executing research, and interpretation of their findings in their scientific context.
- A journal editor will be looking for evidence that the content of the report is suited to the journal's readership. For example, the journal articles related to diabetes mellitus in children and adolescents are published in *Paediatric Diabetes*, whereas the *Journal of Diabetes* publishes articles related to type 1 and type 2 diabetes, which include patients from all age groups.

If a specific readership is the target, it is necessary to select a journal that is aimed at that particular group. In deciding which journal to target, the style and type of articles published should also be considered. If the manuscript categories are specialised topics, a journal that specialises in content relevant to the article should be selected so that the information reaches the appropriate audience. The demographics of the readership should also be considered. If the article has a national focus, it may be better to target a national journal. For example, the article 'Aboriginal research methods and researcher reflections on working two-ways to investigate culturally secure birthing for Aboriginal women', an investigation into the experiences and cultural birthing practices of Aboriginal women giving birth in urban settings and birthing on Country was published in the *Australian Aboriginal Studies* journal (Marriott et al., 2019).

There are two factors that should be kept in mind when selecting a journal: review times and the policies on multiple submissions. Some journals may take months to review an article, delaying the article being accepted for publication. Most, if not all journals, have a policy about not accepting articles that have been submitted to another journal. The main reason why multiple submissions are not permitted is the time commitment of reviewers who are viewed as a valuable resource by the editors of the journal, and are often not paid. It is a waste of their time if the article has been submitted to more than one journal as the article may be withdrawn if it is accepted by another journal. Authors are required to acknowledge that the article has not been previously published or currently being considered by another journal when submitting an article to a journal for review.

Guidelines

Whatever the target readership of the research report, when developing the report, a copy of the guidelines should be obtained and used to guide the layout of the report. In regard to a classroom project, some institutions allocate marks for presentation and referencing, and include the guidelines in a marking rubric to direct the students when preparing their assignment for submission. Universities have guidelines for thesis presentation that students are able to access when completing a thesis or research project as part of a graduate diploma, honours or higher degree. Most university handbooks provide the presentation rules for theses for a research degree, which include margin width, line spacing and submission requirements. Many institutes no longer require students to provide a hard copy of the thesis, with a pdf format required for the examination process and the library copy once the examination process is complete. These instructions should be followed to ensure the expectations of the report are being met.

If an article is being prepared for a journal, a copy of the guidelines for authors, which will detail the format and referencing requirements, should be accessed and should be followed exactly as stipulated. Copies of several articles published in the target journal should be reviewed as examples of the approaches that have been used.

Planning and writing the report

Once the guidelines have been accessed and read, a plan should be developed on the approach that will be adopted for the report. An outline that is as detailed as possible should be developed, including the major topics and subtopics to be included. Each section of the report should then be written according to whatever details have been specified in the guidelines. Once the report is written it should be edited extensively, making correction as necessary. If possible, having someone critique the report is important so that errors are identified prior to submitting the report.

The style of writing used for a research report is generally the same as that used for a research proposal (see Chapter 11); the major points are as follows.

- Use a concise, clear and coherent style.
- Use a writing style that suits the target audience.
  - A quantitative research report is usually written in the formal scientific style to convey objectivity.
  - A qualitative research report may sometimes be written in the personal style to situate the researcher within the research; if this style is used, adherence to formal writing conventions for the literature review, methods, processes and methodology sections is required.
- Use correct English grammar, ensure writing is at a reading level appropriate to the audience, and avoid jargon and sexist language.
- Avoid the use of the passive voice.
- Check spelling using an appropriate spell checker.

Tense is less of a problem in a research report than in a proposal because the report will mainly be written in the past tense. The exception is statements of everyday knowledge, which are written in the present tense.

Structure of the report

The research report has three major components:

1 **preliminaries**: overview and background to the report
2 **body of the report**: contains the main information
3 **supporting materials**: includes references and appendices.

FOR EXAMPLE

COMPONENTS OF THE RESEARCH REPORT

PRELIMINARIES

- Title page
- Required forms*
- Acknowledgements*

ABSTRACT

- Table of contents*
- List of tables*
- List of figures*
- Executive summary⊥

BODY OF REPORT

- Introduction
- Literature review
- Methodology
- Results
- Discussion

SUPPORTING MATERIALS

- References
- Appendices

KEY:

* applicable only to a thesis or long report
⊥ applicable only to a long report

ACTIVITY

Locate two research articles listed in the reference list of any chapter in this book and discuss the nature of the report format used. Consider the following questions when completing this activity.

1 What is the order of the main headings (i.e. title, abstract, aims, objectives, significance and other relevant headings)?
2 Do the main ideas flow well between sections?
3 Do you understand the research methods, processes and outcomes of the study?
4 How has the structure of the report assisted you in understanding the information presented in the research report?

Preliminaries

The preliminaries appear in the first part of the report and include pages that precede the body of the report. A short report only requires the inclusion of a title page and an abstract. A longer report requires additional information, such as a table of contents that includes page numbers for each major section, and separate pages for the list of tables and figures included in the report, both of which will also include page numbers to help the reader easily locate each table and figure.

Title page

The title page should be similar to the title page of a research proposal (see Chapter 11). The title page provides the title of the proposal, as well as the author's name, position, qualifications and affiliation details. Some reports will require details of postal and email addresses of the researcher to be included, as well as a telephone number.

Title

The title of the report should be written as a mini report, or thumbnail sketch, of the work that conveys the essence of the report while stimulating interest in the study. The title can be a statement or a question and should reflect the major theme of the report and the type of investigation. This can be achieved by using keywords. Students often err on the side of excessive length when developing titles for their theses because they want to convey everything about the project, but a more acceptable title will be a concise statement, or question, of no more than 10 to 15 words.

For a journal article, it is important to use keywords that can be indexed so that the article can be retrieved by researchers when undertaking a literature search (refer to Chapter 2).

TIP Compose a title that reflects the most up-to-date material that would be included in a report. Avoid expressions such as 'An investigation of …' and similar. Such expressions are self-evident, take up space and are unexciting, so are unlikely to attract the interest of the reader. More importantly, these expressions are problematic in terms of cataloguing, and they make searches more difficult.

An example of a good title, which will be used as the quantitative example in this chapter, is: 'Lower-limb biomechanics in football players with and without hip-related pain' (King et al., 2020). This study employs a cross-sectional methods approach; that is, quantitative data were collected during the study.

Research by Marriott and colleagues (2019) entitled '"Our culture, how it is to be us": Listening to Aboriginal women about on Country urban birthing' will be used as the qualitative example in this chapter.

Although extracts from these articles are used throughout this chapter, it is advisable to access the full papers listed below so that the associated activities can be completed.

- King, M. G., Semciw, A. I., Schache, A. G., Middleton, K. J., Heerey, J. J., Sritharan, P., Scholes, M. J., Mentiplay, B. F., & Crossley, K. M. (2020). Lower-limb biomechanics in football players with and without hip-related pain. *Medicine and Science in Sports and Exercise*, 52(8), 1776–84. https://doi.org/10.1249/MSS.0000000000002297
- Marriott, R., Reibel, T., Coffin, J., Gliddon, J., Griffin, D., Robinson, M., Eades, A.-M., & Maddox, J. (2019). 'Our culture, how it is to be us': Listening to Aboriginal women about on Country urban birthing. *Women and Birth*, 32(5), 391–403. https://doi.org/10.1016/j.wombi.2019.06.017

Abstract

The abstract for a research article is very similar to the abstract of a research proposal with the addition of the main results. It is a succinct and accurate description of the project, which is written either near or upon completion of the project; an introduction to the research report provides a summary of the project for the reader and highlights the major themes. A well-written abstract essentially presents a good thumbnail sketch of the project.

Usually located between the title and the body of the report, the abstract is one of the most important parts of the report because it should be discoverable when searching for research articles using search engines, such as Google Scholar, and scientific databases, such as SCOPUS (Sanganyado, 2019).

It also helps the person completing a literature search decide whether to access and include the article. An abstract summarises the objectives, methodology, major findings and implications of the project. This section should be concise as it usually has a 250- to 300-word limit; that is, no more than one double-spaced page. It should not require the reader to refer to supporting materials in order to understand the content. The abstract should include four critical components, a brief background that presents the problem that was addressed in the study, the theoretical framework (if one was used), an explanation of the design of the study, including the sample and data collection methods, major findings that show what the author found and the significance of the results. If appropriate, the abstract should conclude with any recommendations (Sanganyado, 2019). Publishers require authors to include three to five key words that portray an accurate representation of the publication. These key words are also important when using search engines to find the most relevant articles during a literature search.

FOR EXAMPLE

ABSTRACT – QUANTITATIVE STUDY

Purpose

This study aimed to evaluate the differences in lower-limb biomechanics between adult sub-elite competitive football players with, and without, hip-related pain during two contrasting tasks. The researchers also explored whether potential differences, if present, were sex dependent.

Method

Eighty-eight football players with hip-related pain (23 women, 65 men) and 30 asymptomatic control football players (13 women, 17 men) who were participating in competitive sport were recruited. Biomechanical data were collected for the stance phase of walking and single-leg drop jump (SLDJ). Differences between groups and sex-specific effects were calculated using linear regression models.

Results

Compared with their asymptomatic counterparts, football players with hip-related pain displayed a lower average pelvic drop angle during walking ($p = 0.03$) and a greater average pelvic hike angle during SLDJ ($p < 0.05$). Women with hip-related pain displayed a greater total range of motion (excursion) for the sagittal plane knee angle ($p = 0.01$) during walking compared with asymptomatic women.

Conclusion

Overall, few differences were observed in lower-limb biomechanics between football players with and without hip-related pain, irrespective of the task. This outcome suggests that, despite the presence of symptoms, impairments in lower-limb biomechanics during function do not appear to be a prominent feature of people with hip-related pain who are still participating in sport.

Source: King, M. G., Semciw, A. I., Schache, A. G., Middleton, K. J., Heerey, J. J., Sritharan, P., Scholes, M. J., Mentiplay, B. F., & Crossley, K. M. (2020). Lower-limb biomechanics in football players with and without hip-related pain. *Medicine & Science in Sports & Exercise, 52*(8), 1776–84.

FOR EXAMPLE

ABSTRACT – QUALITATIVE STUDY

Background

Birth on Country is often assumed as relevant to Aboriginal women in rural/remote locations and not usually associated with urban environments. In Western Australia, one-third of the Aboriginal population live in the greater metropolitan area. We wanted to know Aboriginal women's experiences of on Country urban births.

Methods

Indigenous qualitative data collection and analysis methods were used to learn about Aboriginal women's stories of contemporary and past experiences of maternity care and cultural practices associated with birth on Country.

Results

Aboriginal Birthing, Senior and Elder women consistently reported ongoing cultural practices associated with childbirth including knowledge sharing across generations and family support, observance of extended family present at the time of or shortly after birth, and how their cultural security was improved when Aboriginal staff were present. Also noted, were the inflexibility of health systems to meet their needs and midwives lack of cultural awareness and understanding of the importance of Aboriginal kinship.

Conclusion

In terms of on Country urban birth, the women collectively expressed a strong desire to maintain cultural practices associated with childbirth, including birthing close to home (on Country); having family acknowledged and included throughout the perinatal period; and, having access to Aboriginal midwives, nurses, doctors and other healthcare workers to support their cultural security.

Source: Marriott, R., Reibel, T., Coffin, J., Gliddon, J., Griffin, D., Robinson, M., Eades, A.-M., & Maddox, J. (2019). 'Our culture, how it is to be us': Listening to Aboriginal women about on Country urban birthing. *Women & Birth, 32*(5), 391–403.

ACTIVITY

Critique the abstract reproduced in this section and explain whether the characteristics of an acceptable abstract, as described in this section, have been presented.

Aims and objectives

The aims and objectives are the same as those written for the proposal, with the sentences written in the past tense.

FOR EXAMPLE

AIMS AND OBJECTIVES – QUANTITATIVE STUDY

The aims of this exploratory study were twofold: 1) to evaluate lower-limb biomechanical variables, in low (walking) and high (single-leg drop jump [SLDJ]) impact tasks, in people with and without hip-related pain … and 2) to determine whether differences in lower-limb biomechanics, if present, were sex specific.

Source: King, M. G., Semciw, A. I., Schache, A. G., Middleton, K. J., Heerey, J. J., Sritharan, P., Scholes, M. J., Mentiplay, B. F., & Crossley, K. M. (2020). Lower-Limb biomechanics in football players with and without hip-related pain. *Medicine & Science in Sports & Exercise, 52*(8), 1776–84.

FOR EXAMPLE

AIMS AND OBJECTIVES — QUALITATIVE STUDY

The Birthing on Noongar Boodjar (BONB) project set out to understand the contemporary birth practices of Aboriginal women dwelling and/or giving birth on the lands of the Noongar Nation.

Source: Marriott, R., Reibel, T., Coffin, J., Gliddon, J., Griffin, D., Robinson, M., Eades, A.-M., & Maddox, J. (2019). 'Our culture, how it is to be us': Listening to Aboriginal women about on Country urban birthing. *Women & Birth, 32*(5), 391–403.

Body of the report

The body of the report should include a straightforward description of the problem, methodology and findings, as well as the interpretation of the findings. Also included is an assessment of the significance and the adequacy of the study design, and recommendations for further research. There are four major sections in the body of a research report (Lambie et al., 2008, p. 21):

1 the introduction, or 'Why I did it'
2 the methodology, or 'What I did'
3 the results, or 'What I found'
4 the discussion, or 'What it means'.

The introduction and methodology sections of the research report are similar to the sections presented in the research proposal, with some minor variations in the format.

Introduction and literature review

The introduction and literature review set the scene for a report and justify the reason for conducting the study, providing a theoretical rationale for the importance or significance of the study. The introduction goes from the general to the specific and sets the scene for the research question or problem. The research problem or research question is stated and should answer the questions: 'What problem was investigated?' and 'Why was it done?'

The introduction emphasises the study's importance and sets it in the context of previous work in the area.

An acceptable quantitative research report will contain in its introduction an adequate review of the theoretical and empirical literature. However, this section may be refined so that the literature review is congruent with the findings included in the report. For example, if one part of the findings is not able to be included for some reason, and it is removed from the report, the literature relating to those results is redundant. When writing for a journal, space restrictions require that the literature review only includes the most relevant studies. The findings are emphasised and a critique is included only where it is relevant to the methodology presented.

FOR EXAMPLE

INTRODUCTION AND LITERATURE REVIEW – QUANTITATIVE STUDY

Hip joint pathology has been found to be the most common clinical entity present in a sporting population with longstanding pain in the hip and groin region (Rankin, Bleakley & Cullen, 2015). Hip-related pain often results in reduced physical function, activity levels, family and work participation, and quality of life for young to middle-age adults (Heerey, et al. 2018; Thorborg, Rathleff, Petersen, Branci, & Holmich, 2017).......... To develop more effective treatments for people with hip-related pain, we need a better understanding of the functional impairments associated with this condition ... To date, most studies of biomechanical impairments in people with hip joint conditions have focused on those with more severe pathology, including people with femoroacetabular impingement syndrome (FAIS) awaiting surgery (Diamond, Wrigley, Bennell, Hinman, O'Donnell & Hodges, 2016; Brisson, Lamontagne, Kennedy & Beaulé, 2013; Rylander, Shu, Favre, Safran & Andriacchi, 2013; Hunt, Guenther & Gilbart, 2013) and those with end-stage joint disease (hip osteoarthritis [OA]) (Diamond, Allison, Dobson & Hall, 2018; Meyer, et al. 2018; Hurwitz, Hulet, Andriacchi, Rosenberg & Galante, 1997; Beaulieu, Lamontagne & Beaulé, 2010).

Source: King, M. G., Semciw, A. I., Schache, A. G., Middleton, K. J., Heerey, J. J., Sritharan, P., Scholes, M. J., Mentiplay, B. F., & Crossley, K. M. (2020). Lower-Limb biomechanics in football players with and without hip-related pain. *Medicine & Science in Sports & Exercise*, 52(8), 1776–84.

ACTIVITY

Evaluate the extent to which the literature review just presented achieves the characteristics of an acceptable literature review, as described in this section.

The literature review for the qualitative report will be an amalgam of the literature presented in the proposal, together with that which has been published since the project began. In some projects, such as those involving grounded theory, the literature review may be completed after the data collection and analysis phase of the study. In other collaborative and participatory approaches, such as action research, the literature is reviewed as thematic themes emerge throughout the research processes.

The literature review is important because it alerts the researcher to disagreements, gaps, silences and contradictions in research findings, supporting the claims that the project is significant in its focus and findings. The literature review can also show the extent to which other researchers have made similar conclusions, thereby fortifying the impact of the implications of the project. It is important to check that the literature review contains all the elements of an acceptable literature review as described in this chapter when writing the report (see also Chapter 2).

FOR EXAMPLE

LITERATURE REVIEW – QUALITATIVE STUDY

There is a lack of evidence in the literature about the birth practices of Aboriginal women whose Country is urbanised to the extent that development has impacted on access to traditional birth sites. Nonetheless, Aboriginal culture is dynamic, diverse and thriving; resulting in Aboriginal families and communities maintaining longstanding cultural birth practices despite the changed circumstances in which Aboriginal communities find themselves. According to Bertilone et al. (2017) these birth practices are known to include: knowledge sharing, family involvement and kinship support and family attendance at the time of birth. Furthermore, the practices have survived alongside the necessity to manage circumstances imposed by the requirements of contemporary maternity services, such as restrictions on numbers of support people in attendance at the time of childbirth, the absence of flexible care arrangements or ready access to transport to attend appointments during pregnancy, all of which are known to impact Aboriginal women's engagement in antenatal services (Kildea, Stapleton, Murphy, Low & Gibbons, 2012; Minniecon, Parker & Cadet-James, 2003; Reibel & Walker, 2010; Reibel, Morrison, Griffin, Chapman & Woods, 2015; Kildea et al., 2018).

Source: Marriott, R., Reibel, T., Coffin, J., Gliddon, J., Griffin, D., Robinson, M., Eades, A.-M., & Maddox, J. (2019). 'Our culture, how it is to be us': Listening to Aboriginal women about on Country urban birthing. *Women & Birth, 32*(5), 391–403.

ACTIVITY

Explain what is meant by a critical review of the literature. Does the example just presented provide a critical review of the literature? Discuss your answer.

The design

The principle of this section is that a description of the framework, methods and processes is presented in enough detail to enable another researcher to replicate the study; that is, to conduct another study using the same approach. Therefore, it must include the design, setting, participants, sampling, instruments and procedures for the study. It is important to report the methodology accurately because it helps the reader to evaluate the validity and the researcher's interpretation of the findings. It not only facilitates comparison with other studies on the subject (Pearson et al., 2015; Smagorinsky, 2008), but also facilitates inclusion in systematic reviews and clinical guidelines that inform clinical practice (Pearson et al., 2015). In the following section, the differences in the presentation of the design section for quantitative and qualitative reports are presented.

Elements of quantitative and qualitative research designs

Quantitative research designs

This section should include a statement about the type of research design required and an explanation about why that design was appropriate for the research question (see Chapter 5). Table 12.1 gives an overview of quantitative research designs.

▶ **Table 12.1**   Quantitative research designs: overview

Format	Rationale
The research question or hypothesis	• A description of the purpose of the study showing the relationships between the variables stated in measurable terms is included. If appropriate, the independent and dependent variables are identified and detailed in measurable terms
The setting for the research	• It is not appropriate to include the names of the agencies where the research has been conducted unless they have given permission, but details about the type of setting are included
The participants	• The characteristics of the selected participants and where these participants were recruited from are described; a rationale for selecting this particular group of participants is reported • The size of the sample group included in the study is detailed. Calculating the sample size for the study is stated so that precise and accurate conclusions can be elicited • The sampling method used (see Chapter 5) and any steps taken to prevent bias in the sample is detailed
The criteria	• The criteria for participant selection is described, as well as the rationale for the inclusion and exclusion criteria • Details of how the participants were recruited – by letter, telephone, social media or through personal contact such as email – is provided • The sampling procedure, the number of groups and the number of participants in each group, and how they were allocated to the groups, are described
The instruments or materials used, including any tools or questionnaires	• It is not necessary to explain any standard tests, but any unconventional techniques, tests or instruments should be explained • If an instrument is new, details of how it was developed and tested before use should be included. If the instrument has been used before, details of its origin, how it has been used in other studies, and the reliability and validity should also be reported • Any instrument used to collect data and how the instrument is scored or measured (e.g. on a Likert scale) is described • Diagrams or photographs of an instrument can be included to avoid long descriptions and to stimulate interest. Permission is required if the image is copyrighted • An explanation of why the instrument was suitable for the acquisition of reliable, valid data should be provided • Any questionnaire is described. If the report is a thesis or a student research project, a copy of the questionnaire should be included as an appendix. This may not be necessary for a journal article (see Chapter 5 for a discussion of these concepts)

Format	Rationale
The procedures section	• The procedures that were used in the study are described. If it was an experiment, an explanation of how an experimental treatment was applied is necessary • An explanation of how, when and where the data were collected should provide enough detail for someone to replicate the procedure • Procedures such as participant observation, questionnaire administration and application of an instrument or experimental treatment are reported • Calibration of the instruments or any training given to data collectors prior to data collection is described • For questionnaire administration, details about how these were distributed and how they were returned are provided. Details about anonymity must also be included. The start and completion of data collection is also noted • If any of the procedures were important to the design of the study, particulars concerning the exact time they were carried out are detailed
The data analysis section	• Recording and management of the data, including the coordination of data management if multiple sites are involved, are described • Data entry into a computer, including coding of data, is noted • Data analysis in relation to the research question or hypotheses is detailed, including the data analysis package and procedures used • Statistical tests that were carried out to test each hypothesis are stated
Ethical considerations	• It is not necessary to go into a great deal of detail about the ethical considerations. It should be stated that permission was given by the relevant ethics committees with names included. The reader will thus be assured that reasonable ethical procedures were in place. Journals may require that the human research and ethics reference number be included in the manuscript • Any procedures that were implemented to protect participants from harm are briefly discussed. In a short report, this can be integrated with the appropriate parts of the report, such as the procedures section • If a pilot study was completed, a brief description should be provided. Any changes in the methodology that resulted from the pilot study should be detailed and justified

FOR EXAMPLE

STUDY DESIGN – QUANTITATIVE STUDY

This cross-sectional study involved the Melbourne-based subset of football players participating in an ongoing longitudinal cohort study being conducted in Australia (Crossley et al., 2018). Current sub-elite football players (soccer or Australian Football), who were still actively participating in their chosen sport, were eligible to participate under specific criteria. Participants were recruited via social media advertisement campaigns, mail outs, and direct communication with football organizations and clubs. As the study was exploratory in nature, no formal power analysis was conducted. Ethical approval for the research was obtained from the La Trobe University Human Ethics Committee (HEC 15-019 and HEC 16-045), and all participants provided written informed consent.

Source: King, M. G., Semciw, A. I., Schache, A. G., Middleton, K. J., Heerey, J. J., Sritharan, P., Scholes, M. J., Mentiplay, B. F., & Crossley, K. M. (2020). Lower-Limb biomechanics in football players with and without hip-related pain. *Medicine & Science in Sports & Exercise, 52*(8), 1776–84.

ACTIVITY

Explain the extent to which the sample research design presented achieves the characteristics of an acceptable research design, as described in this section.

Qualitative research design

The body of a qualitative report contains sections on the study's methodology, methods and processes (see Chapter 7 for definitions of each of these sections as they apply to qualitative research). Figure 12.1 provides some questions to guide writing the methodology section of the report.

In a report on a project (e.g. a thesis), the methodology may take part or all of a chapter, which is important to remember when using the examples provided in this chapter to structure the report. The research report must be appropriate for the audience.

At this point, a small section that outlines some key assumptions about qualitative research approaches may be inserted, depending on the intended audience. If there is a chance that the audience will be relatively uninformed about qualitative research, particularly when a design that is not well known has been used, it might be advisable to include a short summary.

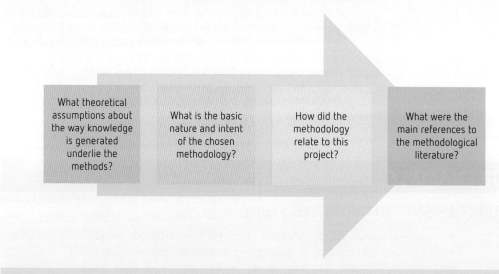

What theoretical assumptions about the way knowledge is generated underlie the methods?

What is the basic nature and intent of the chosen methodology?

How did the methodology relate to this project?

What were the main references to the methodological literature?

▶ **Figure 12.1** Questions for the methodology section

Ethical requirements

The ways that the ethical rights of the participants were safeguarded throughout the project should be reported and the following questions about ethical requirements should be addressed in the report.

• Which committees granted ethical approval?
• What were the ethical considerations?
• How were informed consent, privacy and anonymity honoured?

Ethics

Methods and processes

The method and processes used in the project are reported. If these varied from what was proposed, this should be noted. The following are some questions that may guide the writing of the methods section.

- How were participants enlisted into the project?
- What was the sequence of the research methods?
- What interpersonal processes were involved in undertaking the methods?

If there was no variation from the research intentions, parts of this section may be inserted from the research proposal by changing the sentences to the past tense.

FOR EXAMPLE

METHODS AND PROCESSES – QUALITATIVE STUDY

Study design

The Birthing on Noongar Boodjar (BONB) project's qualitative study design was purposefully developed using Indigenous theoretical concepts to frame culturally secure research processes. The approach incorporated research methods drawn from Indigenist research practices ... combining these with selected mainstream qualitative practices compatible with Indigenous research practice and values. Ethics approval was sought from: WA Aboriginal Health Ethics Committee, and the Murdoch University, South Metropolitan Health Service and North Metropolitan Health Service and WA Health Country Health Service Ethics Committees.

Recruitment method

Recruitment of Aboriginal women participants was purposefully targeted and largely relied on a purposive and organic process of informing Aboriginal community networks and with ACG [Aboriginal Consultative Group] members speaking with women in the community. Women who were interested in yarning with the researchers contacted the project's Research Coordinator, a well-known Noongar woman, and a few Aboriginal women responded to posters displayed in selected maternity services.

Data collection

Yarning is an Indigenist research practice (Bessarab & Ng'andu, 2010; Lin, Green & Bessarab, 2016), which involves different types ('social', 'research', 'collaborative', 'therapeutic', 'clinical', 'diagnostic') to collect stories (information) from Aboriginal research participants (or patients). Yarning used in research or clinical contexts draws on this established cultural practice in a specific way; with the listener respectfully guiding the storyteller towards the topic of interest or enquiry. In a research process, this usually starts with 'social yarning', which relies on a storyteller and story listener developing a rapport, often based on cultural exchange. All yarns and yarning circles were audio recorded, transcribed verbatim and de-identified for analysis.

Data storage and confidentiality

All project participants received an information sheet and provided written consent for their information collected in yarns/yarning circles or interviews to be audio recorded and transcribed for inclusion in project data for analysis. All data was de-identified prior to analysis.

Source: Marriott, R., Reibel, T., Coffin, J., Gliddon, J., Griffin, D., Robinson, M., Eades, A.-M., & Maddox, J. (2019). 'Our culture, how it is to be us': Listening to Aboriginal women about on Country urban birthing. *Women & Birth, 32*(5), 391–403.

The results

In this section, an account of what the investigators found is reported. The results tell a story, but they should be presented in order of their importance (Smagorinsky, 2008) as it is viewed as the heart of the report (Labanu, Wadhwa & Asthana, 2017). The results should also be presented in such a way that they address the research question with data summarised in the form of tables, graphs or numbers (Labani, Wadhwa & Asthana, 2017). Raw data or the data analysis should not be presented in the results section. Although the researcher has the responsibility of deciding which results should be reported, in a student report or thesis it is customary to present all findings, whether or not they are important or noteworthy. For other reports, trimming this section to only include the key findings will be necessary to meet the criteria for the word limit of a journal.

According to Smagorinsky (2008), researchers often err on the side of over-reporting for two reasons:

- they believe that every finding is equally important
- it is felt that if they have gone to the trouble of doing the procedure, it must be reported.

Irrelevant detail in a report can obscure the important findings (Baydekar, 2015). The aim is to make the key findings stand out. If there are many results on several subtopics, the use of headings would be appropriate with all the results on each subtopic presented together, even mixing qualitative and quantitative findings if both approaches have been included in the study.

Quantitative report results comprise the text and supporting illustrations, such as tables, graphs, charts, photographs and models derived from the data.

The statistical tests must be reported with the appropriate result, giving the test, the result of the test and the probability value. Some journals or bodies require that the degrees of freedom are also presented. The statistical test is usually presented in parentheses after the result has been reported. Note that the letters representing the statistical test (e.g. t and the probability p) should be cited in italics. The exact reporting of the p value enables readers to see how close to significance the results were. If the computer gives a p value of 0.0136, then round off the number to two decimal places 0.01. There is a range of software packages used for analysing data, such as SPSS for statistical analysis of quantitative data or NVivo for qualitative data analysis. Many of these programs include resources, such as a user manual, to help with selecting the right data analysis technique as well as how the results should be reported.

The results should be presented in a logical sequence to support the hypotheses, or answer the question stated in the introduction. Negative results should be reported, even if the results do not support the hypothesis, as they may be of importance to other researchers. Important discoveries have been made from data when results obtained were

TIP

It is never appropriate to present only findings that support your hypotheses or beliefs.

TIP

The results section is purely for the presentation of the findings. Interpretation of the data should be reported in the discussion section.

contrary to what was expected (Labani et al., 2017). In experimental and quasi-experimental research reports, a statement of whether a hypothesis was supported is included with each result, including a statement about the null hypothesis and the research hypothesis. The possibilities are that the null hypothesis was:

- rejected, in which case the research hypothesis was supported
- not rejected, in which case the research hypothesis was not supported
- rejected but the findings were in the opposite direction from those predicted by the research hypothesis, which was not supported.

Supporting illustrations

A number of devices can be used to present results in ways other than using words (see Figure 12.2), including photographs, diagrams, models, flow charts, graphs and tables. Tables are simply referred to as 'tables'; the rest are collectively referred to as 'figures'. They provide an economical method of presenting information in ways that are reader-friendly.

An example of a results section is presented below. Note that all the tables have been removed from these results; access the article to view them. Results pertaining to the qualitative data of the study have also been removed.

FOR EXAMPLE

RESULTS SECTION – QUANTITATIVE STUDY

Primary aim

Hip-related pain group versus asymptomatic controls. There was a significant difference in the average frontal plane pelvis angle during the stance phase of SLDJ between football players with and without hip-related pain. Specifically, football players with hip-related pain displayed more pelvic hike (i.e., more lateral tilt of the pelvis toward the ipsilateral side) compared with asymptomatic controls .

Secondary aim

Sex–group interactions. No significant sex–group interactions were found for any of the biomechanical variables during SLDJ.

Source: King, M. G., Semciw, A. I., Schache, A. G., Middleton, K. J., Heerey, J. J., Sritharan, P., Scholes, M. J., Mentiplay, B. F., & Crossley, K. M. (2020). Lower-Limb biomechanics in football players with and without hip-related pain. *Medicine & Science in Sports & Exercise, 52*(8), 1776–84.

ACTIVITY

Explain the extent to which this example of a results section achieves the characteristics of an acceptable results section in a research report.

Introduce illustrative devices in the text before they are presented

- Give each illustrative device a caption and a number; put the caption of a table at the top of the table and the caption of a figure below the figure
- The caption informs the reader about the findings in the table or figure but does not include the name of the statistical test. In short reports, number the figures and tables consecutively throughout, but for larger reports and theses, which have chapters, use the number of each chapter as part of the numbering system (e.g. Table 1.1, Table 1.2, Figure 2.3, Figure 2.4 etc.)

When using tables, avoid giving too much detail

- Keep in mind what information you want your reader to extract, and build the table to make the extraction as easy as possible (Johnson & Green 2009)

Round off numbers to the level of their significance

- If, say, your number is 572 out of 1000, or 57.2 per cent, but the standard deviation is 10 per cent, your figure is accurate only to 57 per cent at best and 60 per cent is really close enough
- Round off all numbers to the same number of decimal places and align the decimal points under each other in the column
- Make sure that your columns and rows have top and side headings. If inferential statistics are used, present the results at the bottom of the table

A figure is a pictorial representation: a photograph, a model, a flowchart or a graph

- Most journals have requirements concerning the presentation of photographs, such as permission to publish the photograph and its size

Graphs are the most commonly used figures in a research report

- When preparing graphs, it pays to frame the graph, use visually prominent symbols, place labels for the values outside the graph and choose a scale that is appropriate for the data
- A graph will usually compare findings for groups or within a group; it might compare the results of two groups on the dependent variable
- When preparing graphs, the dependent variable is usually on the X, the horizontal axis, and the independent variable on the Y, the vertical axis
- Label the axes. Different types of graphs are useful for different purposes; consider the results you want to show when selecting which type of graph to use (see Chapter 6 for examples)

Tests of significance can be reported at the bottom of the figure or in the text

- Tests of significance and other data-analysis particulars are included in the results section along with the actual result
- Data analysis may be put in the results section, but it should be comprehensive and give the reader enough detail to understand exactly what you did

▶ **Figure 12.2**   Devices to present reader-friendly information

The analysis

In a qualitative report, the results section provides a description of how the analysis and interpretation of data were done. The reader needs to be able to see how the data was organised and analysed, so this section should be clearly described. The report should reflect the roles and contributions of all the people in the research phase in regard to the analysis and interpretation of the data. Excerpts of actual dialogue between researchers, co-researchers and participants as sources of data should also be reported to assist in validating interpretations and to act as a decision trail for readers.

Figure 12.3 provides some guiding questions to help write the analysis and interpretation phases of the project. Responses to these questions will differ considerably depending on whether the report is describing a qualitative interpretive or qualitative critical project. The report is organised into sections, or chapters, in which the analysis and interpretation can be demonstrated. The report should demonstrate how individuals' accounts relate to those of other participants and, if it is appropriate to the methodology chosen, also discuss the common themes that emerged from the data analysis and interpretation phases. The following is an example of how to write the analysis and interpretation section. The article in question should be read for the complete information.

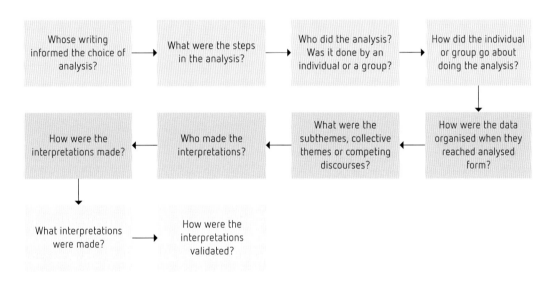

▸ **Figure 12.3** Guiding questions for writing the analysis and interpretation phases

FOR EXAMPLE

DATA ANALYSIS – QUALITATIVE STUDY

Data analysis

Data was analysed using multi-layered, iterative processes, based on decolonising research methods (Laycock, Walker, Harrison, Brands, 2019; Rigney, 1997; Smith, 1999; Saunders, West & Usher, 2010), which support rigorous and culturally informed and meaningful analysis outcomes (Kovach, 2009; Prior, 2007; Simonds & Christopher, 2013; Geia, Hayes & Usher, 2013). The methods were applied, for example, to coding which was undertaken individually by multiple investigators and in collective investigator coding and analysis small group sessions or large group workshops. In sessions and workshops, coding and theme discussions were supported by using NVivo which enabled visual display of coding and themes as these were discussed and changes were being made, which also meant these were able to be collectively validated in real time.

Results

The BONB project findings summarised in this article represent the voices and insights expressed by Aboriginal Birthing, Senior and Elder women participants. From their data, we established that the importance of cultural practices associated with Birthing on Country which has been highly urbanised is not diminished, but has been interrupted and altered. This is most evident in the loss of access to birth sites and loss of Elder women who were traditional (bush) midwives. The findings reported here are a summary of the analysis undertaken for the three Aboriginal women data groups, presented as: [1] Birthing on Country and Cultural Security; [2] System Inflexibility, Continuity and Trauma; [3] Care encounters and Aboriginal Staff; [4] Care Experiences and Racism; [5] Intergenerational Sharing; and, [6] Stories of Old Ways.

Source: Marriott, R., Reibel, T., Coffin, J., Gliddon, J., Griffin, D., Robinson, M., Eades, A.-M., & Maddox, J. (2019). 'Our culture, how it is to be us': Listening to Aboriginal women about on Country urban birthing. *Women & Birth*, *32*(5), 391–403.

The discussion

The discussion section, the last part of the body of the report, explains the importance and relevance of the findings. In this section, the researcher has the opportunity to demonstrate their ability to showcase the study and interpret the meaning of the findings (Bavdekar, 2015). The most important findings are highlighted, data are interpreted in relation to issues raised in the introduction section and placed in the context of the previously published relevant literature (Bavdekar, 2015; Johnson & Green, 2009). The strengths and weaknesses of the study, as well as the impact of the results should be explained. Recommendations for the future research should be specified. Common pitfalls when writing the discussion chapter include:

1 reporting results in great detail – only the gist of the results is required to provide the context for the discussion that is to follow

2 discussing outcomes that were not reported in the results section – only outcomes reported in the results section should be discussed

3 not discussing unexpected results – this detail could stimulate further research

4 the discussion includes the same or similar information presented in the introduction section – these sections should complement one another

5 inclusion of long wordy arguments – focused arguments should be presented

6 not mentioning the limitations of the study – reviewers will indicate the limitations when the article is being reviewed for publication

7 conclusions not supported by data or over-inflating the results – a balanced and honest point of view is necessary when writing the discussion section (Bavdekar, 2015).

It should be noted that there are some differences between a quantitative and qualitative report as discussed below.

Quantitative research

In the results section of a quantitative research report, a statement should be given about whether the null hypotheses have been rejected and the research hypotheses have been supported. The result and interpretation is briefly reiterated for the reader. If the research hypothesis is supported, this is easy to report. If it is not supported, the researcher is left with the task of explaining why not. This is usually either because the design was flawed, the prediction was not valid, or the sample size was too small and undermined the reliability of the study (Button et al., 2013). Sometimes, negative findings are just as important as positive findings and can have just as significant an impact on practice. Borderline findings can stimulate further research, as can reports with a design flaw, which can prevent other researchers from making the same mistakes. Another important factor when findings are being interpreted is to distinguish between statistical significance and clinical significance, which should be reported in the discussion section (Mellis, 2017).

Results are sometimes statistically significant but not clinically significant. This occurs when the p values are less than 0.05 (or whatever level of significance has been set) but the difference between the means of the two groups is low. This can occur because as the sample size increases, the difference required for statistical significance decreases. In other words, with large numbers of participants, the difference required to reach statistical significance is small. To reach clinical significance, a difference should be at least 10 per cent, preferably a difference of 20 per cent should be reached.

> **TIP**
>
> If results are not statistically significant, they cannot be clinically significant.

FOR EXAMPLE

CLINICAL SIGNIFICANCE

Suppose that you compared the dependent variable of the tidal volumes of two groups on two different types of pillows. A normal tidal volume is 500 millilitres. Unless you found a difference of more than 50 millilitres between the mean tidal volumes of each group, the result would not be clinically significant, although with a large-enough sample it may be statistically significant.

The results must relate to the research discussed in the literature review, comparing what was found to that reported previously by other researchers. The findings may support or refute previous findings reported in the literature. These findings are integrated into the interpretation of the findings in the report.

The research should be related to the theoretical or conceptual framework stated earlier in the report. If a theory is being tested, it should be stated whether the findings support, modify or refute the theory. If a theoretical framework was used as a conceptual framework without testing the theory, how the findings are related to the theory should also be described.

The statement on the significance of the study is then presented, the importance of why the study was worth doing is reported, the question 'So what?' is answered, and how the results of this study advance knowledge or practice in nursing and/or healthcare are also demonstrated. If there are possible applications of the results of this study, these should also be stated.

At the end of the discussion section, conclusions are presented, recommendations for further research are made and the clinical implementation of the findings is discussed. In the era of evidence-based practice, being able to generalise findings from one study to a whole population is important; therefore, limitations of the research should also be detailed.

FOR EXAMPLE

DISCUSSION SECTION – QUANTITATIVE STUDY

This study investigated lower-limb biomechanics during walking and SLDJ in football players with and without hip-related pain. Substantial differences between groups were not revealed, irrespective of the task. A small number of biomechanical variables were found to be significantly different, with some having significant sex–group interactions during walking, but in all instances, the magnitude of these differences was small, questioning how meaningful these differences are from a clinical perspective. We also did not find between-group differences in lower-limb biomechanics to be more apparent for SLDJ compared with walking. Thus, overall our hypothesis was not supported.

Sources: King, M. G., Semciw, A. I., Schache, A. G., Middleton, K. J., Heerey, J. J., Sritharan, P., Scholes, M. J., Mentiplay, B. F., & Crossley, K. M. (2020). Lower-Limb biomechanics in football players with and without hip-related pain. *Medicine & Science in Sports & Exercise, 52*(8), 1776–84.

Qualitative research

The final stage of a qualitative research report documents any pertinent discussions of the findings and offers suggestions for nursing, midwifery and allied health practice. Projects can conclude the report by offering suggestions for practice, education and research. At times, and in line with the lack of certainty in qualitative research related to the relativity of truth, tentative statements are made.

Qualitative reports will differ in the concluding section, depending on the particular approaches taken. The report should demonstrate that the final discussion and conclusions are congruent with the overall plan, methods and processes of the research.

FOR EXAMPLE

DISCUSSION SECTION – QUALITATIVE STUDY

The overall dataset from three Aboriginal women's data groups have been synthesised, with findings then summarised to focus on the collective experiences of four or more generations of Aboriginal women. In doing so we have highlighted the issues Aboriginal women clearly identified as related to longstanding cultural birth practices maintained in relation to birthing on

Country in urban contexts and how women have adapted to changes brought about by necessity due to the requirements of the healthcare system they use for their maternity care.

The Birthing on Noongar Boodjar project has generated evidence which provides comprehensive insight into what Birthing on Country in urban settings means to Aboriginal women and represents four generations of women's experiences which describe both continuing cultural practices and the changed circumstances which impact on Aboriginal women and their families and how they have adapted to these. Overall, the Aboriginal women's data provided critical insights into the changes needed in health systems to embed and sustain models of care within existing operational budgets. These models, if based on the evidence in this and other similar recent studies, will ensure Aboriginal women have access to maternity care which is culturally safe, and thus contributes to maintaining their culturally security.

Source: Marriott, R., Reibel, T., Coffin, J., Gliddon, J., Griffin, D., Robinson, M., Eades, A.-M., & Maddox, J. (2019). 'Our culture, how it is to be us': Listening to Aboriginal women about on Country urban birthing. *Women & Birth*, *32*(5), 391–403.

ACTIVITY

Discuss how the results section of a research report differs from the discussion section.

Supporting materials

Referencing

Whatever system is used, it is important to be accurate, particularly in a report that is going to be disseminated. If a report is being written for an organisation that requires a particular referencing style, it is necessary to follow the guidelines. Sloppiness in referencing will give the reader the impression that the research was sloppy too. Even worse, errors in a journal name, volume or issue number could prevent the reader from locating the reference, which negates a major reason for including references. The use of a reference manager such as EndNote (refer to Chapter 2) will help to prevent mismatches between the in-text citations and the reference list.

Appendices

Appendices are used to include material that is too cumbersome for the main text. These should be used wisely. The rationale includes avoiding filling the report with unnecessary detail and interrupting the flow of the main text. Only material that supports or expands on the information in the body of the text should be included.

Items that might be located in an appendix include questionnaires, tools or tests, diagrams of instruments, literature summary tables, consent forms and letters of support. Some disciplines may require the raw data be included in an appendix for a thesis. Each appendix should be presented on a new page and indexed alphabetically.

Putting it together

The mechanics of assembling the report are the same as for a proposal (see Chapter 11).

- It is important to use an appropriate heading system.
- Construct a table of contents; for a long report, the table of contents should include a list of tables and a list of figures, each of which should be displayed on a new page.
- Insert the page numbers of major sections of the report and, if using lists of tables and figures, the page number on which each of these appear is inserted.
- Use the same system of numbering in the table of contents as used in the headings in the text; if, for example, Chapter 1 is used in the text, this should be used in the contents list. Ensure all parts of the report are included.
- If it is a longer report, some form of temporary or permanent binding will be required.
- Check the guidelines to ensure the report conforms with the requirements of the organisation. Check thoroughly for any errors.
- Check grammar and spelling.
- Double-check that the numbers in the tables and figures are accurate and that the numbering of pages and table and figure captions is correct. This is especially important if tables and figures have been moved around in the document.
- It is essential to check that all references are included and are formatted correctly according to the instructed reference style.
- Proofread before submitting the report to correct any remaining errors.

Preparing and presenting for a conference or seminar

Oral presentations

Researchers may be required to deliver an oral presentation of a report to an audience, such as a whole research class, or invited to present a paper at a seminar or conference after submitting an abstract for consideration by the conference organisers (Happell, 2008; Jerger, 2020; Reumann, 2012).

Preparation is essential for an oral presentation. A copy of the full report, preferably double-spaced in a larger typeface to enable easy and unobtrusive reading, can be used during the presentation. In most cases the researcher will be familiar with the topic and could use, for example, Microsoft PowerPoint speaker notes to allow for more eye contact with the audience. It is important to practise presenting the paper to colleagues, friends or relatives so that feedback can be provided. Practice also enables the person to gauge the timing and to become accustomed to using any equipment. Any questions or criticisms can be anticipated and a reply can be prepared.

The audience will not normally have access to the written paper at the time of the presentation, so clarity is essential. Visual aids are useful to add interest to oral presentations; PowerPoint presentations are the norm at professional conferences and can be embellished with special effects, including interesting transitions between slides and the separate introduction of individual points. Musical effects and hypertext links to Internet sites can be included, although the emphasis of the presentation is on content and not technology. Handouts for the audience can also be provided.

The major errors made with this type of media include having too much information on the slide, having too many slides or presenting type that is too small. The latter is usually a consequence of the former. A large font size should be selected with enough room on the slide to accommodate it. A general rule of presentations is to have six lines of text per slide and six words per line (Carnegie Coach, n.d.), or no more than seven lines of text on any slide. This is the limit for effectively communicating ideas during the brief time that a slide is presented. The size of the room should also be considered when creating the slides. If possible, the readability of the print from the back of the room should be checked before the presentation.

Oral presentations have time restriction and should not exceed the time allocated by the organisers. The presenter should be selective about what content to include and plan the timing, which should include time allowed for questions and responses; however, time may be allocated by the event organisers for this, so be sure to check the guidelines for the presentation.

The presentation should be organised in a logical manner, following a similar format to that of a written report. Audience members will be far more interested in the results and implications than in the literature review and methodology, so a brief introduction to the purpose of the study and any previous findings should be presented, with the main focus on results and the implications of the research. See Boullata and Mancuso (2007), Happell (2007, 2008, 2012) and Reumann (2012) for more detail on conference presentation. 'The exhaustive guide to preparing conference presentations', includes a number of great resources; for example, how to write a speech or how to design a presentation. This resource can be accessed from https://24slides.com/presentbetter/preparing-conference-presentation/

Preparing and presenting a poster

A poster is usually presented during the poster session of a conference. Posters are an important part of a conference program and provide an opportunity to communicate complex research results or clinical/educational developments or initiatives (Boullata & Mancuso, 2007; Erren & Bourne, 2007; Goldman & Schmalz, 2010; Grech, 2018; Miller, 2007).

The purpose of the poster presentation is to communicate the major points of the research project to a number of people who have the opportunity to talk to the researcher about the project. Usually there is a group of posters, with the presenters in attendance by their creations. The delegates walk around the room looking at the posters, stopping to talk to the researchers whose presentations interest them. The researchers can then discuss the finer details of their projects with the delegates. It is therefore imperative to capture their attention by ensuring the poster is readable from a distance of 1.5 metres (Lefor & Maeno, 2016).

A poster presentation can be described as a storyboard of information (Boullata & Mancuso, 2007; Miller, 2007). It is important to have a poster that will attract the attention of the delegates, so the title of the project should be read like a newspaper headline; that is, be snappy, stimulating and intriguing to encourage the reader to stop and review the poster (Grech, 2018)

A key approach when designing a poster is the KISS principle. Posters can provide publicity for the research and result in the presenter acquiring valuable ideas from colleagues. When developing a poster, strictly adhere to the conference organisers' guidelines.

TIP

Organise your poster on the KISS principle: Keep it short and simple. A good poster design should balance text and white space, only include two or three colours and only contain good quality images.

Text and images for a poster can be created using a computer program such as PowerPoint (see the example in Figure 12.4). If there are no financial constraints, the poster can be created using a graphics program and printed professionally. Elements of a poster should include:

- the title of the project
- name of the researcher
- purpose of the study
- research question
- method/methodology
- results
- conclusions
- implications.

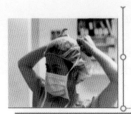

THE USE OF SCORING RUBRICS TO DETERMINE CLINICAL PERFORMANCE IN THE OPERATING SUITE

Project Description
Pat Nicholson, PhD Candidate, Graduate School of Education
The University of Melbourne

THE UNIVERSITY OF
MELBOURNE

Introduction-Aims

- This research evolved out of the need to design and validate an instrument for the assessment of competencies in the specialised area of the operating suite.
- Objectivity is difficult to achieve in the assessment of nursing competency, and while there are numerous tools available, the establishment of an effective measure remains illusive
- Due to the complexity of the specialty areas within nursing, there is a requirement for the assessment of competencies, in particular, the identification of knowledge, skills and attributes required of the specialist nurse
- There is little empirical nursing research into factors that influence the reliability and validity of assessment tools

The aim of this study was to examine the validity and inter-rater reliability of a set of performance-based scoring rubrics that were designed to measure the competency '*the instrument nurse*'

Research questions

- To what extent are ratings of the nurse educators consistent when using analytical and holistic rubrics to judge the performance levels of perioperative nurses?
- What is the relationship between perceived competence and performance levels as defined by the Dreyfuss Model of Skill Acquisition?
- Does the use of analytical scoring rubrics in determining varying levels of clinical performance produce sufficient measures of inter-rater reliability?
- What are the psychometric properties of the Analytical Observation Form?

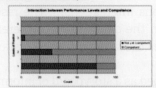

Methodology

Quasi-experimental design
- Instrument development (ACORN NR4 standard, 2006)
  - Analytical Observation Form
  - Holistic Performance Level Rubrics & Competence Rubrics
- Development of video clips (3) of instrument nurses in the operating suite used as a prompts for the survey
- Quantitative data – Survey method involving nurse educators observing video clips using the Rubrics (n = 40)
- Calibration of the Instrument using the Item Response Modelling (IRM) (Rash, 1960)

Sample of Item Scoring Rubric from the Analytical Observation Form

Item	Quality Indicator				
	0	1	2	3	4
Demonstrates knowledge of legal aspects of perioperative nursing practice	Not observed	Verifies correct patient identification	Verifies correct procedure including correct site / side	Verifies consent and patient identification according to approved protocol	Liaises with multidisciplinary team members about legal aspect of perioperative care against patient assessment and admission data

Results

Acceptable reliability estimates were achieved, as well as empirical support for content, construct and criterion validity for the Performance Based Scoring Rubric;
In exploring the relationship between the demographic factors of the raters and rating accuracy, only one background factor was found to be significant.

Interaction between Performance Levels and Competence

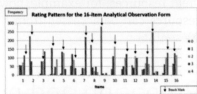

Conclusions / Implications

Rating Pattern for the 16-item Analytical Observation Form (N=313)

- The Holistic Rubrics led to more consistent judgement than the Analytical Observation Form
- The Analytical Observation Form had sufficient construct reliability as determined by the Item Separation Index
- Greater inter-rater reliability could be improved if the average ratings of multiple assessors is used

Key References

Gonczi, A. (1994). Competency based assessment in the professions in Australia Assessment in Education: Principles, policy and practice 1(1), 27 - 44.

Nicholson, P., Gillis, S., & Dunning, T. (2009). The use of scoring rubrics to determine clinical performance in the operating suite Nurse Education Today, 29, 73 - 82.

Nicholson, P., Griffin, P., Gillis, S., Wu, M., & Dunning, T. Measuring nursing competencies: Instrument development and psychometric analysis using Item Response Theory. Nurse Education Today, 33, 1088 – 1093.

Contact Details:

[Name]

[Organisation]

[email]

Photo

▶ Figure 12.4 Poster design

Source: Nicholson, P. (2011). Measuring nursing competencies in the operating theatre: conceptualisation, instrument development, and psychometric analysis using Item Response theory. Unpublished doctoral thesis. Graduate School of Education, The University of Melbourne.

The poster should have visual appeal with a strong impact that will enable the researcher to get the main points across without being wordy. It is important to remember that less is more. The most common mistake is including too much information on the poster. A small amount of text that stands out is acceptable, but most of the space should be filled with well-designed illustrations (Grech, 2018; Miller, 2007).

The poster should be easy to read from a distance of about 1.5 metres, which will encourage people to stop at the display. Letters need to be at least 2.5 centimetres high, which is on average a 72-point font. Information presented as bullet points is easier to read than paragraphs and should take less than 10 minutes to read (Grech, 2018). Remember that people are unlikely to bend down to read any material that is below knee level.

The contrast of colours, including those used for the type, should be pleasing; however, too many colours should be avoided as they may overwhelm the viewer.

Care should be taken when transporting a poster to a conference. It should be packed in a tube and carried during the journey. It may become lost when travelling by air if it is checked in with the luggage.

Many conferences now include electronic posters in conference proceedings, so hard copies are no longer required, eliminating the burden of expensive printing costs. There are many sites that offer free programs for developing an electronic poster; for example, http://www.posterpresentations.com/html/free_poster_templates.html.

After submitting a poster abstract, if accepted, details about the poster presentation will be provided by the conference organising committee including (Grech, 2018):

- the required poster size with height and width clearly specified
- instructions for set-up including date, time and venue
- instructions for timing of the poster session, when the presenter is expected to attend the poster for viewing and discussion by a judging panel
- when the poster must be removed from the poster display area.
  Common errors that are made when preparing a poster include (Grech, 2018):
- the objective/main point of the poster is not instantly obvious
- the text is too small
- poor quality graphics
- poorly organised poster components
- chaotic or an untidy layout of material
- use of too much colour (8% of males are colourblind)
- a dark or black background.

More detail about the content and format of posters can be found in Scarsbrook and colleagues (2006), Grech (2018), Lefor & Maeno (2016), Briggs (2009), Erren and Bourne (2007), Goldman and Schmalz (2010), Ickes and Gambescia (2011) and Miller (2007).

Journal articles and monographs

Research is also intended for public consumption so that it can be scrutinised and have beneficial effects. An important feature of scholarship is inviting the open discussion and critique of original work to verify the usefulness or otherwise of the new information it presents. Although research is open to anyone who shows interest in it, targeting the people most directly associated with it makes the most sense. Effective ways of doing so are through journal articles and **monographs**.

Writing a journal article

The prerequisites

Journals are a medium for communication, and in healthcare fields there are many opportunities to choose a journal that is best able to communicate the results of a research project. There are journals that represent different disciplines, so taking the audience into consideration is important when selecting a journal.

The authors' guide is usually found on the inside front or back cover of the journal, or on what is called the 'imprint page', located on the second or fourth page. Most journals also have guidelines for authors on their website. Notes to contributors are a practical guide from the journal editor as to what is expected of an author in preparing a manuscript for submission. A copy should be accessed and used as a guide when writing the article. The original research report that documents the whole of the research will need to be adjusted to suit the requirements of the journal. There are also word limits for categories of articles that should be noted. Once a journal has been identified, it is important to check the type of articles that have been published, as well as how they have been structured, to increase the chance of having an article accepted for publication.

The writing phase

The manuscript should be prepared to present the information the researcher views as being important in the article. A synopsis of the entire project may be presented, or certain themes or sections from the project may be extracted and elaborated in the article.

If a synopsis of the entire project is being presented, one of the challenges will be keeping to the word limit, which means decisions will have to be made about what content to remove from the manuscript. It is important to ensure the essential features of the project remain intact according to the particular approach taken. A reference on critiquing research, such as this book, can be used to guide the process. This will give an indication of what clinicians are looking for when they read research articles.

If certain parts of the project are extracted for further elaboration, it is worth spending time to decide how this will be done. Clearly identify the focus of the article and consider whether it is a good fit with the current content of the journal being considered for submission. When extracting the section from the research report it will need a new introduction, some extra work in the body of the text and an appropriate conclusion.

Final preparations

The final article must comply with the journal's requirements for content and format. Ideas should flow between sections, and the discussion and conclusion sections should be well substantiated. When the writing phase is over, check for spelling and grammatical errors. The manuscript should follow the journal's referencing conventions and be set out clearly with appropriate headings and subheadings. When the manuscript is ready for submission, colleagues should be approached to read for content, grammar, flow of ideas and any adjustments to the manuscript made according to their feedback. Other details as specified, such as a title page and contact details, must be added and checked for correctness.

A cover letter is included with the article, which is submitted online. Feedback from reviewers will be provided once the article has been reviewed to direct any amendments that are required before the article is published. An alternative outcome may inform the researcher that the manuscript is not suitable for publication in that particular journal. In this case, once the article has been reviewed and the feedback received has been incorporated, the manuscript can then be submitted to another journal. With a few amendments, the article may meet the requirements of another journal.

Two excellent starting points for further reading to learn more about publishing in journals are Busse and August (2020), Lefor (2015), Swann (2009) and Johnson and Green (2009).

> **TIP**
>
> Don't take rejections too much to heart, and above all, don't give up.

Writing a monograph

Definitions for a monograph differ, but it is generally agreed that a monograph is smaller than a book, usually presented as a soft-cover A5 (half an A4) document that contains approximately 50 pages. It is usual for academic organisations to have their own printing facilities that publish their own monographs.

Preparing a monograph appears to be a larger task than preparing for submission to a journal, yet in some ways it can be easier. For one thing, the word limit will be larger so it is easier to present the research intact. Having completed much of the work required for a report, the content can be transferred to the monograph. It will then be a matter of setting out the text in a way that gives the manuscript a good flow of ideas. Once this is done, areas for further elaboration are identified as the main foci for writing.

As is the case with writing for any other publication, it is important to follow the publisher's requirements and thoroughly check and recheck before submission. A copy is then sent to the publisher with a covering letter. Once feedback has been received, adjustments should be made as directed by the publisher. If the manuscript is not appropriate for publication by that publisher, consider submitting the document elsewhere. Rejection is not a comment directed at a person, it is a comment about a piece of written work and what changes are required for it to be published.

Using social media

Communicating research outcomes using a network of social media platforms has provided new opportunities for researchers to disseminate their work (Willis, 2020). A wide range of social media platforms are available to facilitate two-way interactions and allow for dissemination of information (Collins, Shiffman & Rock, 2016), with each platform working in different ways (Willis, 2020). The choice of social media ultimately depends on the utility of the platform and personal preference, with many researchers using social media to facilitate the exchange of knowledge within and among researcher communities, as well as engage with the public (Collins, Shiffman & Rock, 2016).

Common reasons for using social media include (The Research Impact Academy, n.d.):
- sharing ideas
- recognition and exposure of research projects
- access to other areas of research

- opportunities to engage with other audiences (government, service provision, industry experts, policy makers, the public)
- building connections with funders, and industry partners
- availability of tools to and platforms to make processes more collaborative and easier.

▶ Table 12.2   Social media platforms

Facebook	Useful for presenting and discussing research (Willis, 2020)
ResearchGate	Social networking site for scientists and researchers to share research articles, ask and answer questions and find collaborators (Webster, 2016)
Twitter	An interactive social media platform that health researchers use to capture data about health topics or for study recruitment or interventions (Sinnenberg et al., 2017)
LinkedIn	Primarily used for professional networking and developing networks or research specific groups offering a place to communicate about projects
Google Scholar	A simple way of collating publications (and citations) so that the work can be accessed and cited by potential collaborators or other published articles of interest can be accessed

SUMMARY

This chapter discussed the importance of research findings and how to disseminate them, which is the final step in the research cycle.

1	Explain the purpose of preparing a research report	• The purpose of a research report is to communicate key aspects of the project to research consumers so that they can: — replicate the study — undertake a literature review — plan a new study — help find a solution for a clinical practice problem
2	Describe how to write a research report	• When writing a report the writing style is generally the same as for a research proposal: — identify the target audience — develop a plan before writing the report — write in a concise, clear and coherent style — use good English language and avoid jargon — write in the past tense — avoid using passive voice — check spelling and grammar • Content includes: — preliminaries, which introduce the report — body of the report, which contains the main information — supporting materials, which includes references and appendices • Submission of a research report: — access the authors' guide — adhere to the format and style of the journal
3	Identify the elements of a quantitative and qualitative research report	• The structure of a quantitative report is the same as for the proposal: — preliminaries — introduction — methodology and methods — include results, discussion and conclusions • A qualitative report has many similarities with a quantitative report, including a research plan that covers methodology, methods and processes
4	Explain how to prepare and present a conference or seminar presentation	• In developing oral presentations: — consider the audience — be dynamic and interesting — use visual aids — prepare and practise — keep to time during the presentation
5	Explain how to prepare and present a poster	• Posters communicate the major points of the research project to colleagues, and give them an opportunity to talk to the researcher. • In preparing a poster: — adhere strictly to the guidelines — create visual appeal and impact • Elements of a poster are: — title of the project — name of the researcher — purpose of the study — research question — method/methodology — results — conclusions — implications

6	Describe how to write a journal article for publication	• Select the target journal • Obtain and follow the journal author guidelines • Prepare the manuscript • Submit the article with a covering letter to the editor • Colleagues should be approached to read for content, grammar and flow of ideas • Other details as specified, such as a title page and contact details, must be added and checked for correctness
7	Describe how to prepare monographs	• Present the manuscript in its best possible version • Incorporate feedback from colleagues before submitting the document

REVIEW QUESTIONS

1 Outline the common features of both a qualitative and a quantitative report.
2 Discuss how you would prepare a research project article for peer review.
3 Explain how you would prepare a poster for a conference presentation.
4 Explain how you would develop a conference presentation that would include graphs and tables in the presentation.

CHALLENGING REVIEW QUESTIONS

1 You have recently submitted your honours thesis and your supervisor now expects you to start writing an article for publication. Having never published before, you are unsure of the process involved. Discuss how you are going to write the article and what resources are necessary to guide the process.
2 You are required to submit a research report to the funding body who provided funding for the project. Explain what information should be included in the report and discuss how this information will be presented.

CASE STUDY 1

Prisha is an undergraduate nursing student beginning her third year. Prisha is considering her options for a graduate position after she completes her course. As a student nurse, Prisha is aware that stress and burnout are important considerations for hospital nurses and would like to ensure she is fully prepared.

Prisha's friend, who is a student midwife, has experienced hostile and aggressive patients and their families while on clinical placement at the women's hospital. Prisha and her friend have been discussing how research into this unfortunate workplace experience (Hasan & Tumah, 2019) could be disseminated.

1 What considerations should you make before disseminating research?
2 What are the important factors to consider when publishing a quantitative research article?
3 Can you find any research related to student nurse/midwife experiences of hostile and aggressive persons on the variety of social media platforms? Are the authors Hasan and Tumah on professional social media?

CASE STUDY 2

In this case study, we return to Angela, a physiotherapist in a multidisciplinary team in a large city hospital (introduced in Chapter 4 and last read about in Chapter 7). Angela is enrolled in a Master of Physiotherapy Studies and is interested in the issue of elderly women's invisibility to the multidisciplinary team. She has used a mixed-method approach to explore the issue, collect the necessary evidence and analyse the qualitative data. She has just been given approval to present her findings at an international conference in England and must now prepare her paper.

1   Describe the key points that Angela should consider when preparing her oral presentation.

2   Explain what visual aids could be included in the presentation.

3   Identify the mistakes presenters make when preparing an oral presentation.

REFERENCES

Adams, S., Farrington, M., & Cullen, L. (2012). Evidence into practice: Publishing an evidence-based practice project. *Journal of PeriAnesthesia Nursing, 27*(3), 193–202.

Bavdekar, S. B. (2015). Writing the discussion section: Describing the significance of the study findings. *Journal of Association of Physicians of India, 63*, 40–2.

Blake, G., & Bly, R.W. (2000). *The Elements of Technical Writing.* United States: Pearson Education.

Boullata, B., & Manusco, C. (2007). A 'how-to' guide in preparing abstracts and poster presentations. *Nutrition in Clinical Practice, 22*, 641–6.

Briggs, B. J. (2009). A practical guide to designing a poster for presentation. *Nursing Standard, 23*(34), 35–9.

Busse, C., & August, E. (2020). How to write and publish a research paper for a peer-reviewed journal. *Journal of Cancer Education.* https://doi.org/10.1007/s13187-020-01751-z

Button, K. S., Ioannidis, J. A., Mokrysz, C., Nosek, B. A., Flint, J., Robinson, E. J., & Munafò, M. R. (2013). Power failure: Why small sample size undermines the reliability of neuroscience. *Nature Reviews Neuroscience, 14*(5), 365–76.

Carnegie Coach (n.d.). 2 ways to avoid death by PowerPoint. http://carnegiecoach.com/avoid-death-by-powerpoint/

Collins, K., Shiffman, D., & Rock, J. (2016). How are scientists using social media in the workplace? *PLoS ONE, 11*(10), 1–10. https://doi.org/10.1371/journal.pone.0162680

Erren, T. C., & Bourne, P. E. (2007). Ten simple rules for a good poster presentation. *PLoS Computational Biology, 3*(5), e102.

Goldman, K., & Schmalz, K. (2010). Poster session fundamentals: Becoming a proficient 'poster child' for health education. *Health Promotion Practice, 11*(4), 445–9.

Grech, V. (2018). WASP (Write a Scientific Paper): Preparing a poster. *Early Human Development, 125*, 57–9. https://doi.org/10.1016/j.earlhumdev.2018.06.007

Happell, B. (2007). Conference presentations: Developing nursing knowledge by disseminating research findings. *Nurse Researcher, 15*(1), 70–7.

Happell, B. (2008). Conference presentations: A guide to writing the abstract. *Nurse Researcher, 15*(4), 79–87.

Happell, B. (2012). A practical guide to writing clinical articles for publications. *Nursing Older People, 24*(3), 30–4.

Hasan, A. A., & Tumah, H. (2019). The correlation between occupational stress, coping strategies and the levels of psychological distress among nurses working in mental health hospital in Jordan. *Perspectives in Psychiatric Care, 55*, 153–60. https://doi.10.1111/ppc.12292

Hoogenboom, B. J. & Manske, R. C. (2012). Invited commentary: How to write a scientific article. *The International Journal of Sports Physical Therapy, 7*(5), 512–17.

Ickes, M. J., & Gambescia, S. F. (2011). Abstract art: How to write competitive conference and journal abstracts. *Health Promotion Practice, 12*(4), 493–6.

Jerger, J. (2020). How to give a better Powerpoint talk: Dr Jerger's 9 rules for a more effective slide presentation. *The Hearing Review, 2*, 16.

Johnson, C., & Green, B. (2009). Submitting manuscripts to biomedical journals: Common errors and helpful solutions. *Journal of Manipulative Physiology Therapy*, *32*, 1–12.

Ketefian, S. (2018). Editorial: Why do we do research and publish? *Pacific Rim International Journal of Nursing Research*, *22*(2), 91–2.

King, M. G., Semciw, A. I., Schache, A. G., Middleton, K. J., Heerey, J. J., Sritharan, P., Scholes, M. J., Mentipay, B. F., & Crossley, K. M. (2020). Lower-limb biomechanics in football players with and without hip-related pain. *Medicine & Science in Sports & Exercise*, *52*(8), 1776–84.

Labani, S., Wadhwa, K., & Asthana, S. (2017). Basic approach to data analysis and writing of results and discussion sections. *MAMC Journal of Medical Sciences*, *1*.

Lambie, G., Sias, S., Davis, K., Lawson, G., & Akos, P. (2008). A scholarly writing resource for counselor educators and their students. *Journal of Counseling & Development*, *86*, p. 21.

Lefor, A. K., & Maeno, M. (2016). Preparing scientific papers, posters, and slides. *Journal of Surgical Education*, *73*(2), 286–90. https://doi.org/10.1016/j.jsurg.2015.09.020

Marriott, R., Reibel, T., Coffin, J., Gliddon, J., Griffin, D., Robinson, M., Eades, A.-M., & Maddox, J. (2019). 'Our culture, how it is to be us': Listening to Aboriginal women about on Country urban birthing. *Women & Birth*, *32*(5), 391–403.

Marriott, R., Reibel, T., Gliddon, J., Griffin, D., Coffin, J., Eades, A.-M., Robinson, M., Bowen, A., Kendall, S., Martin, T., Monterosso, L., Stanley, F., & Walker, R. (2019). Aboriginal research methods and researcher reflections on working two-ways to investigate culturally secure birthing for Aboriginal women [online]. *Australian Aboriginal Studies*, *32*, 36–53.

Mellis, C. (2017). Mini-symposium: Interpreting clinical research: Lies, damned lies and statistics: Clinical importance versus statistical significance in research. *Paediatric Respiratory Reviews*, doi:10.1016/j.prrv.2017.02.002.

Miller, J. E. (2007). Preparing and presenting effective research posters. *HSR: Health Services Research*, *42*(1), 311–28.

Pearson, A., Jordan, Z., Lockwood, C., & Aromataris, E. (2015). Notions of quality and standards for qualitative research reporting. *International Journal of Nursing Practice*, *21*(5), 670–6.

Reumann, M. (2012). Preparing for conferences-basic presentation skills [GOLD]. *IEEE Pulse*, *3*(3), 6–12. https://doi.org/10.1109/MPUL.2012.2189645

Sanganyado, E. (2019). How to write an honest but effective abstract for scientific papers. *Scientific African*, *6*. https://doi.org/10.1016/j.sciaf.2019.e00170

Scarsbrook, A. F., Graham, R. N. J., & Perriss, R. W. (2006). Expanding the use of Microsoft PowerPoint. An overview for radiologists. *Clinical Radiology*, *61*(2), 113–23. https://doi.org/10.1016/j.crad.2005.10.004

Sinnenberg, L., Buttenheim, A.M., Padrez, K., Mancheno, C., Ungar, L., & Merchant, R M. (2017). Twitter as a tool for health research: A systematic review. *American Journal of Public Health*, *107*(1), e1–8.

Smagorinsky, P. (2008). The method section as conceptual epicenter in constructing social science research reports. *Written Communication*, *25*(3), 389–411.

Swann, J. (2009). Writing for publication: Sharing ideas and information. *Nursing & Residential Care*, *11*(4), 204–6.

The Research Impact Academy. (n.d.). Top 4 social platforms for researchers – what, why and how. https://researchimpactacademy.com/

Webster, P. (2016). Gaining the benefits of scholarly social networks. *IATUL Annual Conference Proceedings*, *37*, 95–104.

Willis, P. (2020). How social media can create impact for research. *Australian Zoologist*, *40*(3), 462–7. https://doi.org/10.7882/AZ.2019.020

FURTHER READINGS

Bailey, S., & Handu, D. (2012). *Introduction to Epidemiologic Research Methods in Public Health Practice*. Burlington, MA: James & Bartlett Learning.

Jackson, K., & Bazeley, P. (2019). *Qualitative Data Analysis with NVivo* (3rd edition.). Thousand Oaks: SAGE.

Pallant, J. F. (2020). *SPSS Survival Manual: A Step by Step Guide to Data Analysis using IBM SPSS* (7th edition.). Allen & Unwin.

Wager, E. (2009). Why you should not submit your work to more than one journal at a time. *African Journal of Traditional Complementary and Alternative Medicines*, *7*(2), 160–1.

13 EVIDENCE-BASED PRACTICE

Chapter learning objectives

The material presented in this chapter will assist you to:

1 define evidence-based practice
2 describe the steps and skills necessary for evidence-based practice
3 describe the relationship between research, practice and education
4 apply research to clinical practice
5 examine the barriers to applying research findings to practice
6 describe strategies for educating clinicians about evidence-based practice.

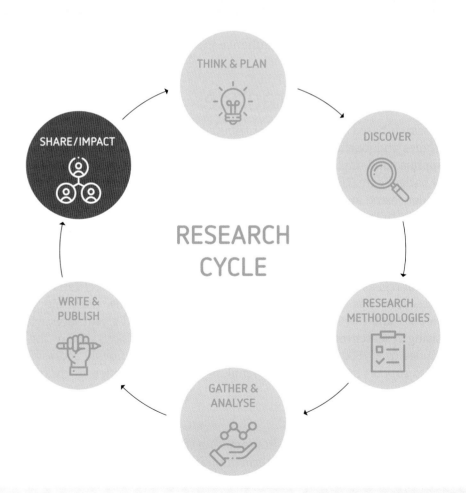

Research cycle

The primary focus of this chapter is evidence-based practice (EBP), describing its origins, the definitions and criteria used when judging levels of evidence, and how research can be implemented into practice. The clinical use of research in practice is highlighted in the research framework diagram above.

Introduction

This last chapter of the book focuses on using evidence accessed from research and applying it to practice. In writing this chapter, certain assumptions have been made:

- evidence-based practice (EBP) bases current practice on research
- it is not always easy for clinicians to apply research outcomes in their practice
- senior clinicians and educators need to use research in their work to show clinicians how to become consumers of research.

With these assumptions in mind, this chapter provides strategies for applying research findings, through practices such as national governance, the establishment of effective change measures and **clinical practice guidelines**. Policy and procedure manuals are also described as a means of ensuring that research guides practice. A number of barriers to research utilisation in clinical practice have been identified, including lack of time and the need for further education about the use of research (Lehane et al., 2019; Hewitt-Taylor, Heaslip & Rowe, 2012); therefore, accessibility should be facilitated to increase evidence utilisation. Some strategies to increase accessibility include creating a **research culture** in clinical settings, enhancing research–practice links and undertaking collaborative interdisciplinary research.

If research is to be used in clinical settings, education that prepares clinicians for research-based practice is necessary. This chapter offers strategies to assist educators prepare evidence-based clinicians and enhance their own teaching strategies.

Evidence-based practice

Although research-based evidence has contributed to clinical decisions, the proliferation of research studies and journal publications presents a challenge for clinicians to be able to critically appraise and implement evidence that supports best possible treatment options and quality patient care. This highlights the importance of clinicians being about to source scientific evidence and apply it to their practice.

Dr Archie Cochrane, a British epidemiologist and visionary leader, founded the EBP movement. In his publication 'Effectiveness and efficiency' (Cochrane, 1972), Cochrane strongly criticised commonly accepted healthcare interventions that were not supported by reliable evidence. Although not achieved in his life time, the importance of developing an international register of randomised controlled trials and explicit criteria for appraising published research was strongly advocated by Cochrane. The Cochrane Centre was launched in 1992 and the Cochrane Collaboration was founded a year later, with the goal of synthesising research evidence to inform healthcare decisions. Today the Cochrane Library includes over 7500 Cochrane systematic reviews that provide accessible, credible information to support informed decision making in clinical practice (Cochrane, n.d.).

Research and practice

Perhaps the most powerful influence in promoting the use of research in clinical practice has been the introduction of EBP. As the term implies, EBP bases current practice on research evidence, which has evolved from a scientifically grounded evidence-based medicine (EBM) model (Thoma & Eaves, 2015). The most common definition, developed by Dr David Sackett, a physician considered to be the father of EBM, describes it as 'the conscientious, explicit, and judicious use of current best evidence in making decisions about the care of individual patients' (Sackett et al., 1996, p. 71). This is further elaborated to include the importance individual expertise, including the proficiency and judgement that is acquired through clinical experience and clinical practice as well as taking into consideration the patients' values (Sackett et al., 1996).

A number of definitions of EBP can be found in the literature with a contemporary definition provided by Melnyk and colleagues (2010). Evidence-based practice is defined as:

> a problem-solving approach to the delivery of healthcare that integrates best evidence from studies and patient care data with clinician expertise and patient preferences and values. When delivered in a contest of caring and in a supportive organizational culture, the highest quality of care and best patient outcomes can be achieved.

(Melnyk et al., 2010, p. 51)

The EBP triad illustrates an approach to decision making that integrates the clinician's clinical expertise with the best available research-based evidence while taking into account the patient's values and expectation of care (see Figure 13.1).

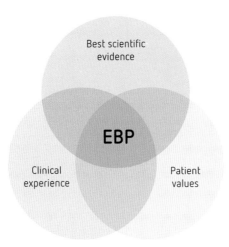

▶ **Figure 13.1**   Evidence-based practice triad

Source: The Regents of the University of California, Davis campus. Available for re-use under CC BY.

This definition prompts the following questions.
- What is the best possible evidence?
- How is the evidence evaluated and critiqued?
- Why is it necessary to critique the evidence?
- How can the evidence be applied?
- Under what circumstances can the evidence be used?

Clinicians who are curious about using the best possible evidence to guide their clinical decisions are unlikely to support EBP in an unsupportive healthcare culture. In fact, in an effort to accelerate the use of EBP by clinicians, hospitals are no longer being reimbursed for treating preventable hospital-acquired injuries or infections, such as pressure injuries. Healthcare providers are therefore required to develop a comprehensive approach to measuring quality patient outcomes and support an EBP environment (Melnyk et al., 2009).

Figure 13.2 presents EBP within the context of caring and EBP culture.

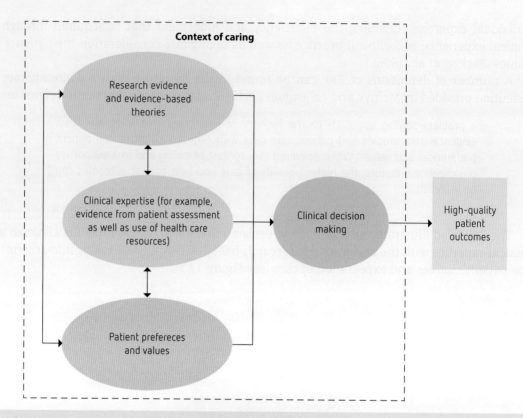

▶ **Figure 13.2** Evidence-based practice organisational culture

Source: Adapted with permission from Wolters Kluwer Health, Inc.: Melnyk, B. M., Fineout-Overholt, E., Stillwell, S. B., et al., Evidence-Based Practice: Step by Step: Igniting a Spirit of Inquiry, *American Journal of Nursing*, *109*(11), pp 49–52, doi: 10.1097/01.NAJ.0000363354.53883.58

Dawes (2005, p. 4) suggests that EBP 'aims to provide the best possible evidence at the point of clinical (or management) contact'. Implicit in the definitions of EBP is the use of research in decision making about patient care. Evidence-based clinical practice is the incorporation of 'the 'best' research evidence 'blended with approved policies and clinical practice guidelines, clinical expertise and judgment, and patient preferences' (Penz & Bassendowski, 2006, p. 250). In other words, EBP involves clinical decision making that uses the best research evidence and practice knowledge available to provide patient-centred care. This requires that clinicians can locate, evaluate, interpret and then apply evidence to their practice. In the current healthcare arena, the demand for transparency, accountability and efficiency is increasing, therefore paving the way for EBP (Cookson, 2005).

ACTIVITY

Think about your professional group and discuss with colleagues the extent to which clinicians use research to inform their practice.

Origins

Although EBP has been established in medicine for decades, with the increasing public and professional demand for accountability, the impact of EBP has echoed across allied health disciplines. The United States medical profession began to develop EBM after a study reported that few current medical procedures had been shown by clinical trials to be effective. It was also stimulated by evidence of substantial variation in clinical practice patterns, increased financial pressure and the difficulty that clinicians have in incorporating rapidly evolving evidence into their practice.

The medical profession has set up an international initiative to facilitate the retrieval and synthesis of literature relevant to EBP. The Cochrane Collaboration, based in Oxford, has established specialised databases of systematic reviews to promote EBP. These reviews are disseminated through medical journals and the internet. There are Cochrane Centres in several countries, including Canada, the United States and Australia. EBM has grown rapidly in the United Kingdom, Canada and the United States. It is a growth industry that has almost become a medical specialty on its own and includes the establishment of the *Journal of Evidence-based Medicine*.

The **Joanna Briggs Institute (JBI)** was established in Adelaide to promote evidence-based nursing practice, initially by the production and dissemination of systematic reviews through best-practice sheets (Perry, 2006). Similarly, the New Zealand Centre for Evidence-based Nursing (NZCEBN) was established by Auckland Healthcare and Auckland University, in collaboration with JBI, to provide evidence-based information for practice (Lu, 2008).

Nevertheless, some notes of caution have been sounded. Holmes and colleagues (2006) suggest that the Cochrane Collaboration, among others, has created a hierarchy that has been endorsed by many academic institutions and that serves to (re)produce the exclusion of certain forms of research. Because regimes of truth, such as the evidence-based movement, currently enjoy a privileged status, scholars not only have a scientific duty, but also an ethical obligation to deconstruct these regimes of power. Koehn and Lehman (2008) and Nolan (2008) have found clinicians hesitant to implement findings from populations and settings different to their own.

EBP has become firmly established in the United States, most of Western Europe, including the United Kingdom, and many countries in the southern hemisphere, including Australia and New Zealand. Key EBP organisations are the National Institute of Clinical Studies (NICS), the JBI, Cochrane Collaboration, the National Institute for Health and Care Excellence (NICE), the Agency for Healthcare Research and Quality (AHRQ), the Canadian Centre for Evidence-based Nursing (CCEBN) and the New Zealand Guidelines Group (NZGG).

Sackett and colleagues (1996) have attributed the worldwide spread of EBP to the need for research-based clinical decisions, guidelines and protocols, and the knowledge explosion in new journals, and among the general public, in preference to textbook information. Finding the evidence involves the logistics of a literature search, including the databases to be searched, the people to do the work and the assistance anticipated from librarians. Finding the evidence also includes conducting the literature search, which is a complex and skilful undertaking performed by people experienced in the activity. Appraisal of the evidence is also required to be undertaken according to specific criteria.

Evidence-based practice criteria

The Australian National Health and Medical Research Council (NHMRC) provides a guide for developing, implementing and evaluating clinical practice guidelines (CPGs), to support the inclusion of best possible evidence in the recommendations (NHMRC, 1999). Table 13.1 indicates the levels of evidence that are preferred when developing EBP guidelines, from the highest, most valued (Level I) to the lowest, least valued (Level IV).

▶ **Table 13.1** Guidelines for the development, implementation and evaluation of clinical practice

Level I	Evidence obtained from a systematic review of all relevant randomised controlled trials (RCTs)
Level II	Evidence obtained from at least one properly designed randomised controlled trial
Level III–I	Evidence obtained from well-designed pseudorandomised controlled trials (alternate allocation or some other method)
Level III–II	Evidence obtained from comparative studies with concurrent controls and allocation not randomised (cohort studies), case-control studies or interrupted time-series with a control group
Level III–III	Evidence obtained from comparative studies with historical control, two or more single arm studies or interrupted time-series without a parallel control group
Level IV	Evidence obtained from case series (either post-test or pretest and post-test)

Source: National Health and Medical Research Council (NHMRC) (1999). *A Guide to the Development, Implementation and Evaluation of Clinical Practice Guidelines.* Canberra: Australian Government Publishing Service, p. 56.

The levels shown in this table indicate the types of research that are deemed the best sources of information, with quantitative research methods dominating because of their fit with the generation and validation of biomedical science. EBP grew out of the discipline of medicine and therefore reflects biomedical values about what constitutes knowledge that can be valued and trusted. Historically, nurses have found that the limited qualitative research data as evidence has impacted on their use of EBP, a deficit that the JBI has attempted to address. A hierarchy of four levels of evidence, which is inclusive of qualitative research under the acronym FAME (as outlined in Table 13.2), was developed by JBI (and has since been updated), so that clinicians can make a preliminary judgement on the methodological quality and rigour of the evidence according to feasibility, appropriateness, meaningfulness and effectiveness.

▶ **Table 13.2** The Joanna Briggs Institute levels of evidence

Levels of evidence	Feasibility F (1–4)	Appropriateness A (1–4)	Meaningfulness M (1–4)	Effectiveness E (1–4)
1	Metasynthesis of research with unequivocal synthesised findings	Metasynthesis of research with unequivocal synthesised findings	Metasynthesis of research with unequivocal synthesised findings	Meta-analysis (with homogeneity) of experimental studies (e.g. RCT with concealed randomisation) OR one or more large experimental studies with narrow confidence intervals

Levels of evidence	Feasibility F (1–4)	Appropriateness A (1–4)	Meaningfulness M (1–4)	Effectiveness E (1–4)
2	Metasynthesis of research with credible synthesised findings	Metasynthesis of research with credible synthesised findings	Metasynthesis of research with credible synthesised findings	One or more smaller RCTs with wider confidence intervals OR quasi-experimental studies (without randomisation)
3	Metasynthesis of text/opinion with credible synthesised findings One or more single research studies of high quality	Metasynthesis of text/opinion with credible synthesised findings One or more single research studies of high quality	Metasynthesis of text/opinion with credible synthesised findings One or more single research studies of high quality	Cohort studies (with control group) Case-controlled Observational studies (without control group)
4	Expert opinion	Expert opinion	Expert opinion	Expert opinion, physiology bench research or consensus

Source: The Joanna Briggs Institute Levels of Evidence and Grades of Recommendation Working Party (2014). Supporting Document for the Joanna Briggs Institute Levels of Evidence and Grades of Recommendation. The Joanna Briggs Institute. https://wkhealth.force.com/ovidsupport/s/article/The-JBI-Hierarchy-of-Evidence-Model-FAME-1489081397984. The latest versions of JBI resources can be found at: https://jbi-global-wiki.refined.site/space/JED/2089386646/Resources,+Forms+and+Templates. Reproduced with permission.

Even though the overwhelming consensus is that EBP is essential for current practice, busy clinicians have many pressures competing for their attention. Numerous barriers to the implementation of research evidence into practice have been presented in the literature (Bonner, 2008; Hewitt-Taylor, Heaslip & Rowe, 2012; Higgins et al., 2010; Houlston, 2012; Johnston et al., 2016; Jordan, Bowers & Morton, 2016; Lu, 2008; Majid et al., 2011; Penz & Bassendowski, 2006; Sherriff, Wallis & Chaboyer, 2007). These barriers have been reported at a personal, professional and organisational level (Johnston et al., 2016). The predominant barriers included time factors, inadequate resources to access information, lack of familiarity with EBP and the complexity of research reports, clinicians' research knowledge and critical appraisal skills, resistance to change and the current healthcare culture. Time constraints, especially when facing the demands of patient caseloads and staff shortages, are also mentioned.

ACTIVITY

Ask your co-workers how they would define evidence-based practice and whether they think it is implemented in their clinical settings.

Busy clinicians have many pressures competing for their attention; if they are required to base their practice on recent research, practical strategies should be implemented in the clinical context to ensure that EBP happens. If clinicians ignore, avoid or otherwise obstruct EBP, no research-based practice changes will occur. As noted above, a number of authors have identified factors that contribute to clinical nurses conducting research as well as implementing research findings in their practice (Bonner, 2008; Hewitt-Taylor, Heaslip & Rowe, 2012; Higgins et al., 2010; Houlston, 2012; Lu, 2008; Majid et al., 2011; Penz & Bassendowski, 2006; Sherriff, Wallis & Chaboyer, 2007). Challenges and uptake of evidence in allied health disciplines have also been identified (Ekeland, Bergem & Myklebust, 2019; Foster et al., 2015; Grimmer et al., 2004; Haider, Dunstan & Bhullar, 2019).

Various research uptake and change strategies are discussed in the literature, including national governance (Griffiths & Clark, 2004), health policy (Grady & Hinshaw, 2017; Regan et al., 2015), the establishment of effective change measures (Dawes et al., 2005; Fairbrother, Jones & Rivas, 2010) and CPGs (Taylor et al., 2010; Turner et al., 2019).

ACTIVITY

Explain why it is difficult for clinicians to use research to guide their practice.

If clinicians are required to base their practice on recent research, practical strategies need to be implemented in the clinical context to ensure that the delivery of care is based on quality research-based evidence.

The steps of evidence-based practice

Although researchers have described the importance and process of EBP, less has been written about how to integrate evidence into practice. Melnyk and colleagues (2010) describe a multistep EBP process that provides clinicians with the resources to successfully integrate evidence at the point of care. These steps are detailed in the following sections.

Step 0: Cultivate a spirit of inquiry

This step refers to an ongoing curiosity about the best evidence that should be used to guide clinical decision making. Questions include whether an intervention is necessary (e.g. preoperative fasting among surgical patients), whether the evidence supports a clinical practice such as 2-hourly vital signs or if there is better evidence supporting treatment options (e.g. administration of aspirin for a patient experiencing chest pain).

Questions that may spark a spirit of inquiry include:
- *Who* can I seek out to assist me in enhancing my evidence-based practice (EBP) knowledge and skills and serve as my EBP mentor?
- *Which* of my practices are currently evidence based and which don't have any evidence to support them?
- *When* is the best time to question my current clinical practices and with whom?
- *Where* can I find the best evidence to answer my clinical questions?
- *Why* am I doing what I do with my patients?
- *How* can I become more skilled in EBP and mentor others to implement evidence-based care? (Melnyk et al., 2009, p. 51).

Step 1: Ask clinical questions in PICOT format

Asking answerable questions in relation to EBP is a skill that comes with experience. It is important to pose clear and focused questions based on the participants, activities, interventions, outcomes of interest and relevant studies. Rather than asking background questions, such as who, what, when, how and why (Sackett et al., 2000), specific questions that affect treatment, referred to as foreground questions, should be used following the PICOT format.

Melnyk and colleagues (2010) suggest that 'the PICOT format provides an efficient framework for searching electronic databases, one designed to retrieve only those articles relevant to the clinical question' (p. 52). Planning the use of questions or inquiries can be assisted by using the PICOT system, outlined in Table 13.3.

▶ **Table 13.3** PICOT system

P	Population, patient or problem of interest
I/E	Intervention or area of interest or exposure
C	Comparison intervention of group
O	Outcome
T	Time

Sources: Sackett, D. L., Richardson, W. S., Rosenbery, W., & Haynes, R. B. (1997). *Evidence-based medicine: How to practice and teach EBM.* New York: Churchill Livingstone. Melnyk, B. M., Fineout-Overholt, E., Stillwell, S. B., Williamson, K .M. (2010). Evidence-based practice step by step: The seven steps of evidence-based practice. *The American Journal of Nursing*, 110(1), 51–3.

For humanistic study, PICOT may be adapted to include more subjective parameters. In addition to the person who is motivated to ask the question, there needs to be a reference group that explores, critiques and expands issues where appropriate before the question is formulated. These groups may include experts, relevant community groups of persons experiencing a condition under discussion and business personnel.

Step 2: Search for the best evidence

Using the PICOT format can streamline the search for evidence, with key words or phrases identified, that when entered into the search engine should retrieve a list of articles relevant to the question posed (Melnyk et al., 2010). A comprehensive overview of searching the literature has been presented in Chapter 2.

Step 3: Critically appraise the evidence

Once articles have been retrieved, a rapid appraisal using three key questions is undertaken to determine which articles are most relevant, valid and applicable to the clinical question. These questions are used when completing a rapid critical appraisal of the articles.

1 Are the results of the study valid? This question is to determine whether the research methods were rigorous enough to produce results that are credible.
2 What are the results and are they important? This question is to establish whether similar results will be achieved if the study was conducted in the clinician's practice setting.

3   Will the results help me care for my patients? This question explores the considerations of whether the population is similar to the clinicians' own patients, whether the benefits outweigh the risks, as well as the feasibility and cost effectiveness of the intervention (Melnyk et al., 2010).

A comprehensive overview of conducting a critical appraisal of the literature is presented in Chapter 3.

Step 4: Integrate the evidence with clinical expertise and patient preferences and values

Research-based evidence is not sufficient on its own to justify a change in practice. An integration of patient data, including patient assessment data, laboratory results and patients' preferences and values, are taken into consideration and combined with clinical judgement when implementing EBPs (Melnyk et al., 2010).

Step 5: Evaluate the outcomes of the practice decisions or changes based on evidence

Monitoring the effects of EBP change is important so that any changes in outcomes are either supported or resolved. Patients most likely to benefit from the EBP practice change can also be identified. As stated by Melnyk and colleagues (2010), 'just because an intervention was effective in a rigorously controlled trial doesn't mean it will work exactly the same way in the clinical setting' (p. 53).

Step 6: Disseminate EBP results

One of the most important aspects of EBP includes dissemination of outcomes as a way of reducing the duplication of practices, and perpetuating practices that are not evidence based. Unfortunately, clinicians who have achieved successful outcomes don't always share their experiences. Dissemination of successful initiatives can be at an organisational, regional or national level, such as presenting at events within the institution, at national conferences or publishing in peer-reviewed journals or a professional newsletter (Melnyk et al., 2010).

Linking research, practice and education

Research and education

Research books are geared towards developing research skills in healthcare professionals. Books and journal articles comprise the main teaching tools for educators conveying the essentials of research models, methods and processes. Studies have found a statistically significant improvement in research knowledge and ability (Black et al., 2016); however, despite having completed research training many clinicians feel overwhelmed and ill prepared for addressing health-related questions (Blanchard, Artino & Visintainer, 2014).

Undergraduate degrees in tertiary education organisations set up comprehensive research programs at honours, postgraduate diploma, master and doctoral levels. Such programs are studded with generic and specialised information relative to the level of education and geared specifically to fine-tuning research knowledge and skills.

Other educational sites where research is offered include professional development and clinical education programs within hospitals and health departments, and professional bodies such as colleges of professional disciplines (e.g. the Australian College of Physiotherapy).

In the United Kingdom, Australia and New Zealand, an increased focus on research in healthcare has come about since the 1980s, the time when the practice discipline of nursing and midwifery moved to the tertiary sector and the impetus for EBP was first being felt in healthcare generally.

Research is a subject taught in many places for different purposes. In relation to healthcare, research education must have clinical relevance to be of use to patients whose good it intends to serve. The following are three articles that are worthy of further reading.

- Lehane, E., Leahy-Warren, P., O'Riordan, C., Savage, E., Drennan, J., O'Tuathaigh, C., O'Connor, M., Corrigan, M., Burke, F., Hayes, M., Lynch, H., Sahm, L., Heffernan, E., O'Keeffe, E., Blake, C., Horgan, F., & Hegarty, J. (2019). Evidence-based practice education for healthcare professions: An expert view. *Evidence-Based Medicine*, 24(3), 103.
- Holbrook, A. M., Tennille, J., & Buck, P. W. (2017). Building capacity for evidence-based practice together. *Social Work in Public Health*, 32(7), 421–431. https://doi.org/10.1080/1937 1918.2017.1344601
- Fineout-Overholt, E. & Johnston, L. (2005). Teaching EBP: A challenge for educators in the 21st century. *Worldviews on Evidence-Based Nursing*, 2(1), 37–9.

Applying research to practice

While the general consensus is that EBP is necessary in healthcare, there does not seem to be an equal degree of confidence and conviction applied to ensuring that the evidence actually finds its way into practice. Zeitz and McCutcheon (2003, p. 272) ask a very pertinent question: 'Rather than focusing on EBP as the solution to the development of best practice, is it not time to change the focus to real strategies that will assist in achieving best practice?' The authors argue that applying research into practice involves 'the creation of rigorous, relevant evidence, the valuing of clinical expertise and the changing of cultures' in which clinicians 'develop and practice' (Zeitz & McCutcheon, 2003). McClosky (2008) suggests that 'identifying perceptions and documenting the factors affecting nurses' abilities to conduct or utilise research is the first step. Once the factors have been identified, strategies should be developed to improve upon or eliminate those that are not effective'.

Effective change measures

Research can also find its way into practice through the establishment of effective change measures. Dawes and colleagues (2005) suggest that it is important to be aware of how change happens in individuals and organisations, and the levels of change from micro to macro that are negotiated as the culture of the workplace adapts gradually to research-based changes. They also describe ways to bring about effective change, such as for opinion leaders to make personal contact with clinicians in their workplaces to influence them to be willing to drop their practice fads and traditions in favour of embracing and establishing evidence-based changes.

Davies (2005, pp. 225–6) reminds us that change:

> can take place at [the] macro and micro level of health care, at the national and local level, at the strategic level and the operational level … It is important that healthcare practitioners clarify at the outset the level at which they are operating, the types of innovation that are appropriate and feasible at that level, and the systems, individuals and groups that they are likely, and unlikely, to be able to influence.

ACTIVITY

Would you be encouraged to use research if a renowned nurse researcher made special contact with you in your workplace and described the new research-based practices? Explain your answer. Discuss what other ideas you envisage would help your colleagues to become more willing to use EBP.

EBP

Constant changes are being introduced into healthcare services across the world and while clinicians need to be flexible and accommodating, some may not be aware of new research evidence being available. This results in a gap between interventions that have been shown to be effective and the translation of evidence into practice (Kent, 2019). In an effort to bridge the gap, evidence from research, CPGs and standards of practice provide a foundation on which clinicians can develop their capacity as consumers of research, as well as integrate EBP into their clinical practice (Kristensen, Nymann & Konradsen, 2016).

National health imperatives

In response to the World Health Organization's global strategy 'Health for all by the year 2000', the National Health Priority Areas (NHPA) initiative was developed to address specific diseases and conditions that contribute significantly to the burden of illness and injury in Australia. Further information about health priorities can be found on the Australian Institute of Health and Welfare website (http://www.aihw.gov.au/national-health-priority-areas).

In Australia, the federal government has a health portfolio and the ministers for this portfolio take advice from key leaders in the health field when planning **national health initiatives** developed to help improve the health of all Australians. The government also connects with health researchers through peak bodies on an organisational level, such as through the NHMRC and key hospital and university medical departments. Government funding goes to high-priority healthcare areas with EBP considered a high priority; therefore, researchers and developers apply an EBP focus to their work and ensure that the outcomes are reflected in current practice.

Connected to national governance is the imperative that health research benefits the population and has international marketability, so the research projects funded through government-sponsored agencies are usually those projects of immense importance, such as cures for diseases and innovative diagnostic and treatment advances. This places medical researchers in the ideal position to pursue their research while altruistically serving the good of society. Unsurprisingly, the positive effects of medical research are rewarded with the highest proportion of government funding for further projects. Change reaches clinical areas, then, when medical and health research findings are introduced into practice for the good of the patient.

Clinical practice guidelines

It is at the level of basic clinical practice that EBP needs to be fostered. Clinicians have problems in applying research for a number of reasons, including a lack of evidence, a lack of time to acquire the evidence and a lack of research skills and experience to critically evaluate the evidence. Even if clinicians are able to access and appraise evidence, they may have difficulty in recalling it when required. This situation has led to the development of clinical practice guidelines (CPGs) or evidence-based protocols. The latter half of the 1990s saw the development of hundreds of sets of CPGs.

As defined by the NHMRC (n.d.), 'clinical practice guidelines are evidence-based statements that include recommendations intended to optimise patient care and assist healthcare practitioners to make decisions about appropriate healthcare for specific clinical circumstances'. CPGs were introduced to try to reduce the marked variability in clinical practice; that is, to provide the healthcare team with a consistent approach to patient care. Evidence-based CPGs normally comprise a set of statements related to a specific condition or patient problem and are developed from systematic reviews. They are prepared by a committee of experts who translate the evidence into formulae for practice. Clinicians then implement the guidelines rather than distilling the research findings and making decisions based on the evidence.

Essentially, a clinical guideline will appear in hard copy as a sheet of paper in a procedures or CPG book or folder, or in electronic form on a computer database. They can also appear as algorithms, clinical pathways, protocols and practice policies. A clinical guideline is a helpful, practical and sequential guide for clinicians in how to safely and effectively go about a clinical procedure. A clinical guideline may, for example, be about caring for a patient with confusion or undertaking the care of a patient receiving chemotherapy. If clinicians accept well-prepared and researched CPG, the research-based information included in the document can find its way into practice. The following examples in the 'Evidence for best practice' box are of collaborative projects undertaken to develop CPG for practice.

EVIDENCE FOR BEST PRACTICE

CLINICAL PRACTICE GUIDELINES DEVELOPED FROM RESEARCH

A multidisciplinary collaborative project using a suite of evidence-based interventions was undertaken to improve warfarin management at St Vincent's Private Hospital in Sydney. The project used 'clinical indicator data and a practice improvement methodology' to transfer knowledge of best practice warfarin therapy into clinical practice. Two warfarin protocols were developed, a new warfarin clinical pathway was successfully integrated into the hospital's existing processes, and an online self-paced education module enabled ongoing staff education (Duff & Walker, 2010).

The Victorian Day Surgery Special Interest Group (DSSIG) developed guidelines from the results of three systematic reviews carried out by researchers at La Trobe University in collaboration with members of the DSSIG. An expert panel was established and consensus reached on practice knowledge. Primary research topics were identified by a lack of evidence in the development of the systematic reviews (Pearson, Richardson & Cairns, 2004; Pearson et al., 2004a, 2004b).

CPGs bridge the gap between research and practice by providing practice recommendations based on rigorously developed systematic reviews and consensus among clinical experts and key stakeholders. That is, they can comprise knowledge synthesised from variable study designs and consensus of expert opinion. As a result, the knowledge contained within CPGs could be limited as expert opinion does not always reflect the state of current medical knowledge. CPGs can be adapted to be context-specific, and in that sense, they guide clinicians rather than mandate practice. Acceptance of a CPG is likely to depend on the quality of the evidence on which it is based, development of the CPG and whether it is perceived as being useful.

Four examples of the use of CPG can be found in the following articles which review Australian general practitioners' views on the impact of CPG on practice.

- Mazza & Russell (2001). Are GPs using clinical practice guidelines? *Australian Family Physician*, *30*(8), 817–21.
- Carlsen, Glenton & Pope (2007). Thou shalt versus thou shalt not: A meta-synthesis of GPs' attitudes to clinical practice guidelines. *British Journal of General Practice*, *57*(545), 971–8.
- Slade, S. C., Kent, P., Patel, S., Bucknall, T., & Buchbinder, R. (2016). Barriers to primary care clinician adherence to clinical guidelines for the management of low back pain: A systematic review and meta-synthesis of qualitative studies. *The Clinical Journal of Pain*, *32*(9), 800–16. https://doi.org/10.1097/AJP.0000000000000324
- Baynouna Al Ketbi, L. M., & Zein Al Deen, S. (2018). The attitudes and beliefs of general practitioners towards clinical practice guidelines: A qualitative study in Al Ain, United Arab Emirates. *Asia Pacific Family Medicine*, *17*(5). https://doi.org/10.1186/s12930-018-0041-2

TIP

CPGs, while useful, do not replace the knowledge, skills and expertise of the clinician or the preferences of the patient and family.

In Australia, the NHMRC has set up a preferred process for CPG development. Further detail can be accessed via the Australian Clinical Practice Guidelines website (https://www.clinicalguidelines.gov.au/portal). As stated previously, the JBI issues regular CPGs in the form of best practice sheets. Some practice matters include pressure injuries, falls in hospitals and the management of peripheral intravascular devices.

Problems in applying research to practice

On the surface, CPGs seem to be the best way of ensuring that research is implemented into clinical practice. However, there are numerous issues identified with CPGs. One issue is the extent to which clinicians feel they have been imposed on in their practice. When non-discipline specific groups impose guidelines (e.g. in nursing), it can be problematic. They might try to encourage nurses to use a non-nursing framework and rate randomised controlled trials as the highest form of evidence and expert opinion as the lowest form. Enshrining clinical trials as the highest form of evidence does not promote qualitative research, neither is its value understood by nurses themselves. Information from qualitative studies is also vital as it relates to the human element of nursing practice. Results from these studies provide information with which to extend a nurse's understanding of the effects of a phenomenon and how it impacts on a patient or family. The scientific and human elements of patient care are inextricably linked and should not be confused as being the same. Clinicians need to be involved in developing CPGs and decide what evidence they deem appropriate for sound practice. This requires clinicians to break down the barriers that prevent the implementation of research in the clinical setting, upgrade their skills concerning the consumption and practice of research, and identify research priorities.

Another problem is that CPGs address only discrete parts of care and could be inappropriate for complex problems. This approach supports a reductionist view of patients and dismisses other holistic considerations of them as people. It is important that clinicians set up some criteria for judging the quality of CPGs and remain open to broader views of caring for people beyond the scripted guidelines for practice. The Appraisal of Guidelines for Research and Evaluation (AGREE) tool was developed in 2003 to assist with critically appraising CPGs, with a revised and updated version published in 2009. AGREE II is an international collaboration of researchers and policymakers who seek to improve the quality and effectiveness of CPGs by establishing a shared framework for their development, reporting and to be used as an evaluation tool. Another issue concerning CPGs is whether they will have the expected impact.

FOR EXAMPLE

ISSUES IN DEVELOPING EVIDENCE-BASED TOOLS

Results from an observational study of the development of multidisciplinary evidence-based clinical management tools (Hutchinson & Johnston, 2008) identified three major themes.

- Nurses assumed responsibility for coordination of the development of the clinical management tools that focused on describing current practice.
- The forms of evidence used included experiential knowledge, opinions and knowledge of the context, as well as research evidence. Reference to research evidence was limited and infrequently incorporated into the clinical management tools.
- Use of research evidence during the development of the clinical management tools emerged in relation to how such evidence was employed. The nurses relied on the research knowledge of the medical practitioners and allied health professionals; they did not actively search for research evidence.

It will come as no surprise, then, that the best-laid plans of change agents can go awry when they are faced with the culture of a workplace resistant to evidence-based change. Change is often imposed in the planning stages, without the involvement of clinicians or those expected to implement and use the change. Change processes themselves can often be implicated in the success or failure of change. Even so, the predominance of EBP in healthcare and concerted and sustained efforts by governments and leaders in research and development will ensure that more and more research quickly finds its way into practice and creates a new and effective EBP culture. Countering this is the argument put forward by Holmes and colleagues (2008) that nursing best practice guidelines threaten to supplant the reality of patient healthcare by impeding nurses' critical thinking and serving as disciplinary technologies to govern nursing work.

Policy and procedure manuals

Policy and procedure manuals play an important part in establishing the ways in which health professionals practise. These documents are found in hospital wards and departments in accessible areas for clinicians to access and read quickly. Policy and procedure manuals are written according to the latest evidence on the practice discipline. The presence and use of these manuals by staff may in fact be essential in ensuring that the organisation retains its accreditation as a healthcare facility; therefore, much emphasis is placed on maintaining policy and procedure manuals with up-to-date information that staff can use in practice and refer to if and when problems arise.

For the information in policy and procedure manuals to be clinically relevant and contemporary, the documents must reflect best practice principles. In turn, the best practice that professionals can give is based on the latest research evidence. Practice procedures are based on directives and policies from the respective health departments that are prepared for operation clinically, legally and ethically. This evidence is derived from research projects reported in refereed journal articles that have been subjected to a systematic review process. The process involves developing the review protocol, asking answerable questions, finding and appraising the evidence, and judging the applicability of the evidence (Pearson & Field, 2005).

Obvious disadvantages of policy and procedure manuals are that they are only as effective as the information within them and the extent to which clinicians apply this information to practice. The information within these manuals must be generated from the most recent and best research as determined by a systematic review process. To be transparent in the process, manuals must cite the authors of the research and provide full referencing details for clinicians to access and be able to read the research projects in full.

ACTIVITY

Locate the policy and procedural manuals in your workplace. Are they research-based? Are the research projects fully referenced in the manuals? Explain your answers.

The many barriers to clinicians applying research into practice are described in this chapter. But barriers notwithstanding, the culture of hospitals places great faith in, and reliance on, the use of succinct information in policy and procedure manuals. If information is accessible and easy to read, there is a very good chance that busy clinicians will be attentive to the information contained in the policy.

Creating a research culture in clinical settings

The funding provided to healthcare organisations caters to the establishment of research positions such as joint appointments between the health sector and universities, and/or research and professional development roles conducted solely within the healthcare organisation. Project-based funding is also available through the respective health departments. Regardless of how these research positions are established, they will only be effective if they meet the needs of clinicians and improve clinical practice.

A *research culture* refers to a group of people who are knowledgeable about the fundamentals of research methods and processes and are confident in promoting and sharing the practice and application of research. Such knowledge and confidence only comes with regular exposure to doing research and to understanding and applying its outcomes. If research activity is local and logical, it can be learned and conducted by clinicians who have an interest in research.

There are many practical measures for creating a research culture in clinical settings.

- Researchers can involve wards and departments in manageable projects of clinical relevance to their daily work.
- Management can give staff time off from work to attend hospital-organised research talks and seminars and/or to attend relevant national and international professional conferences.
- Clinicians can become conversant with research language through professional development seminars and conferences, and by talking and reading about research often and openly in familiar places, such as ward meetings and tearooms.

Bonner (2008) undertook research to examine the knowledge, attitude and use of research by nurses. The results of this study showed that:

- senior nurses were more likely to have a positive attitude towards research
- completion of university subjects on nursing research was significant in determining attitudes and knowledge of research
- all nurses, regardless of position, identified barriers to performing research.

Bonner (2008) asserted that a positive attitude towards research by senior nurse managers has the potential to influence other nurses in establishing an active research culture.

The development of clinical schools has provided opportunities for conducting clinical research. The development and evaluation of a multidisciplinary critical appraisal and research utilisation training program is one initiative undertaken as an approach to the challenge of ensuring that practice is evidence based (Milne et al., 2007). One issue of note in the evaluation of the program was that 'implementation of practice change does not occur unless clinicians feel they "own" the practice issue and are part of the process undertaken to investigate the issue and identify potential changes' (Milne et al., 2007, p. 1638).

Research (theory)–practice links

One of the biggest challenges for health professionals is to put theory into practice. Theory comes from research: theory is knowledge and research creates and validates knowledge. If it is assumed that research and theory are inextricably linked, all that remains is to ensure that research (theory) and practice become linked just as firmly. The debates of the 1980s covered the area of the theory–practice gap, and it comes as no surprise that this was also the decade in which the education of practice disciplines, such as midwifery, nursing and physiotherapy, entered tertiary settings. It is not the intention of this chapter to breathe new life into those old debates; suffice it to say here that, essentially, it was recognised that the translation of theory into practice was not as good as it could be and that certain strategies could be helpful in strengthening theory–practice links.

In the practice discipline of nursing in Australia, the 1980s saw the arrival of a number of initiatives. Nursing units were established in hospitals and health agencies to provide primary nursing care and to research its effectiveness. Joint appointments, funded by universities and clinical organisations, were set up to undertake research and establish that evidence in practice. Faculty practice was established to ensure that nursing educators had clinical relevance to teach from experience by being up-to-date with clinical policies, procedures and practices. Postgraduate research degrees previously taken in other disciplines, such as education, psychology and sociology, were taken in nursing.

There are many incentives and strategies for clinicians to use research in their practice. Clinical research can be made easy and accessible by using the research (theory)–practice links described already and by other simple and effective means, such as:

- sharing research information in ward discussions
- seminars and conferences, which can strengthen practice links
- clinical research in which university researchers can become involved, not only through their own research interests, but also in supervising undergraduate and postgraduate degrees that focus on clinical issues.

Collaborative research

Collaborative research processes can be oriented to the needs of clinicians. The easiest and most accessible clinical research involves clinicians researching their own practice to answer their own clinical problems. In the process, clinicians can choose to gain academic recognition through attaining research awards for their practice-centred research.

Any research project can become collaborative if it is undertaken in partnership with other professionals within and across practice disciplines. Examples of collaborative research projects include Black et al. (2015), Cleary et al. (2008), Delany et al. (2016b), Hill et al. (2009), Kain et al. (2006), McMurray et al. (2010), Ullrich, McCutcheon and Parker (2011) and Wynaden et al. (2006).

EVIDENCE FOR BEST PRACTICE

COLLABORATIVE CLINICAL RESEARCH

The following are two examples of collaborative clinical research undertaken to develop best practice and thus reduce the theory–practice gap.

NATIONAL CONSULTATION INFORMING DEVELOPMENT OF GUIDELINES FOR A PALLIATIVE APPROACH FOR AGED CARE IN THE COMMUNITY SETTING

The aim of the study undertaken by Holloway and colleagues (2015) was to obtain points of view about a palliative approach to aged care in the community setting from key stakeholders to inform the development of Australian national guidelines and identify practice areas for inclusion. Using a descriptive, exploratory qualitative design, data were collected during audiotaped, semi-structured, individual and focus group interviews. Several themes emerged from the data, which underpinned the development of new guideline documents.

DEVELOPING CLINICAL PRACTICE GUIDELINES FOR END-OF-LIFE CARE: BLENDING EVIDENCE AND CONSENSUS

The aim of the study undertaken by Dunning and colleagues (2012) was to develop CPGs for managing diabetes at the end of life, with the process detailed in the article. Individual interviews were conducted with people with diabetes and their carers, using both formative and summative evaluation. Important information about how people wanted their diabetes to be managed was elicited from the interviews. The formative evaluation enabled stakeholders to participate in developing the CPGs. The summative evaluation confirmed the CPGs are easy to use and appropriate to clinical staff.

Any number of variations are possible in using quantitative, qualitative or mixed-methods approaches. The whole idea of collaborative research is open to whatever can be arranged between interested parties in the clinical and academic settings (Loeb et al., 2008).

A collaborative research project, funded by the Australian Office of Learning and Teaching, was undertaken by academics at the University of Melbourne (lead), Flinders University, the University of Sydney, the University of Queensland and the University of Auckland. The aim of this project was to produce a suite of practical resources for academics to design assessments in Indigenous health education at the master's level employing a qualitative approach (Delany et al., 2016a).

> **TIP**
>
> Any research project can reflect collaboration if it is done cooperatively and by sharing workloads and responsibilities.

ACTIVITY

Some ideas for making clinical research easy and accessible include: practical strategies for creating a research culture in clinical settings, research–practice links and types of collaborative research that can be undertaken easily. What other possibilities can you think of for making clinical research easy and accessible?

Educating evidence-based clinicians

This section describes some means for educating evidence-based clinicians to increase the likelihood that research will be put into practice. Ideas are offered to help educators prepare evidence-based clinicians and to enhance their own teaching effectiveness. The suggestions are by no means complete, nor are they exclusive of other possibilities.

Preparing evidence-based clinicians

Starting with the assumptions that clinical practice is complex, changes occur rapidly and clinicians need to be up to date with the latest research, there are many simple strategies for clinical educators to prepare evidence-based clinicians for practice.

Teaching evidence-based care

One way to encourage clinicians to read and use research is to model those behaviours in education. When they cite research sources and use researchers' names and projects, clinical educators model evidence-based behaviours. Students may also be assisted in recognising the importance of current research evidence and other sources of ethical and personal knowledge (Ireland, 2008; Penz & Bassendowski, 2006). These behaviours can be highly influential regarding the ways that clinicians become familiar with and operationalise research in their daily practice.

Lecturers can enlist simple teaching measures on a regular basis, such as always teaching from research and listing the researchers whose work underlies clinical procedures and theories relating to practice. Fully reference researchers' work by name, initials, date, title, journal article, volume, number and pages: full referencing details connect the procedure or theory directly to research and enable students to pursue further reading. Consistent referencing of practice to research strengthens the connection so that the link becomes strong and expected.

Another strategy to incorporate EBP in teaching is by facilitating undergraduate students' skills in accessing and analysing the most relevant evidence to support their beginning practice (Meeker, Jones & Flanagan, 2008; Penz & Bassendowski, 2006). Graduate students require the skill to undertake systematic reviews for the development of CPGs. Krainovich-Miller, Haber and Kaplan Jacobs (2009) present the teaching of EBP components of a research course early, adventurously and differently (TREAD) as a framework for use in graduate research courses. Clinical educators also play a role in the promotion of evidence-based care. The clinical educator can guide students within a framework of systematic observation, experience and reliance on current nursing research to develop sound nursing practices (Penz & Bassendowski, 2006). This does not mean that the clinical educator must know everything; rather, they should know how to search for and evaluate evidence in clinical practice and role-model these skills for students. Students thus develop critical thinking skills through independent, evidence-based methods of clinical decision making.

It follows that clinicians grounded in evidence-based education will transplant the expectations of evidence into clinical practice and demand up-to-date procedures validated by systematic review processes to substantiate clinical decisions.

Encouraging honours and postgraduate research degrees

Research knowledge and skills take time to develop. Rarely would an undergraduate degree provide sufficient preparation in research knowledge and skills to prepare a clinician to undertake independent research. Educators can become involved in career trajectory advice and actively encourage undergraduates to pursue further research programs. Students may feel that they are unable to do research, or may be unaware of the possibilities that a research degree holds for them in the future.

Encouraging research skills

Fostering an inquiring mind underpins the passion for research, which is based on the love of questioning. Educators encourage this passion in students to become researchers and research consumers by teaching them practical skills such as questioning, database skills, critical literature review skills and reflective practice.

Database skills

Database skills are essential for keeping up with the latest research literature. Educators need to emphasise the usefulness of information technology skills directly connected to research (see Chapter 3).

Once literature has been procured through database and library searches, students will need to develop skills in undertaking critical literature reviews, as doing this as an assessment task is common practice in most undergraduate degree courses. Students are also required to produce annotated bibliographies. By being built into academic essay writing and research units of instruction, literature review skills can be enhanced through repeated practice (see Chapter 2).

Reflective practice skills

Reflective practice involves systematic questioning and focuses itself on practice (Taylor, 2006). In a similar fashion to critical thinking, reflective practice has been promoted in health professions for some time. Educators should be reflective practitioners in their teaching, and clinicians should be reflective practitioners in their work. Researchers need to reflect on their practice of research to constantly develop expertise. Educators can encourage reflective practice skills and connect those skills to research (e.g. Duffy, 2007; Forneris & Peden-McAlpine, 2006; Mantzoukas & Watkinson, 2008).

TIP

Research becomes easier and more accessible when it is experienced as doable.

TIP

Educators who encourage students to undertake honours and postgraduate research degrees are likely to be highly influential in increasing research uptake and impact on practice.

SUMMARY

This chapter focused on using research in education and practice.

1	Define evidence-based practice	• Evidence-based practice is a problem-solving approach to clinical care that incorporates three major components: 1. The best evidence from research studies and patient data, 2. The individual practitioner's clinical expertise, and 3. Patient preferences and values.
2	Describe the steps and skills necessary for evidence-based practice	• Step 0: Cultivate a spirit of inquiry • Step 1: Ask clinical questions in PICOT format • Step 2: Search for the best evidence • Step 3: Critically appraise the evidence • Step 4: Integrate the evidence with clinical expertise and patient preferences and values • Step 5: Evaluate the outcomes of the practice decisions or changes based on evidence • Step 6: Disseminate EBP results
3	Describe the relationship between research, practice and education	• Theory comes from research because theory is knowledge and research creates and validates knowledge • If research is to be used in clinical settings, education that prepares clinicians for research-based practice is needed
4	Apply research to clinical practice	• Evidence-based practice involves clinical decision making using the best research evidence available and practice knowledge to provide patient-centred care
5	Examine the barriers to applying research findings to practice	• Busy clinicians have many pressures competing for their attention • Barriers include time constraints, inadequate resources to access information, lack of familiarity with EBP and the complexity of research reports, clinicians' research knowledge and critical appraisal skills, resistance to change and the current healthcare culture.
6	Describe strategies for educating clinicians about evidence-based practice	• Lecturers can enlist simple teaching measures on a regular basis: – teaching from research – listing the researchers whose work underlies clinical procedures and theories relating to practice – facilitating students' skills in accessing and analysing the most relevant evidence to support their beginning practice

REVIEW QUESTIONS

1   Discuss whether your professional practice is considered to be evidence based.
2   Describe the relationship of practice, research and education in relation to evidence-based practice.
3   Discuss three strategies for applying research into practice.
4   Discuss the perceived problems with clinical practice guidelines.
5   Discuss four strategies for educating evidence-based clinicians.

CHALLENGING REVIEW QUESTIONS

1   The manager of the education department approached you to assist with developing a 'more research-focused' department because you have recently completed your honours degree. There is

some funding available so you will be required to prepare a report for the funding to be approved. Explain how you would approach this project and discuss how you could ensure your idea would be successful and achieve the goal of an evidence-based practice department.

2   A call for expressions of interest has been circulated in the hospital for staff to register if they are interested in being involved in the development of clinical practice guidelines (CPGs) for preventing falls in elderly patients. You have been working in the geriatric ward and have become concerned about the lack of consensus with regards to managing this clinical problem, but you are not familiar with the process of developing CPGs. Discuss what information you would need to access to familiarise yourself with the development of CPGs before you volunteer yourself to join the committee.

CASE STUDY 1

Prisha is an undergraduate nursing student beginning her third year. Prisha is considering her options for a graduate position after she completes her course. As a student nurse, Prisha is aware that stress and burnout are important considerations for hospital nurses and would like to ensure she is fully prepared.

Prisha is eager to apply for a graduate position in a healthcare facility that has a good working environment for the staff and is exploring evidence-based practice concepts related to the topic.

1   Is there an Australian clinical guideline to guide healthy working environments for nurses?
2   What is the highest level of evidence related to nurses work environment?
3   What are some challenges Prisha might face if she wanted to implement evidence-based changes to the clinical environment?

CASE STUDY 2

We return to Angela, discussed in 'Case study 2' of Chapter 12. Angela presented her findings at an international conference in England, which were well received. She now wants to implement her findings in clinical practice.

1   Explain whether the results from the study can be used to guide clinical practice.
2   Discuss the importance of disseminating results on completion of a study. Provide examples of how that can be achieved.

REFERENCES

Black, A. T., Balneaves, L. G., Garossino, C., Puyat, J. H., & Hong, Q. (2016). Promoting evidence-based practice through a research training program for point-of-care clinicians. *Journal of Nursing Administration*, S36–42.

Black, J., Gerdtz, M., Nicholson, P., Crellin, D., Browning, L., Simpson, J., Bell, L., & Santamaria, N. (2015). Can simple mobile phone applications provide reliable counts of respiratory rates in sick infants and children? An initial evaluation of three new applications. *International Journal of Nursing Studies*, *52*, 963–9. doi:10.1016/j.ijnurstu.2015.01.016

Blanchard, R. D., Artino, A. J., & Visintainer, P. F. (2014). Applying clinical research skills to conduct education research: Important recommendations for success. *Journal of Graduate Medical Education, 6*(4), 619–22.

Bonner, A. (2008). Examining the knowledge, attitude and use of research by nurses. *Journal of Nursing Management, 16*, 334–43.

Cleary, M., Matheson, S., Walter, G., Malins, G., & Hunt, G. (2008). Demystifying research and evidence-based practice for consumers and carers: Development and evaluation of an educational package. *Issues in Mental Health Nursing, 29*, 131–43.

Cochrane, A. L. (1972). Effectiveness and efficiency: Random reflections on health services. Nuffield Trust. https://www.nuffieldtrust.org.uk/research/effectiveness-and-efficiency-random-reflections-on-health-services

Cochrane. (n.d.). Cochrane. About us. https://www.cochrane.org/about-us

Cookson, R. (2005). Evidence-based policy making in health care: What it is and what it isn't. *Journal of Health Services Research & Policy, 10*(2), 118–21.

Davies, P. (2005). Changing policy and practice. In M. Dawes, P. Davies, A. Gray, J. Mant, K. Seers & R. Snowball, *Evidence-Based Practice: A Primer for Health Care Professionals* (2nd edn, pp. 223–40). Edinburgh: Churchill Livingstone.

Dawes, M. (2005). Evidence-based practice. In M. Dawes, P. Davies, A. Gray, J. Mant, K. Seers & R. Snowball, *Evidence-Based Practice: A Primer for Health Care Professionals* (2nd edn, pp. 1–10). Edinburgh: Churchill Livingstone.

Dawes, M., Davies, P., Gray, A., Mant, J., Seers, K., & Snowball, R. (2005). *Evidence-Based Practice: A Primer for Health Care Professionals* (2nd edn). Edinburgh: Churchill Livingstone.

Delany, C., Ewen, S., Harms, L., Remedios, L., Nicholson, P., Andrews, S., Kosta, L., McCullough, M., Edmondson, W., Bandler, L., Shannon, C., Willis, J., Reid, P., & Doughney, L. (2016a). Guiding assessment for learning in Indigenous health at Level 9 of the Australian Qualifications Framework. http://www.olt.gov.au/project-guiding-assessment-learning-indigenous-health-level-9-australian-qualifications-framework-20

Delany, C., Kosta, L., Ewen, S., Nicholson, P., Remedios, L., & Harms, L. (2016b). Identifying pedagogy and teaching strategies for achieving nationally prescribed learning outcomes. *Higher Education Research & Development, 35*(5), 895–909. doi:10.1080/07294360.2016.1138450

Duff, J., & Walker, K. (2010). Improving the safety and efficacy of warfarin therapy in a metropolitan private hospital: A multidisciplinary practice improvement project. *Contemporary Nurse, 35*(2), 234–44.

Duffy, A. (2007). A concept analysis of reflective practice: Determining its value to nurses. *British Journal of Nursing, 16*(22), 1400–7.

Dunning, T., Savage, S., Duggan, N., & Martin, P. (2012). Developing clinical guidelines for end-of-life care: Blending evidence and consensus. *International Journal of Palliative Nursing, 18*(8), 397–405.

Ekeland, T.-J., Bergem, R., & Myklebust, V. (2019). Evidence-based practice in social work: Perceptions and attitudes among Norwegian social workers. *European Journal of Social Work, 22*(4), 611–22. https://doi.org/10.1080/13691457.2018.1441139

Fairbrother, G., Jones, A., & Rivas, K. (2010). Changing model of nursing care from individual patient allocation to team nursing in the acute inpatient environment. *Contemporary Nurse, 35*(2), 202–20.

Forneris, S., & Peden-McAlpine, C. (2006). Contextual learning: A reflective learning intervention for nursing education. *International Journal of Nursing Scholarship, 3*(1), 1–18.

Foster, A., Worrall, L., Rose, M., & O'Halloran, R. (2015). 'That doesn't translate': The role of evidence-based practice in disempowering speech pathologists in acute aphasia management. *International Journal of Language & Communication Disorders, 50*(4), 547–63. https://doi.org/10.1111/1460-6984.12155

Grady, P. A., & Hinshaw, A. S. (2017). *Using Nursing Research to Shape Health Policy*. Springer Publishing Company.

Griffiths, M., & Clark, J. (2004). Managing the local agenda: Planning to get research/evidence-based care into practice. In C. Clifford & J. Clark (eds) *Getting Research into Practice* (pp. 61–82). Edinburgh: Churchill Livingstone.

Grimmer, K., Bialocerkowski, A., Kumar, S., & Milanese, S. (2004). Implementing evidence in clinical practice: The 'therapies' dilemma. *Physiotherapy, 90*(4), 189–94. https://doi.org/10.1016/j.physio.2004.06.007

Haider, T., Dunstan, D., & Bhullar, N. (2019). Improving psychologists' adherence to evidence-based practice guidelines for treating musculoskeletal injuries: A feasibility study. *Australian Psychologist, 54*(6), 483–93. https://doi.org/10.1111/ap.12395

Hewitt-Taylor, J., Heaslip, V., & Rowe, N. (2012). Applying research to practice: Exploring the barriers. *British Journal of Nursing, 21*(6), 356–9.

Higgins, I., Parker, V., Keatinge, D., Giles, M., Winskill, R., Guest, E., Kepreotes, E., & Phelan, C. (2010). Doing clinical research: The challenges and benefits. *Contemporary Nurse, 35*(2), 171–81.

Hill, K., Middleton, S., O'Brien, E., & Lalor, E. (2009). Implementing clinical guidelines for acute stroke management: Do nurses have a lead role? *Australian Journal of Advanced Nursing, 26*(3), 53–8.

Holloway, K., Toye, C., McConigley, R., Tieman, J., Currow, D., & Hegarty, M. (2015). National consultation informing development of guidelines for a palliative approach for aged care in the community setting. *Australasian Journal on Ageing, 34*(1), 21–6.

Holmes, D., Murray, S., Perron, A., & McCabe, J. (2008). Nursing best practice guidelines: Reflecting on the obscene rise of the void. *Journal of Nursing Management, 16*, 394–403.

Holmes, D., Murray, S., Perron, A., & Rail, G. (2006). Deconstructing the evidence-based discourse in health sciences: Truth, power and fascism. *International Journal of Evidence-based Healthcare, 4*, 180–6.

Houlston, C. (2012). The role of a research nurse in translating evidence into practice. *Nursing Management, 19*(1), 25–8.

Hutchinson, A., & Johnston, L. (2008). An observational study of health professionals' use of evidence to inform the development of clinical management tools. *Journal of Clinical Nursing, 17*(16), 2203–11.

Ireland, M. (2008). Assisting students to use evidence as part of reflection on practice. *Nursing Education Perspectives, 29*(2), 90–3.

Johnston, B., Coole, C., Feakes, R., Whitworth, G., Tyrell, T., & Hardy, B. (2016). Exploring the barriers to and facilitators of implementing research into practice. *British Journal of Community Nursing, 21*(8), 392–8.

Jordan, P., Bowers, C. M., & Morton, D. (2016). Barriers to implementing evidence-based practice in a private intensive care unit in the Eastern Cape. *Southern African Journal of Critical Care, 32*(2), 50. doi:10.7196/SAJCC.2016.v32i2.253

Kain, V., Yates, P., Barrett, L., Bradley, T., Circosta, M., Hall, A., Hardy, J., Israel, F., McLeod, L., Vora, R., & Wheatley, H. (2006). Developing guidelines for syringe driver management. *International Journal of Palliative Nursing, 12*(2), 60–9.

Kent, B. (2019). Implementing research findings into practice: Frameworks and guidance. *International Journal of Evidence-Based Healthcare, 17*(1), S18–21.

Koehn, M. L., & Lehman, K. (2008). Nurses' perceptions of evidence-based nursing practice. *Journal of Advanced Nursing, 62*(2), 209–15.

Krainovich-Miller, B., Haber, J., & Kaplan Jacobs, S. (2009). Evidence-based practice challenge: Teaching critical appraisal of systematic reviews and clinical practice guidelines to graduate students. *Journal of Nursing Education, 48*(4), 186–95.

Kristensen N., Nymann C, & Konradsen H. (2016). Implementing research results in clinical practice – the experiences of healthcare professionals. *BMC Health Services Research*, 16:48.

Lehane, E., Leahy-Warren, P., O'Riordan, C., Savage, E., Drennan, J., O'Tuathaigh, C., O'Connor, M., Corrigan, M., Burke, F., Hayes, M., Lynch, H., Sahm, L., Heffernan, E., O'Keeffe, E., Blake, C., Horgan, F., & Hegarty, J. (2019). Evidence-based practice education for healthcare professions: An expert view. *Evidence-Based Medicine, 24*(3), 103.

Loeb, S., Penrod, J., Kolanowski, A., Hupcey, J., Kopenhaver Haider, K., Fick, D., McGonigle, D., & Yu, F. (2008). Creating cross-disciplinary research alliances to advance nursing science. *Journal of Nursing Scholarship, 40*(2), 195–210.

Lu, X. (2008). Evidence-based practice in nursing: What is it and what is the impact of leadership and management practices on implementation? *Nursing Journal NorthTec, 12*, 6–12.

Majid, S., Foo, S., Luyt, B., Zang, X., Theng., Y., Chang, Y., & Mokhtar, I. (2011). Adopting evidence-based practice in clinical decision making: Nurses' perceptions, knowledge, and barriers. *Journal Medical Library Association, 99*(3), 222–36.

Mantzoukas, S., & Watkinson, S. (2008). Redescribing reflective practice and evidence-based practice discourses. *International Journal of Nursing Practice, 14*, 129–34.

McClosky, D. (2008). Nurses' perceptions of research utilization in a corporate health care system. *Journal of Nursing Scholarship, 40*(1), 44.

McMurray, A., Chaboyer., W., Wallis, M., & Fetherston, C. (2010). Implementing bedside handover: Strategies for change management. *Journal of Clinical Nursing, 19*, 2580–9.

Meeker, M. A., Jones, J. M., & Flanagan, N. A. (2008). Teaching undergraduate nursing research from an evidence-based practice perspective. *Journal of Nursing Education, 47*(8), 376–9.

Melnyk, B. M., Fineout-Overholt, E., Stillwell, S.B., Williamson, K.M. (2009). Evidence-based practice. Step by step: Igniting a spirit of inquiry: An essential foundation for evidence-based practice. *American Journal of Nursing, 109*(11), 49–52.

Melnyk, B. M., Fineout-Overholt, E., Stillwell, S. B., & Williamson, K .M. (2010). Evidence-based practice step by step. The seven steps of evidence-based practice. *American Journal of Nursing, 110*(1), 51–3.

Milne, D., Krishnasamy, M., Johnston, L., & Aranda, S. (2007). Promoting evidence-based care through a clinical research fellowship programme. *Journal of Clinical Nursing, 16*(9), 1629–39.

National Health and Medical Research Council (NHMRC). (1999). *A Guide to the Development, Implementation and Evaluation of Clinical Practice Guidelines*. Canberra: Australian Government Publishing Service.

National Health and Medical Research Council (NHMRC). (n.d.) Clinical Practice Guidelines Portal. https://www.clinicalguidelines.gov.au/portal

Nolan, P. (2008). Evidence-based practice: Implications and concerns. *Journal of Nursing Management, 16*, 388–93.

Pearson, A., & Field, J. (2005). The systematic review process. In M. Courtney (ed). *Evidence for Nursing Practice* (pp. 73–8). Sydney, NSW: Churchill Livingstone.

Pearson, A., Richardson, M., & Cairns, M. (2004). Best practice in day surgery units: A review of the evidence. *Journal of Ambulatory Surgery, 11*, 49–54.

Pearson, A., Richardson, M., Peels, S., & Cairns, M. (2004a). The pre-admission care of patients undergoing day surgery: A systematic review. *Health Care Reports, 2*(1), 1–20.

Pearson, A., Richardson, M., Peels, S., & Cairns, M. (2004b). The care of patients whilst in the day surgery unit: A systematic review. *Health Care Reports, 2*(2), 21–52.

Penz, K., & Bassendowski, S. (2006). Evidence-based nursing in clinical practice: Implications for nurse educators. *Journal of Continuing Education in Nursing, 37*(6), 250–4.

Perry, L. (2006). Promoting evidence-based practice in stroke care in Australia. *Nursing Standard, 20*(34), 35–42.

Regan, M., Gater, R., Rahman, A., & Patel, V. (2015). Mental health research: Developing priorities and promoting its utilization to inform policies and services. *Eastern Mediterranean Health Journal, 21*(7), 547–21.

Sackett, D. L., Rosenberg, W. M., Gray, J. A., Haynes, R. B., & Richardson, W. S. (1996). Evidence based medicine: What it is and what it isn't. *BMJ (Clinical Research Edition), 312*(7023), 71–2.

Sackett, D. L., Straus, S. E., Richardson, W. S., & Haynes, R.B. (2000). *Evidence-Based Medicine: How to Practice and Teach EBM* (2nd edn). New York: Churchill Livingstone.

Sherriff, K., Wallis, M., & Chaboyer, W. (2007). Nurses' attitudes to and perceptions of knowledge and skills regarding evidence-based practice. *International Journal of Nursing Practice, 13*, 363–9.

Taylor, B. J. (2006). *Reflective Practice: A Guide for Nurses and Midwives* (2nd edn). Maidenhead, UK: Open University Press.

Taylor, C., Gribble, K., Sheehan, A., Schmied, V., & Dykes, F. (2010). Staff perceptions and experiences of implementing the Baby Friendly Initiative in neonatal intensive care units in Australia. *Journal of Obstetric, Gynecologic and Neonatal Nursing, 40*, 25–34.

Thoma, A., & Eaves III, F. F. (2015). A brief history of evidence-based medicine (EBM) and the contributions of Dr David Sackett. *Aesthetic Surgery Journal, 35*(8), NP261–3. https://doi.org/10.1093/asj/sjv130

Turner, S., Sharp, C. A., Sheringham, J., Leamon, S., & Fulop, N. J. (2019). Translating academic research into guidance to support healthcare improvement: How should guidance development be reported? *BMC Health Services Research, 19*(1), 1–7. https://doi.org/10.1186/s12913-019-4792-8

Ullrich, S., McCutcheon, H., & Parker, B. (2011). Reclaiming time for nursing practice in nutritional care: Outcomes of implementing protected mealtimes in a residential aged care setting. *Journal of Clinical Nursing, 20*, 1339–48.

Wynaden, D., Landsborough, I., McGowan, S., Baigmohamad, Z., Finn, M., & Pennebaker, D. (2006). Best practice guidelines for the administration of intramuscular injections in the mental health setting. *International Journal of Mental Health Nursing, 15*, 195–200.

Zeitz, K., & McCutcheon, H. (2003). Evidence-based practice: To be or not to be, this is the question! *International Journal of Nursing Practice, 9*(5), 272.

FURTHER READING

Cook, B. G., Landrum, T. J., & Tankersley, M. (2013). *Evidence-Based Practices*. Bingley, UK: Emerald.

Davies, J. (2014). *Evidence-Based Practice*. London: Routledge.

Gupta, L., Ward, J. E., & Hayward, R. S. (1997). Clinical practice guidelines in general practice: A national survey of recall, attitudes and impact. *Medical Journal of Australia, 166*(2), 69–72.

Mead, P. (2000). Clinical guidelines: Promoting clinical effectiveness or a professional minefield?' *Journal of Advanced Nursing, 31*(1), 110–16.

Riddell, T. (2007). Critical assumptions: Thinking critically about critical thinking. *Journal of Nursing Education, 46*(3), 121–6.

Swanberg, S. M., Dennison, C. C., Farrell, A., Machel, V., Marton, C., O'Brien, K. K., Pannabecker, V., Thuna, M., & Holyoke, A. N. (2016). Instructional methods used by health sciences librarians to teach evidence-based practice (EBP): A systematic review. *Journal of the Medical Library Association*, *104*(3), 197–208. doi:10.3163/1536-5050.104.3.004

Tagney, J., & Haines, C. (2009). Using evidence-based practice to address gaps in nursing knowledge. *British Journal of Nursing*, *18*(8), 484–9.

Tilson, J. K., Mickan, S., Howard, R., Sum, J. C., Zibell, M., Cleary, L., Mody, B., & Michener, L. A. (2016). Promoting physical therapists' use of research evidence to inform clinical practice: Part 3 – long term feasibility assessment of the PEAK program. *BMC Medical Education*, *16*, 144. doi:10.1186/s12909-016-0654-9

Turner, T., Misso, M., Harris, C., & Green, S. (2008). Development of evidence-based clinical practice guidelines (CPGs): Comparing approaches. *Implementation Science*, *3*, 45.

van Hooft, S., Gillam, L., & Byrnes, M. (1995). *Facts and Values: An Introduction to Critical Thinking for Nurses*. Sydney, NSW: Maclennan & Petty.

Wu, S., Khan, M., & Legido-Quigley, H. (2020). What steps can researchers take to increase research uptake by policymakers? A case study in China. *Health Policy and Planning*, *35*(6), 665–75. https://doi.org/https://academic.oup.com/heapol/issue

Zwolsman, S., te Pas, E., Hooft, L., Wieringa-de Waard, M., & van Dijk, N. (2012). Barriers to GPs' use of evidence-based medicine: a systematic review. *British Journal of General Practice*, *62*(600), 511–21.

GLOSSARY

abstract
A succinct and accurate description of the project, including the problem statement, the theoretical framework and an explanation of the design of the study that includes the sample and data collection methods, the major findings, conclusions and, if appropriate, any recommendations.

analysis
A systematic review of research data with the intention of sorting and classifying the data into representational groups and patterns.

annotated bibliography
An organised list of references to books, articles, internet-based sources, or other documents. Each reference is followed by an annotation, which is a short description and evaluation, written in paragraph form.

applicability
The degree to which the results of an observation, study or review are likely to hold true in a particular practice setting.

applied research
Knowledge applied to specific situations.

basic research
Develops fundamental knowledge and tests theory.

bias
When a systemic error is introduced that may distort the results of a research study.

body of the report
The main information of a research report, including the introduction, literature review, methodology, results and discussion.

Boolean operators
Specific words used to combine keywords to improve the chances of finding relevant information. The most commonly used Boolean operators are *AND*, *OR* and *NOT*.

bracketing
A process derived from mathematics whereby researchers' presuppositions are put to one side (in brackets) to be attended to separately so they do not impose meaning on the research.

causal relationships
Those relationships that establish cause and effect between variables. They can be inferred only from an experimental design.

central limit theorem
When you draw an infinite number of random samples and take the mean of each, the range of sample means would follow a normal distribution.

CINAHL Complete
Cumulative Index to Nursing and Allied Health Literature, the primary database for identifying publications in these specialities.

clinical guidelines
Systematically developed statements to assist clinician and patient decisions about appropriate healthcare for specific clinical circumstances.

clinical significance
The meaningfulness to clinical practice of your findings, which can be determined using confidence intervals, odds ratios and risk calculations.

Cochrane Australia
An international initiative to facilitate the retrieval and synthesis of literature relevant to evidence-based practice.

comparative descriptive design
Compares the characteristics of one group to those of another group.

concept
An abstract generalised idea that describes a phenomenon or a group of related phenomena.

concept analysis
A general term for several different strategies used to analyse text.

conceptual framework
Elaborates the research problem in relation to relevant literature.

confidence intervals
Identifies a range of values that indicates the true population value of a particular characteristic at a specified probability level (usually 95%).

confidentiality
A human right for private matters to remain secret; it is the researcher's responsibility to keep data confidential so that individuals are not compromised.

confounding variables
A third variable that can adversely affect the relationship between the independent variable and dependent variable, which may distort the results of experimental research.

congruency
In qualitative research this is the fit or correspondence between foundational ideas and the activity phases of the research, such as the project's assumptions, aims, objectives, methods and processes.

constant comparative analysis
A flexible and open-ended feature of grounded theory, in which the researcher works with the data from the beginning of the project in a process of analysis

to constantly compare all new data that emerge from participants' accounts of their experiences in order to identify similarities in codes and categories.

context
The particular features of the research setting that need to be taken into account when planning, undertaking and reporting a research project.

control group
A group of subjects included in an experimental design, who do not receive the treatment being introduced in the study, and who are used for comparison to the experimental group who do receive the treatment.

correlational design
Examines whether one variable is influencing another variable.

critical appraisal
The process of systematic assessment of the outcome of scientific research (evidence) to judge its trustworthiness, value and relevance in a particular context.

critical research
Serves to address societal structures and institutions that oppress and exclude so that transformative actions can be generated that reduce inequitable power conditions.

cross-sectional study
Includes the collection of data on more than one case at a single point in time to detect patterns of association.

culture
A way of life for a group of people, interpreted through their symbols, beliefs, customs, language and life patterns.

data
Numbers and/or words collected by the researcher in order to answer the research question.

dependent variable
A dependent variable is the variable being tested and measured. It is dependent on the independent variable. As the researcher changes the independent variable, the effect on the dependent variable is observed and recorded.

descriptive design
Uses numbers to describe a phenomenon; is not truly experimental.

descriptive statistics
Statistics that describe a phenomenon.

discourse
All that is written and spoken and invites dialogue or conversation.

discourse analysis
Interrogates knowledge and power inherent in spoken and written life texts.

discrete (interval) data
Data that can be counted only as whole numbers.

discursive analysis
An interdisciplinary approach to the study of discourse that views language as a form of social practice and focuses on the ways in which social and political domination are reproduced in text and talk.

empirico-analytical research
Employs the scientific method (and is sometimes referred to by this term) in observation and analysis; referred to as quantitative.

empowerment
In critical research, methods and processes are geared towards helping people to find and accept their own power.

EndNote
The industry-standard software tool for publishing and managing bibliographies, citations and references.

epistemology
The study of knowledge and how it is judged to be true. Questions about what a researcher knows and how they know it is trustworthy are epistemological questions.

ethics
In nursing and healthcare research, ethics concerns moral questions and behaviour in conducting research.

ethics approval
Approval required from the relevant ethics committees for research involving human participants.

ethnography
Provides a portrait of people by describing and raising awareness of a group's cultural characteristics, such as their shared symbols, beliefs, values, rituals and patterns of behaviour.

evidence-based
The integration of clinical expertise, patient values, and the best research evidence into the decision-making process for patient care.

evidence-based practice (EBP)
Current clinical practice based on the best, most recent research.

expanders (*see also* **limiters**)
Tools for expanding the search beyond the results you have received with a current search.

experimental design
Used for establishing cause-and-effect relationships between variables; provides conclusive evidence of causality; considered to be the most powerful quantitative research designs.

experimental group
In an experiment where a variable is being tested, the experimental group

receives the treatment. The group is then compared to a control group to explore differences between the groups.

explicit themes
Those themes that come up easily from the text because they are part of the pattern of answers and insights within the text and are relevant because their identity is clearly and directly connected to the research aims and objectives.

extraneous variables
Extraneous variables are undesirable variables that influence the relationship between the variables that a researcher is examining.

Foucauldian-style discourse analysis
A complex examination of text because it requires careful reading of entire bodies of text and other organising systems (e.g. taxonomies, commentaries and conference transcriptions) in relation to one another in order to interpret patterns, rules, assumptions, contradictions, silences, consequences, implications and inconsistencies.

grounded theory
Starts from the ground of an area of human interest and works up in an inductive fashion to make sense of what people say about their

experiences and to convert these statements into theoretical propositions. It involves simultaneous data collection and analysis when conducting the research study.

Hawthorne effect
When participants in a study change their behaviour because they know they are being studied.

historical research
Reconstructs from primary and secondary sources (with due attention to a rigorous research process) an accurate and truthful record of events, thereby amending previous knowledge and discovering new knowledge in relation to specific areas and interests.

human research ethics committee (HREC)
Plays a central role in the ethical oversight of research involving humans and reviewing research proposals involving human participants, to ensure they are ethically acceptable and in accordance with relevant standards and guidelines.

hypothesis
A statement of what the researcher thinks is going to be the outcome of the investigation.

impact factor
A measure of the frequency with which the average

article in a journal has been cited in a particular year.

implicit themes
These themes lie hidden in the text, not always stated as a direct word or words, or even as an easily recognisable concept.

independent variable
A variable that is presumed to affect or determine a dependent variable. It can be changed as required; its values do not represent a problem requiring explanation in an analysis but are simply taken as given.

inductive
A form of reasoning in which a generalised conclusion is formulated from particular instances.

inferential statistics
Statistics that enable us to make inferences through a process of hypothesis testing about the population from which the data were collected.

informed consent
The agreement of the participant to take part in the research project after having been thoroughly briefed about the project and its possible outcomes.

integrated literature review
A form of research that reviews, critiques and synthesises representative literature on a topic in an integrated way such that new frameworks and

perspectives on the topic are generated.

integrity
In research, integrity is expressed in a commitment to the honest and ethical search for knowledge.

intention to treat (ITT)
ITT analysis includes every participant who is randomised according to the treatment assignment, ignoring non-compliance or withdrawal from the study.

interpretations
In qualitative research reports, can be theories, findings, results, insights, strategies, implications, examples of reflective awareness and changed practice and so on, to reflect the assumptions and intentions of the research methodology.

interpretive research
Aims mainly to generate meaning, to explain and describe in order to make sense of areas of interest.

Joanna Briggs Institute (JBI)
An international not-for-profit research and development organisation specialising in evidence-based resources for healthcare professionals in nursing, midwifery, medicine and allied health.

limiters (*see also* **expanders**)
Ways of narrowing a search to more effectively target your results.

literature
The total body of writing that deals with the topic being researched, mainly comprising theoretical and research papers.

literature review
A description of the literature relevant to a particular field or topic.

lived experience
The knowledge people have of things of interest because they have experienced them through the daily activities of living their lives.

longitudinal study
Data are gathered for the same subjects repeatedly over a period of time and can extend over years or even decades.

measurement
The process of determining a quantitative characteristic of some phenomenon, such as how big, how often or how many.

methodological congruency
The match of epistemological assumptions of a particular methodology to the research methods used to gather that type of knowledge.

methodology
The theoretical assumptions underlying the choice of methods and processes used in generating and validating a particular form of knowledge.

methods
The means or strategies by which data are sought and analysed in a qualitative research project.

mixed methods design
Involves the integration of quantitative and qualitative data collection and analysis in a single study.

monograph
A small book, usually presented as a soft-cover, A5-sized document containing approximately 50 pages, usually produced by academic or professional organisations to publish their research.

multimethod design
Combining more than one method to address a research question.

multiple methodologies
Combinations of methodologies that offer wider frames of reference with a greater likelihood of generating more options for knowledge generation.

narrative analysis
Attempts to find meaning in stories through a variety of methods that best suit the research questions, aims and objectives.

narratives
Views or stories. Postmodernists are opposed to grand or metanarratives or world views based on claims to legitimise their truth; however, mini, micro, local or traditional narratives as stories that make no truth claims are acceptable.

national health initiatives
Health research priorities that originate at national government level and are transmitted in the form of government funding to medical and allied healthcare practices throughout the nation.

naturalistic setting
A place in which people carry out the activities of their daily life.

nominal data
Are data that are observable, not measurable; for example, gender, hair colour or state of residency. Objects or people are assigned to named categories which may be given a numerical value.

non-probability sample
A sample that does not attempt to represent the population.

observational studies
A type of study in which individuals are observed or certain outcomes are measured, and no attempt is made to affect the outcome.

ontology
The study of existence; whenever researchers ask about the nature of the

existence of something or someone, they are asking ontological questions.

p values
The probability of making an error in interpreting your findings because your sample, for some reason, does not accurately reflect the real population parameters.

paradigm
A way of looking at phenomena that encompasses a set of philosophical assumptions and that guide one's approach to inquiry.

parametric data
Data that are collected on at least an interval level scale and that are representative of the population from which they were collected.

peer review
The process involving a critical evaluation of a research proposal by independent experts (peers) for evaluating and assuring the quality of the study before and after it is funded.

peer-reviewed journal articles
Articles judged by at least three peers to be of a high enough standard to be published in a professional journal.

phenomenological reduction
Allows for reflection in research while at the same time ensuring that the findings are not overly influenced or directed by the researcher's agenda.

phenomenology
The study of things within human existence by discovering, exploring and describing the essence of phenomena through directly attending to them.

pilot study
A small-scale 'dress rehearsal' for the main study.

plagiarism
Claiming somebody else's work as your own; failing to formally acknowledge the source of your ideas. Considered to be stealing, plagiarism is also a form of academic or professional fraud.

population
A group whose members have specific common characteristics that you want to investigate in your research study.

positivist
Is based on the view that there is valid knowledge (truth) only in scientific knowledge.

poster
In the context of a conference, a succinct graphic overview of research depicted on a cardboard sheet to communicate the major points of the research project to delegates, who then have the opportunity to talk to the researcher about the project.

pragmatism
The view that the answer to the research question is of prime importance and the researcher should use the best available tools to identify it.

preliminaries
These introduce the research report. They always include the title page and an abstract, as well as forms, acknowledgements, a table of contents, lists of figures and tables and an executive summary.

primary sources
The original theories or findings written by the person or persons involved at the time of the inquiry.

privacy
In a research context, privacy refers to the right of participants to decide which information they want to disclose, particularly concerning their attitudes, beliefs, behaviours and opinions, and records such as diaries and other private papers.

probability sample
A sample that attempts to portray the target population in miniature by representing the broad characteristics of that population.

processes
How data collection and analysis methods are undertaken; involves the embodied values of researchers, such as respecting, being patient and thoughtful, honouring, acknowledging and other ways of being mindful of the human nature of the research.

prospective study
Observes for outcomes during the study period, such as the development of a disease, and relates them to other factors such as suspected risk or protection factor(s).

qualitative analysis
Analysis of participants' words, language and/or images using manual or computer-assisted means.

qualitative critical methodologies
These methodologies interpret meaning by aiming to bring about change and raised awareness by systematic political critique and attempting to expose control, oppression, power and domination.

qualitative interpretive methodologies
Interpret meaning by exploring, explaining and describing items of interest in order to make sense of them.

qualitative research
Research interested in questions that involve human consciousness and subjectivity and that values humans and their experiences in the research process.

quantitative research
Research that focuses on measuring objective variables and the cause-and-effect relationship between them, such as the effects of a drug dose on a patient's blood pressure.

ranked (ordinal) data
Data in the form of names or categories.

ratio (continuous) data
Data that can be collected on a scale with infinitely small graduations of measurement, with an absolute zero.

reliability
The degree to which a quantitative study would have the same results if repeated many times.

research
Literally means 'looking carefully again'; researchers are searching again for new or adapted knowledge to inform them about areas of interest so they can begin or add to a body of knowledge.

research area
In qualitative approaches, a broad or focused interest for research.

research culture
A group of people who are conversant with the fundamentals of research methods and processes and are confident in promoting and sharing the practice and application of research.

research design
The framework by which a project will answer a particular research question.

research objectives
The reasons why a study is being conducted.

research plan
A map or outline of the steps to be taken to achieve the objectives of a research project.

research problem
Is selected within the general area of a discipline, and is particular to that discipline as an issue that needs research inquiry. Is presented as a statement.

research proposal
A formal, structured, written account of a plan for a research project that argues why, how, where, when and at what cost it will be done.

research purpose
A general statement of the purposes, aims, intentions and/or objectives of the study.

research question
A specific question about a problem or issue that guides the study and keeps the research interest in focus.

research report
A formal account of a research project presented variously as a classroom project report, journal article, thesis, dissertation, or seminar or conference paper.

retrospective study
Looks backward in time and examines exposures to suspected risk or protection factors in relation to an outcome that has been established at the start of the study.

review of the literature
To read, sort and analyse the literature, and then put it into some kind of order; a critique of individual research reports.

rigorous
Degree to which research methods are scrupulously and meticulously carried out in order to recognise important influences occurring in an experiment.

rigour
The strictness in judgement and conduct that must be used to ensure that the successive steps in a project have been set out clearly and undertaken with scrupulous attention to detail so that the results, findings or insights can be trusted by people with whom they resonate.

sampling
Extracting a subgroup from within a population in order to study this group through research.

scale of measurement
The level of precision associated with a measurement technique.

scoping review
A review that is done to identify and map the available research literature with the aim of identifying characteristics/concepts using a rigorous and transparent method.

secondary sources
Literature written by others to which an author refers.

seminal
Articles or publications that influence the scholarly community's thinking and, ultimately, the body of knowledge.

simple descriptive design
Used to describe or observe a phenomenon without manipulating the environment.

statistical significance
The probability that a finding is false; expressed as a *p* value.

subjectivity
That which comes from an individual's sense of internal and external things.

supporting materials
The references and appendices in a research report.

systematic review
A literature review focused on a research question that tries to identify, appraise, select and synthesise all high-quality research evidence relevant to that question.

thematic analysis
A method for identifying themes, essences or patterns within a text.

theoretical framework
Guides research to determine what variables to measure and what statistical relationships to look for. Connects the researcher to existing knowledge.

theoretical sampling
The data collection process for theory generation. Grounded theory sampling is an ongoing process of data collection and analysis that directs the researcher to obtain further samples.

theoretical sensitivity
A beginning point in grounded theory for seeking some clarity on the nature of the research area to sensitise the researcher and provide insights.

theory
An attempt to describe, organise or explain a phenomenon or group of phenomena of a discipline in a language appropriate to the discipline.

triangulation
The use of multiple references, such as data, investigations, theories, methods and methodologies, that converge in research

projects to enable the researcher to draw conclusions that may be more confidently claimed as being trustworthy.

trustworthiness
When the argument made based on the results is strong and it is demonstrated that the evidence for the results reported is sound. The trustworthiness of a qualitative study can be increased by maintaining high credibility and objectivity.

trustworthy
The degree to which the findings of qualitative research reflect reality.

validity
The degree to which a quantitative study (or measurement tool) is measuring what it claims to measure.

variable
A factor in a quantitative project that varies.

voice
The modern conception of the author's perspective, but postmodernists question the attribution of privilege or special status to any voice; a public voice is more acceptable to postmodernists because it makes discourse broadly understandable.

INDEX

Aboriginal and Torres Strait
Islander people 191, 321
abstracts
definition 367
and literature searches 31
in research proposals 280
in research reports 312–13
accuracy, importance of 122, 247
action research 91, 176–9, 187,
190, 260, 316
administrative support 87
Agency for Healthcare Research
and Quality (AHRQ) 345
aims statements 87, 289, 314–14
alpha errors 148–9
analysis 258, 367
see also under qualitative data
analysis; quantitative data
analysis
analysis of variance (ANOVA) 63,
158–9, 160–1
analytical designs 100, 103–9
annotated bibliographies 47–8, 367
anonymity 189, 190, 205, 276, 292
appendices 295, 329
applicability 57, 367
applied research 2, 367
Appraisal of Guidelines for
Research and Evaluation
(AGREE) II 58, 355
approval of research proposals 300
archival searches 184–5
artistic expression 185, 192, 199
aspects (themes) 207
associations in findings 151–4,
159–61, 162
attributable risk 254
attrition 114
audio recordings 134, 185, 188,
190, 192, 201, 202, 209
Australia, evidence-based
practice 345, 351, 352–2, 357–7
Australian College of
Perioperative Nurses 300
Australian Institute of Health
and Welfare 352
Australian Research Council
(ARC) 25, 299
axial coding 169, 170

bar graphs 140
basic research 2, 367
beta errors 148–9
bias
and critiquing 57
definition 367
literature reviews 33, 43

qualitative research
methodologies 168
quantitative research
methodologies 106, 112, 116,
117, 119, 120
research questions 85
bibliographies 46
see also annotated
bibliographies
biomedical discourses 216
biomedical science 346
blind studies 111, 115
body of research proposal 279,
280–7
body of research report 310,
315–16, 367
books
in literature reviews 26
monographs 333, 335, 371
for qualitative analysis 219
research training 350
Boolean operators 38, 40–1, 367
borderline findings 327
bracketing 171, 367
brainstorming research problems
80
budgets 85–6, 287, 294–5, 299

Canada, evidence-based practice
345
Canadian Centre for Evidence-
Based Nursing (CCEBN) 345
case-based samples 117
case controlled studies 100
case reports 100
case series 100
case studies 100, 185
cases 130
cataloguing research literature
43–5
categorisation of data 169, 206
causal-comparative research
designs 105
causal relationships 250–1, 367
central limit theorem 146–7, 367
central tendency, measures of
142–4
Centre for Evidence-Based
Medicine (UK) 58
change measures for evidence-
based practice 351–1, 355
chi-square test 156–8
child participants 114, 119
CINAHL Complete 30, 37, 367
classroom research reports 307
clinical education programs 351
clinical educators 360

clinical practice guidelines (CPGs)
216, 345–5, 353–4, 360, 367
clinical schools 357
clinical significance 84, 161, 251–8,
327, 367
clinical use of research 3–4
cluster sampling 117
Cochrane 342, 345
Cochrane, Archie 342
Cochrane Australia 30, 367
codebooks 133, 205
coding 134–8, 169, 170, 205, 207
coding sheets 135, 136
Cohen's d 63
cohort studies 98, 100, 104
collaborative research 4–5, 187,
291, 299, 316, 358–8
colleagues/staff 119, 122, 202, 300
colour-coding in thematic
analysis 209
communication skills 188, 192
comparative descriptive designs
102, 103, 367
computer software
data analysis 134, 135–6, 159,
206, 210, 247, 322
data management 218–19
concept analysis 367
concept mapping 35
concepts 367
conceptual frameworks 14, 368
conclusions from findings 258,
328
concurrent/convergent design
232–3
concurrent embedded design
233, 234
concurrent triangulation design
234
conference presentations 27, 80,
220, 307, 308, 330–32
confidence intervals 57, 64, 161,
253, 368
confidentiality 276, 368
confirmatory phase 229
conflicts of interest 122
confounding variables 115–16, 368
congruency 183, 262–3, 368
consent *see* informed consent
CONSORT 2010 58
CONSORT flow diagram 112
constant comparative analysis
169, 368
constructivist grounded theory
167–8
constructivist theory 167, 226,
227